Listening and Spoken Language Therapy for Children With Hearing Loss

A Practical Auditory-Based Guide

To Angie + Zoe —

We hope this book helps in your family journey + child's success!

Maura Martindale

Sylvia Roefleesch

Listening and Spoken Language Therapy for Children With Hearing Loss

A Practical Auditory-Based Guide

Sylvia Rotfleisch, MSc(A), CCC-A, BSc(OT), LSLS Cert, AVT
Maura Martindale, EdD, LSL Cert, AVEd

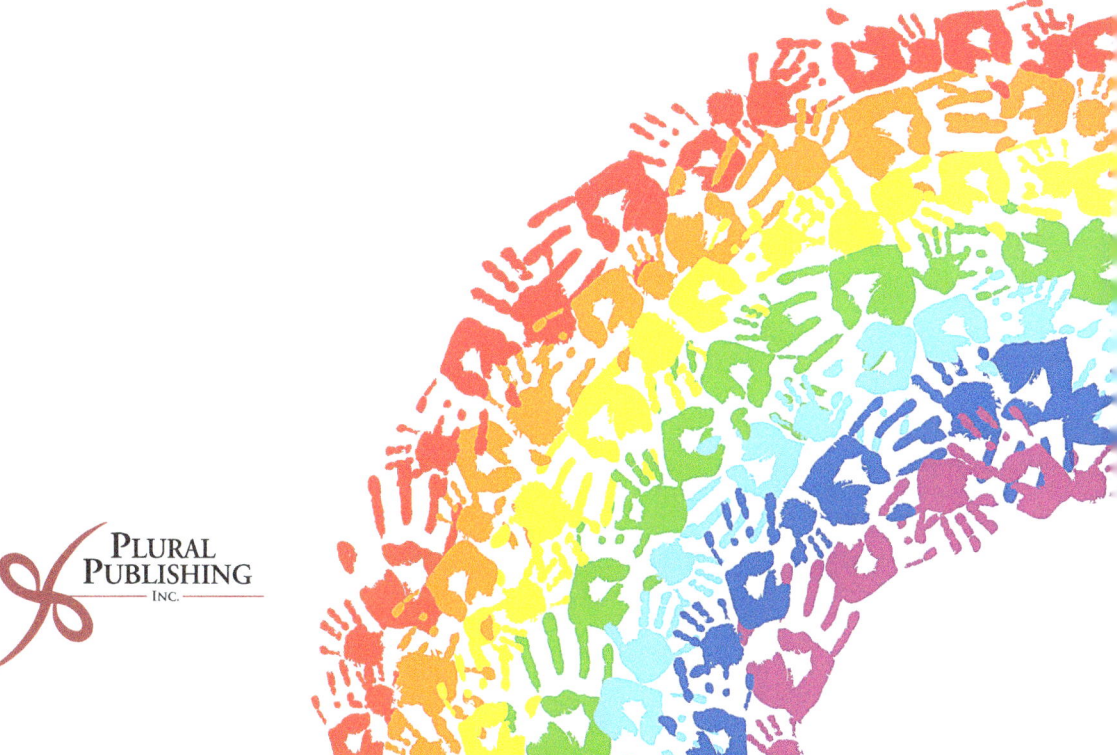

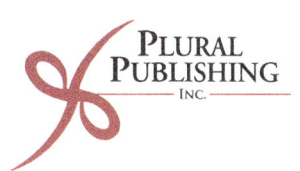

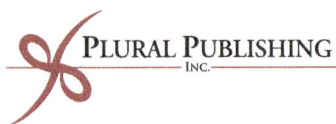

5521 Ruffin Road
San Diego, CA 92123

Email: information@pluralpublishing.com
Website: https://www.pluralpublishing.com

Copyright © 2023 by Plural Publishing, Inc.

Typeset in 10/13 Stone Serif by Flanagan's Publishing Services, Inc.
Printed in the United States of America by Integrated Books International

All rights, including that of translation, reserved. No part of this publication may be reproduced, stored in a retrieval system, or transmitted in any form or by any means, electronic, mechanical, recording, or otherwise, including photocopying, recording, taping, web distribution, or information storage and retrieval systems without the prior written consent of the publisher.

For permission to use material from this text, contact us by
Telephone: (866) 758-7251
Fax: (888) 758-7255
Email: permissions@pluralpublishing.com

Every attempt has been made to contact the copyright holders for material originally printed in another source. If any have been inadvertently overlooked, the publisher will gladly make the necessary arrangements at the first opportunity.

Library of Congress Cataloging-in-Publication Data:
Names: Rotfleisch, Sylvia, author. | Martindale, Maura, author.
Title: Listening and spoken language therapy for children with hearing loss : a practical auditory-based guide / Sylvia Rotfleisch, Maura Martindale.
Description: San Diego, CA : Plural Publishing, Inc., [2023] | Includes bibliographical references and index.
Identifiers: LCCN 2021030778 (print) | LCCN 2021030779 (ebook) | ISBN 9781635503876 (paperback) | ISBN 1635503876 (paperback) | ISBN 9781635503883 (ebook)
Subjects: MESH: Hearing Loss—rehabilitation | Language Therapy—methods | Language Development | Auditory Perception
Classification: LCC RF290 (print) | LCC RF290 (ebook) | NLM WV 270 | DDC 617.8—dc23
LC record available at https://lccn.loc.gov/2021030778
LC ebook record available at https://lccn.loc.gov/2021030779

Contents

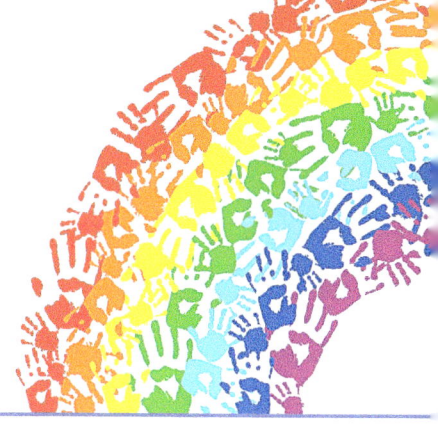

	Introduction	*xiii*
	Acknowledgments	*xix*
	Reviewers	*xxi*
	List of Figures	*xxiii*
	List of Tables	*xxv*
Chapter 1.	**Speech Acoustics: The Gold at the End of the Rainbow Audiogram** **Sylvia Rotfleisch**	**1**

Why Do We Need to Understand Speech Acoustics?	1
Section I. Basics of Sound	2
Key Points	2
Basics of Sound	2
Audiogram	2
A Sound Basis: The Applications	3
Hearing Loss and Detection	3
Modifying the Signal	4
Ear Shot/Speech Bubble	5
Background Noise and Noise Clutter	5
Audible Versus Intelligible	6
The 6-dB Significance	7
The 6-dB Rule	7
Sounds of Speech	9
The Basics	9
Applications	10
Discussion Questions	13
Section II. Speech Features	14
Key Points	14
Speech Features and Acoustic Correlates	14
The Basics	14
The Applications Related to Speech Features	19
Suprasegmentals, Vowels, and Diphthongs	19
Consonants	22
Discussion Questions	26

	Section III. Speech Acoustics Tools and Applications	27
	Key Points	27
	Ling Six-Sound Test	27
	Purpose and Administration	27
	Applications of the Ling Six Sounds	28
	Interpretation of the Ling Six Sounds	28
	The Rainbow Audiogram	30
	Applications of the Rainbow Audiogram	30
	Functional Audiogram	34
	Error Analysis to Determine Perception and Error Patterns	35
	Case Study Application of Speech Acoustics Tools	38
	Speech Acoustics and Hearing Loss Configurations	39
	Speech Acoustics and the Impact on Speech Production	39
	Speech Acoustics and Language Development	45
	Case Study Application of Speech Acoustics for Speech and Language Development	49
	The Gold at the End of the Rainbow Audiogram: Applications for Speech Acoustics	49
	Discussion Questions	52
	References	52
Chapter 2.	**Guiding and Supporting Parents/Caregivers**	**55**
	Maura Martindale	
	Key Points	55
	Why Are Parents Included in Auditory Sessions?	55
	Getting Started: Planning	56
	Emotional Supports for Families	56
	Teaching Parents and Caregivers: Why Are They Part of Every Session?	57
	Family Life: Activities of Daily Living (ADL) as the Foundation of Every Session	60
	Engaging Families in Sessions	62
	Cultural Considerations	62
	Screen Time	64
	Speech Acoustics and Parents	65
	Summary	65
	Discussion Questions	65
	References	66
Chapter 3.	**Stages Not Ages Model**	**69**
	Sylvia Rotfleisch and Maura Martindale	
	Key Points	69
	Stages/Sequence of Development (Flow Chart)	70

Determining Child's Level	72
Expectations for Growth	73
Brain Functions of Audition	76
Auditory Processing	78
Typical Development	78
Language	78
Speech	82
Theory of Mind	84
Self-Advocacy	86
Higher-Order Thinking	86
Summary	87
Discussion Questions:	87
Cases	87
Case 1	87
Case 2	90
Case 3	91
References	93

Chapter 4. Assessment of English Language, Speech, and Listening — 97
Maura Martindale

Key Points	97
Terms and Definitions	97
General Tips for Assessment of Children	98
Formal, Standardized Tests for Assessment	99
Checklists, Observations, and Questionnaires	100
Brain Functions for Listening and Spoken Language	100
Assessing Spoken Language	101
Spoken Vocabulary/Semantics	101
Language Sampling	102
Mean Length of Utterance (MLU)	103
Pragmatic Functions	104
Speech Assessment (Phonetic and Phonologic)	105
How to Align Assessment Data With the Proposed Therapy Model	105
Prelinguistic Stage	106
Single-Word Stage	106
Emerging Word Combinations Stage	106
Communication With Childlike Errors Stage	106
Competent Communicator Stage	106
Advanced Communicator Stage	107
Reporting Your Findings	107
Goal Setting Based on Data Gathered and Analyzed	107
Summary	108

	Discussion Questions	108
	References	108
Chapter 5.	**Therapy Basics**	**113**
	Sylvia Rotfleisch and Maura Martindale	
	Key Points	113
	What Should Therapy Look Like? Fun!	113
	The Chocolate Chip Cookie Theory	113
	General Tips for the Sessions	115
	Tools, Strategies, Building Materials	116
	Turn Taking or Serve and Return	116
	Infant- and Child-Directed Speech (IDS, CDS)	116
	Narrating	117
	The Expectant Pause	117
	Waiting, Waiting, and Sometimes . . . More Waiting . . .	117
	Blah, Blah, Blah Ginger	118
	Joint Attention	118
	Auditory Closure	119
	Auditory Sandwich	119
	Listening Hoop	119
	Enhancing Perception	119
	Acoustic Highlighting	120
	Life in Slow Motion	122
	The Three-Act Play	122
	Expansion	122
	Upping the Ante	123
	Vocabulary Expansion	123
	Summary	126
	Discussion Questions	126
	References	126
Chapter 6.	**The Prelinguistic Stage**	**129**
	Sylvia Rotfleisch	
	Key Points	129
	Basic Characteristics of the Prelinguistic Child	129
	Listening	129
	Language	130
	Speech	131
	Goals for the Prelinguistic Stage	132
	Developing an Appropriate Therapy Plan by Addressing Strengths and Areas of Need	132
	Typical Goals for the Prelinguistic Stage	132
	How Do We Work on These Goals?	134

	Targeting and Incorporating Goals	136
	Auditory Attention, Detection, Memory, and Discrimination	136
	Auditory Feedback and Development of the Speech Production System; Auditory Retrieval and Expressive Communication	139
	Language Comprehension Development of Auditory Recognition, Sequencing, and Comprehension	140
	Putting It All Together: Case History	143
	Auditory Processes for Using Sound Meaningfully	143
	Auditory Processes for Learning to Talk	144
	Auditory Processes for Learning Language	144
	The Intervention Session	144
	Summary	150
	Discussion Questions	150
	References	150
Chapter 7.	**Single-Word Communication Stage**	**153**
	Sylvia Rotfleisch	
	Key Points	153
	Basic Characteristics of the Child at the Single-Word Stage of Communication	153
	Listening	153
	Language	154
	Speech	156
	Goals for the Single-Word Stage	156
	Developing an Appropriate Therapy Plan by Addressing Strengths and Areas of Need	156
	Typical Goals for the Single-Word Communication Stage	157
	How Do We Work on These Goals?	157
	Targeting and Incorporating Goals	161
	Auditory Attention, Detection, Memory, Discrimination, Auditory Recognition, Sequencing, and Comprehension	161
	Auditory Feedback and Speech Production Development of the Speech Production System, Auditory Retrieval, and Expressive Communication	164
	Putting It All Together: Case History	166
	Auditory Processes for Using Sound Meaningfully	166
	Auditory Processes for Learning to Talk	167
	Auditory Processes for Learning Language	168
	The Intervention Session	168
	Summary	178
	Discussion Questions	178
	References	179

Chapter 8. Emerging Word Combinations Stage — 181
Sylvia Rotfleisch

Key Points	181
Basic Characteristics of the Child With Emerging Word Combinations	181
Listening	181
Language	182
Speech	184
Goals for the Emerging Word Combinations Stage	184
Developing an Appropriate Therapy Plan by Addressing Strengths and Areas of Need	184
Typical Goals for the Emerging Word Combinations Stage	185
How Do We Work on These Goals?	185
Targeting and Incorporating Goals	189
Auditory Attention, Detection, Memory, Discrimination, Auditory Recognition, Sequencing, and Comprehension	189
Targeting and Meeting Goals for Development of the Speech Production System: Auditory Retrieval and Expressive Communication	193
Putting It All Together: Case History	197
Auditory Processes for Using Sound Meaningfully	198
Auditory Processes for Learning to Talk	198
Auditory Processes for Learning Language	199
Summary	201
The Intervention Session	201
Summary	207
Discussion Questions	208
References	208

Chapter 9. Communication With Typical Childlike Errors Stage — 211
Sylvia Rotfleisch

Key Points	211
Basic Characteristics of the Child Who Communicates With Typical Childlike Errors	211
Listening	211
Language	212
Speech	213
Goals for the Stage of Communication With Errors	214
Developing an Appropriate Therapy Plan by Addressing Strengths and Areas of Need	214
Typical Goals for the Communication With Errors Stage	214

How Do We Work on These Goals?	215
Targeting and Incorporating Goals	219
Auditory Attention, Detection, Memory, Discrimination, Auditory Recognition, Sequencing, and Comprehension	219
Auditory Retrieval and Expressive Communication	219
Putting It All Together: Case History	226
Auditory Processes for Using Sound Meaningfully	227
Auditory Processes for Learning to Talk	228
Auditory Processes for Learning Language	228
Diagnostic Therapy and Informal Assessment	229
Progress in AVT Sessions	231
Summary	231
The Intervention Session	232
Summary	237
Discussion Questions	238
References	238

Chapter 10. Competent Communicator Stage — 241
Sylvia Rotfleisch

Key Points	241
Basic Characteristics of the Child Who Is a Competent Communicator	241
Listening	241
Language	242
Speech	243
Goals for the Competent Communicator Stage	244
Developing an Appropriate Therapy Plan by Addressing Strengths and Areas of Need	244
Typical Goals for the Stage of Competent Communicator	244
How Do We Work on These Goals?	246
Targeting and Incorporating Goals	247
Auditory Attention, Detection, Memory, Discrimination, Auditory Recognition, Sequencing, and Comprehension	247
Auditory Retrieval and Expressive Communication	247
Putting It All Together: Case History	257
Auditory Processes for Using Sound Meaningfully	258
Auditory Processes for Learning to Talk	259
Auditory Processes for Learning Language	259
Summary	263
The Intervention Session	263
Summary	268
Discussion Questions	268
References	268

Chapter 11 Advanced Communicator Stage   271
Sylvia Rotfleisch

Key Points	271
Basic Characteristics of the Child at the Advanced Communicator Stage	271
Listening	271
Language	272
Speech	272
Goals for the Advanced Communicator	274
Developing an Appropriate Therapy Plan by Addressing Strengths and Areas of Need	274
Typical Goals for the Advanced Communicator Stage	274
How Do We Work on These Goals?	276
Targeting and Incorporating Goals	279
Auditory Attention, Selection, Memory, Discrimination, Auditory Recognition, Sequencing, and Comprehension	279
Auditory Retrieval and Expressive Communication	279
Putting It All Together: Case History	283
Auditory Processes for Using Sound Meaningfully	283
Auditory Processes for Learning Language	285
Summary	288
Progress Over Time With Intervention	288
The Intervention Session	292
Summary	299
Discussion Questions	300
References	300
Index	*303*

Introduction

Sylvia Rotfleisch and Maura Martindale

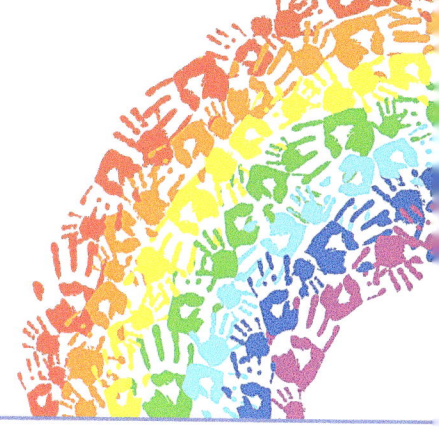

What Was the Vision and Intended Audience for This Book?

Our vision for this book was to create a highly practical guide for professionals who are providing auditory-based listening and spoken language (LSL) therapy for children with hearing loss. The textbook provides educators with a specific model of language, speech, and listening, viewed through the theoretical lens of social interaction theory (Vygotsky, 1962). The approach presented here assumes that children's language is acquired through meaningful social interactions with language models in their environment coupled with their natural innate potential to communicate via a language system. We present a stages approach, as opposed to the more traditional approach using children's ages. It is designed for new, beginning, or experienced professionals, as well as instructors of college-level courses.

Here are some other questions that readers may have about the book.

What Is the Best Way to Use This Book?

- The book's chapters are designed and sequenced for children's success in learning spoken language through listening. It is recommended that the reader use the chapters in sequence as the chapters build on previously covered materials.
- We begin with a chapter on speech acoustics. It is essential for professionals to have a thorough understanding of speech acoustics for an auditory-based therapy approach to be successful and to ensure that children with hearing loss have access to and use all the sounds of spoken language. It is the first order of business.
- Use the table of contents, and the lists of tables and figures, to help you find relevant sections. Flip back and forth to locate information relevant to your work or caseload.
- The model is presented using a color-coded system of stages, consistent presentation of content and tables, and a comprehensive case study for each stage.

What Resources Accompany This Book?

- There is a companion website that includes supports for instructors (e.g., quizzes, lecture slides). On the website, all readers will also find printable handouts from the numerous tables.

- Videos of the different stages that are presented in the model are available and captioned.
- There is an abundance of tables and figures throughout the book to be used as resources for establishing goals and planning sessions. For ease of use, tables for the different stages (Chapters 6 to 11) are consistently organized.
- There are case histories, intervention sessions with scripts, and session analyses.
- A discussion on supporting and guiding parents is presented for readers in the second chapter since the approach is based on the premise that parents will be included in every session. Parents will take on the majority of the therapy at home and in sessions over time.

Why Are the Terms for Strategies Used Here Not Universal in the Field?

- We know that some strategy terms (Chapter 5) do not have consistent names within the LSL field.
- In reading the therapy-specific chapters (Chapters 6 to 11), you may need to refer back to earlier chapters for terms and definitions. The index will assist you.

What Is the Scope of This Book?

- This therapy model is applicable for professionals who teach children with hearing loss, regardless of the type or degree of loss, and these children's parents.
- Professionals working with children with additional disabilities would benefit by using the model with adaptations and in collaboration with the child's multidisciplinary team.
- This model of spoken-language acquisition can be used with children who are English learners, who are from diverse cultures, and are late starters. Use the model in collaboration with the child's multidisciplinary team.
- Professionals currently providing LSL therapy will also find this model very useful in setting goals and planning for individualized lessons for children in their caseloads.
- Typical language milestones presented here are just that—milestones. Numerous tables, figures, and case histories are located within the chapters, which incorporate these milestones and beyond. There are many other textbooks on language development that are more comprehensive and include an in-depth coverage of typical language development.

What Topics Are Included in Previously Published Books?

- There are numerous books that have been published on pediatric audiology, cochlear implants, auditory management, general theory of auditory-verbal practice, and literacy. This book is therapy centered.
- There are other resources, organizations, and published materials for professionals and parents who are providing language instruction in sign

language. We recommend that readers research these resources as it is outside the scope of this book.
- There are numerous audiology textbooks that cover topics such as the anatomy of the ear, and types of assistive hearing technologies, so these topics will not be included here.
- It is assumed that the reader or instructor has a basic understanding of audiology and has some knowledge of the International Phonetic Alphabet (English) or IPA.
- Literacy is promoted by increasing the child's listening and spoken language level to one that is commensurate with hearing peers (Geers et al., 2017; Dettman et al., 2013). Achieving literacy for children is primarily based on their oral language development, abilities, vocabulary development, fluency, access to and discrimination of the sounds of speech, and comprehension of spoken language (Adams, 1994). These are discussed in every therapy chapter as they relate to listening and speaking, but literacy is not a specific focus here in and of itself.

What Terms Are Used for Consistency?

- "Professionals" will be used to refer to teachers, therapists, pathologists, clinicians, interventionists, and any practitioners and/or educators who teach, or will teach, children with hearing loss in homes, schools, centers, and therapy settings.
- "Children" or "child" will be used to refer to young people who have hearing loss and who are infants, preschoolers, and elementary and secondary schoolers in need of therapy intervention to learn spoken language via audition.
- "Hearing loss" will be used to refer to children who have been identified with any and all degrees and types of loss, including those with unilateral losses.
- The term "parents" is used to refer to mothers, fathers, grandparents, guardians, caregivers, adult siblings, or other adults who assume primary responsibility for raising the child.
- We employed both formal and informal language depending on the chapter's topics. For example, the chapter on speech acoustics contains information that requires formal, scientific language, while the chapter that addresses working with parents lends itself to a more informal discussion.

What Is the Sequence of the Chapters?

- In Chapter 1, we begin with a comprehensive chapter on speech acoustics, which is broken down into three sections. This allows the instructor to check for understanding via activities, quizzes, discussion questions, and videos before moving on to the next section. Within each section the reader will find helpful tables and figures that assist in comprehension of rather challenging concepts and content. It is written so that even new professionals will understand how knowledge of this content can be directly related to the child's learning of spoken language via audition using today's hearing technology.

- Chapter 2 discusses how to support and guide parents through the process of assuming the important role of naturally incorporating listening into daily living. Suggestions and ideas on talking to parents about their feelings are discussed, as they are an essential aspect of sessions.
- Chapter 3 includes an explanation of the model, and serves as a guidepost to the rest of the book. In the succeeding chapters, each stage is delineated with an abundance of strategies. The model represents a developmental approach with expectations that children will progress from one stage to the other, following the same trajectory as their typically hearing peers.
- Chapter 4 focuses on assessment, stressing the use of language sampling as a way to monitor a child's progress through the model, plus an overview of other assessments commonly used.
- Chapter 5 provides professionals abundant strategies to include in any auditory-based session with a child with hearing loss and their parents. In other words, the basics of therapy.
- Chapter 6: The Prelinguistic Stage chapter contains a detailed description and strategies for speech, language, and listening at the prelinguistic stage. Well-developed goals for the prelinguistic stage in listening, receptive and expressive language, and speech are presented for use in developing therapy lessons as well as reports. Numerous tables support the content for practical application. An extensive dialogue between the parent, child, and professional provides an example of a typical session at this stage of development.
- Chapter 7: The Single-Word Stage. Once a child has advanced to the single-word stage, this chapter provides a road map of what to expect in the domains of listening, language, and speech. Numerous tables and figures incorporate the basic strategies from Chapter 5 into this stage of development.
- Chapter 8: The Emerging Word Combinations Stage. The child is now able to understand more complex directions, to combine single words into short phrases, and to ask simple questions. Goals are presented in all relevant domains, along with a description of the therapy plan moving forward. An extensive case history of the child and parent, as well as a dialogue of a session at this level, is included. We see the parent taking more of a leadership role in the session with continued support from the professional.
- Chapter 9: The Communication With Childlike Errors Stage. This chapter targets the language user whose expressive language contains errors similar to those of the typically hearing child who is learning to talk. The child's listening skills have advanced considerably and longer conversations are possible, even with unfamiliar adults. A list of engaging games is included, along with suggestions on what skills to incorporate within each game. The parent is taking the lead during the extensive case history and intervention session. Tables of practical information and goals assist the reader in planning therapy sessions.
- Chapter 10: The Competent Communicator Stage. While able to hold more extensive conversation and to continue to build an expanding vocabulary, this child may experience some

difficulties in larger groups and in noisy backgrounds. Auditory abilities are at a very high functional level and the student is able to participate in most social situations where language is essential. The case history, with a language sample and intervention session, aim to deal with communication breakdowns and hold the student to an even higher level of linguistic knowledge. More complex assessments are conducted and illustrate the expectation of growth in all domains.

- Chapter 11: The Advanced Communicator Stage. The reader will become familiar with a student who is at or above typical levels of language usage in social and academic settings. Easy-to-use tables assist the reader in guiding students to linguistic independence, the ability to acquire complex academic vocabulary, and becoming comfortable in social situations with adults and peers using verbal and nonverbal clues. Goals are complex and lead the parent and student to becoming responsible for their own growth. It should be noted that most children at this stage would no longer require weekly therapy or any therapy at all, just occasional check-ins a few times a year as needed.

The authors thank you for joining us in learning how to support children with hearing loss and their parents. We hope this book will add to your professional journey.

References

Adams, M. J. (1994). *Beginning to read: Thinking and learning about print*. MIT Press.

Brown, R. (1973). *A first language: The early stages*. George Allen & Unwin.

Dettman, S., Wall, E., Constantinescu, G., & Dowell, R. (2013). Communication outcomes for groups of children using cochlear implants enrolled in auditory-verbal, aural-oral, and bilingual-bicultural early intervention programs. *Otology and Neurotology, 34*(3), 451–459. https://europepmc.org/article/PMC/PMC7998424#free-full-text

Dornan, D., Hickson, L., Murdoch, B., & Houston, T. (2009). Longitudinal study of speech perception, speech, and language for children with hearing loss in an auditory-verbal therapy program. *The Volta Review, 109*(2–3), 61–85.

Geers, A., Mitchell, C. M. Warner-Czyz, A., Wang, N. Y, & Eisenberg, L. S. (2017). Early sign language exposure and cochlear implantation benefits. *Pediatrics, 140*, 1–11, https://pediatrics.aappublications.org/content/pediatrics/140/1/e20163489.full.pdf

Roberson, L. (2009). *Literacy and deafness: Listening and spoken language*. Plural Publishing.

Vygotsky, L. (1962). *Thought and language*. MIT Press.

Acknowledgments

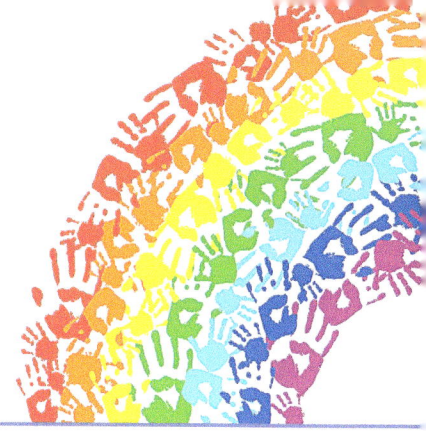

We would like to thank all the families who have let us be part of their journey over the years. It is through that work and your encouragement that this book went from a seed of an idea to a reality.

To our amazing teachers, Dr. Daniel Ling, Dr. Arthur Boothroyd, Judy Simser, and Mary McGinnis, who opened our eyes to all that could be for children with hearing loss. We thank them for allowing us to learn from them and stand on the shoulders of giants.

Special thanks and gratitude to our husbands, Don Kossman and Rich Martindale, and our children, Rachel and Jacob Kossman and Liz Martindale, for supporting us while we were absorbed by our work and encouraging us to complete this book. Through thick and thin, you were there for us.

We owe a debt of gratitude to Jacob Kossman for his creative and original graphics, Daniel Fishkin for his support and counsel, and Beth Walker Wooten for insights and edits.

Sylvia would like to thank the many in her village for getting her through to the light at the end of the tunnel and especially Susan Bercovitch, Jessica Bercovitch, Melinda Gillinger, and Karen Hyder.

Last, but certainly not least, we would like to thank the entire team at Plural Publishing who helped us make this book a reality.

Reviewers

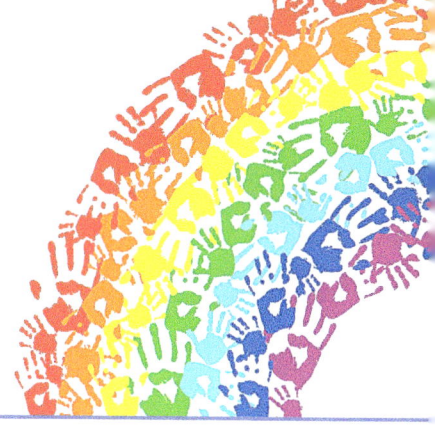

Plural Publishing and the authors thank the following reviewers for taking the time to provide their valuable feedback during the manuscript development process. Additional anonymous feedback was provided by other expert reviewers.

Jennifer B. Boyd, MA, CCC-SLP, LSLS, Cert AVT
Speech-Language Pathologist
Certified Listening and Spoken Language Specialist
LSLS Certification Mentor
Independent Consultant
Hearts for Hearing and Hearing First
Oklahoma City, Oklahoma

Jodi Cottrell, AuD, CCC-A, LSLS Cert. AVEd
Associate Professor and Program Director
The Luke Lee Listening, Language, and Learning Lab
Marshall University
Huntington, West Virginia

Susan Dillmuth-Miller, AuD, CCC-A
Associate Professor in Communication Sciences and Disorders
East Stroudsburg University
East Stroudsburg, Pennsylvania

Cynthia Gonzalez, MSEd, LSLS Cert. AVEd
Deaf and Hard of Hearing Education Specialist
Ontario, California

Paula Gross, MA, CED, ABD
Undergraduate Deaf Education Program Director
Fontbonne University
St. Louis, Missouri

Julie Heimler, MEd, LSLS Cert. AVEd
Deaf and Hard of Hearing Teacher
Los Angeles, California

Nicole Jacobson, MS, CCC-SLP, LSLS Cert. AVEd
Director of Sound Beginnings
Clinical Assistant Professor
Utah State University
Logan, Utah

Sarah Law, MEd
Clinical Assistant Professor
Utah State University
Logan, Utah

Raschelle Neild, PhD
Associate Professor
Ball State University
Muncie, Indiana

Bridget Scott-Weich, EdD, LSLS Cert. AVEd
Director of Graduate Programs and Administration
Mount Saint Mary's University/John Tracy Center
Los Angeles, California

Karen Schwartz, AuD, CCC-A, F-AAA
Assistant Professor
Touro College Graduate Program in Speech-Language Pathology
Brooklyn, New York

Cindy Sendor, MA, CCC-SLP
Assistant Professor of Communication Sciences and Disorders
California Baptist University
Riverside, California

Joanna L. Stith, PhD, CCC-SLP, LSLS Cert. AVT
Owner
Listening for Life
Broomfield, Colorado

Marguerite Vasconcellos, EdD, LSLS Cert. AVT
Adjunct Professor
Department of Special Education Language and Literacy
The College of New Jersey
Ewing, New Jersey

Michelle A. Veyvoda, PhD, CCC-SLP
Assistant Professor
Iona College
New Rochelle, New York

Jennifer Wickesberg-Summers, AuD, CCC-A, LSLS Cert. AVT
Director of Audiology
Texas Hearing Institute
Houston, Texas

List of Figures

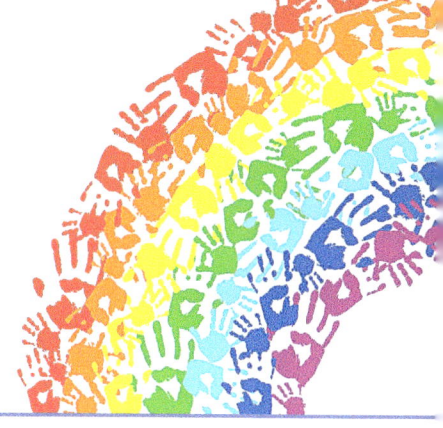

Figure 1–1. Audiogram representing normal hearing levels. — 4
Figure 1–2. Audiogram representing a hearing loss. — 5
Figure 1–3. Application of the 6 dB rule. — 8–9
Figure 1–4. 90/10 dilemma. — 12
Figure 1–5. A diagram showing the approximate frequency range of the first and second formants of the English vowels as spoken by adult males. — 16
Figure 1–6. Rainbow audiogram. — 31
Figure 1–7. Downward sloped audiogram. — 40
Figure 1–8. Corner audiogram. — 40
Figure 1–9. Cookie bite audiogram. — 41
Figure 1–10. Reverse slope audiogram. — 41
Figure 1–11. A. Low-frequency speech features. B. Mid-frequency speech features. C. High-frequency speech features. — 43–44
Figure 1–12. A. Low-frequency language structures. B. Mid-frequency language structures. C. High-frequency language structures. — 47–48

List of Tables

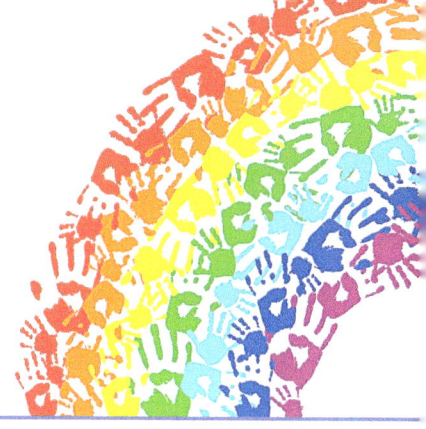

Chapter 1. Speech Acoustics: The Gold at the End of the Rainbow Audiogram

Table 1–1. General Principles Related to Low and High Frequencies	11
Table 1–2. Speech Features Related to Low and High Frequencies	11
Table 1–3. Speech Features	15
Table 1–4. Consonant Classification Chart	18
Table 1–5. International Phonetic Alphabet Key	19
Table 1–6. Acoustic Cues for Speech Features	20
Table 1–7. Suprasegmentals: Important Factors and Applications	23
Table 1–8. Vowels: Important Factors and Applications	23
Table 1–9. Consonants: Important Factors and Applications	26
Table 1–10. Ling Six Sounds	27
Table 1–11. Administration of the Ling Six-Sound Test	28
Table 1–12. Applications of the Ling Six-Sound Test	28
Table 1–13. Interpretation of the Ling Six-Sound Test	29
Table 1–14. Rainbow Audiogram Features	32
Table 1–15. The Steps for a Systematic Task Analysis	35
Table 1–16. Task Analysis: Consonant Manner of Production	36
Table 1–17. Task Analysis: Consonant Voicing	37
Table 1–18. Task Analysis: Consonant Place of Production	37
Table 1–19. Prognostic Indications Based on Downward Sloping Audiogram Configuration	40
Table 1–20. Prognostic Indications Based on Corner Audiogram Configuration	40
Table 1–21. Prognostic Indications Based on Cookie Bite Audiogram Configuration	41
Table 1–22. Prognostic Indications Based on Reverse Slope Audiogram Configuration	41
Table 1–23. Babbling Stages Related to Speech Features and Acoustic Correlates	42
Table 1–24. Speech Acoustics Applied to Speech Production Patterns	44
Table 1–25. Speech Feature Availability Based on Audition	45
Table 1–26. Speech Acoustics Analysis of Morphemic Functions	46
Table 1–27. Speech Acoustics Analysis of Language Structures	47
Table 1–28. Applications of Speech Acoustics	50–51

Chapter 2. Guiding and Supporting Parents/Caregivers

Table 2–1. Increasing Engagement With Families	63
Table 2–2. Connecting With Families and Their Cultures	64

Chapter 3. Stages Not Ages Model

Table 3–1. Model for Intervention	70
Table 3–2. Indication for Placement Into Stage	71
Table 3–3. Basic Indications of Progression Through Stages of Intervention	74–75
Table 3–4. Organization of Table Content in Intervention Chapters	75
Table 3–5. Brain Functions for Listening and Spoken Language	77
Table 3–6. Language Development Milestones	79–80
Table 3–7. Mastery of Morphemes	81
Table 3–8. Number of Receptive Words to Expect at Different Ages	81
Table 3–9. Tiers Framework of Vocabulary Acquisition	82
Table 3–10. Babble Skills Typically Evidenced at the Prelinguistic Stage	83
Table 3–11. Sequence of Development of Consonants in Children	84
Table 3–12. Theory of Mind Developmental Timeline	85
Table 3–13. Cognitive and Higher-Order Thinking Activities for Therapy: Aligned With Bloom's Taxonomy Levels—Cognitive Domain	88–89
Table 3–14. CELF-P Scores	92

Chapter 5. Therapy Basics

Table 5–1. Sample Acoustic Highlighting Strategies Illustrated by Speech Feature	121
Table 5–2. Preventing Vocabulary Stagnation	124–125

Chapter 6. The Prelinguistic Stage

Table 6–1. Auditory Abilities Evidenced in the Prelinguistic Stage	130
Table 6–2. Language and Speech Skills Evidenced in the Prelinguistic Stage	131
Table 6–3. Auditory Goals for Understanding Sound as Meaningful in the Prelinguistic Stage	133
Table 6–4. Auditory Feedback and Speech Production Goals in the Prelinguistic Stage	133
Table 6–5. Auditory Goals for Language Comprehension in the Prelinguistic Stage	134
Table 6–6. Auditory Goals for Developing Expressive Language in the Prelinguistic Stage	134
Table 6–7. Knowledge Areas in the Prelinguistic Stage	135
Table 6–8. Optimal Strategies to Implement in the Prelinguistic Stage	135
Table 6–9. Guide and Coach Parents To:	137
Table 6–10. Tips for Encouraging Initial Use of Technology	138
Table 6–11. Factors to Consider When Assessing Initial Responses to Sounds	138
Table 6–12. Stereotypic Phrases	141
Table 6–13. Preliminary Words: Examples to Use at the Prelinguistic Stage	142

Table 6–14. Sound-Object Associations	143
Table 6–15. By the End of the Prelinguistic Stage, the Child Should:	150

Chapter 7. Single-Word Communication Stage

Table 7–1. Auditory Abilities Evidenced in the Single-Word Stage	154
Table 7–2. Language and Speech Skills Evidenced in the Single-Word Stage	155
Table 7–3. Auditory Goals for Understanding Sound as Meaningful in the Single-Word Stage	158
Table 7–4. Auditory Feedback and Speech Production Goals in the Single-Word Stage	159
Table 7–5. Auditory Goals for Language Comprehension in the Single-Word Stage	159
Table 7–6. Auditory Goals for Developing Expressive Language in the Single-Word Stage	160
Table 7–7. Knowledge Areas in the Single-Word Stage	161
Table 7–8. Optimal Strategies to Implement in the Single-Word Stage	161
Table 7–9. Guide and Coach Parents To:	162
Table 7–10. By the End of the Single-Word Stage, the Child Should:	178

Chapter 8. Emerging Word Combinations Stage

Table 8–1. Auditory Abilities Evidenced in the Emerging Word Combinations Stage	182
Table 8–2. Language and Speech Skills Evidenced in the Emerging Word Combinations Stage	183
Table 8–3. Auditory Goals for Understanding Sound as Meaningful in the Emerging Word Combinations Stage	186
Table 8–4. Auditory Feedback and Speech Production Goals in the Emerging Word Combinations Stage	187
Table 8–5. Auditory Goals for Language Comprehension in the Emerging Word Combinations Stage	187
Table 8–6. Auditory Goals for Developing Expressive Language in the Emerging Word Combinations Stage	188
Table 8–7. Knowledge Areas in the Emerging Word Combinations Stage	188
Table 8–8. Optimal Strategies to Implement in the Emerging Word Combinations Stage	188
Table 8–9. Guide and Coach Parents To:	190–191
Table 8–10. LittlEARS Scores	198
Table 8–11. Receptive-Expressive Emergent Language Scale-3 (REEL-3) Scores	199
Table 8–12. Pre-School Language Scale-4 (PLS-4) Scores	200
Table 8–13. By the End of the Emerging Word Combinations Stage, the Child Should:	208

Chapter 9. Communication With Typical Childlike Errors Stage

Table 9–1. Auditory Abilities Evidenced in the Communication With Childlike Errors Stage	212
Table 9–2. Language and Speech Skills Evidenced in the Communication With Childlike Errors Stage	213

Table 9–3. Auditory Goals for Understanding Sound as Meaningful in the Communication With Childlike Errors Stage — 215

Table 9–4. Auditory Feedback and Speech Production Goals in the Communication With Childlike Errors Stage — 216

Table 9–5. Auditory Goals for Language Comprehension in the Communication With Childlike Errors Stage — 216

Table 9–6. Auditory Goals for Developing Expressive Language in the Communication With Childlike Errors Stage — 217

Table 9–7. Knowledge Areas in the Communication With Childlike Errors Stage — 217

Table 9–8. Optimal Strategies to Implement in the Communication With Childlike Errors Stage — 217

Table 9–9. Guide and Coach Parents To: — 220–221

Table 9–10. Test for Auditory Comprehension of Language–3 (TACL-3) Age-Equivalent Test Scores — 227

Table 9–11. Test of Auditory Processing Skills-3 (TAPS-3) Scores — 228

Table 9–12. Pre-School Language Scale-5 (PLS-5) Scores — 229

Table 9–13. By the End of the Communication With Childlike Errors Stage, the Child Should: — 238

Chapter 10. Competent Communicator Stage

Table 10–1. Auditory Abilities Evidenced by a Child Who Is a Competent Communicator — 242

Table 10–2. Language and Speech Skills Evidenced in the Competent Communicator Stage — 243

Table 10–3. Auditory Goals for Understanding Sound as Meaningful in the Competent Communicator Stage — 245

Table 10–4. Auditory Feedback and Speech Production Goals in the Competent Communicator Stage — 245

Table 10–5. Auditory Goals for Language Comprehension in the Competent Communicator Stage — 245

Table 10–6. Auditory Goals for Developing Expressive Language in the Competent Communicator Stage — 246

Table 10–7. Knowledge Areas in the Competent Communicator Stage — 246

Table 10–8. Optimal Strategies to Implement in the Competent Communicator Stage — 247

Table 10–9. Guide and Coach Parents To: — 248–249

Table 10–10. Life Skills to Teach Children — 250

Table 10–11. CELF-P Sentence Structure — 260

Table 10–12. CELF-P Word Structure — 260

Table 10–13. CELF-P Expressive Vocabulary — 260

Table 10–14. CELF-P Concepts and Following Directions — 260

Table 10–15. CELF-P Recalling Sentences — 261

Table 10–16. CELF-P Word Classes—Receptive — 261

Table 10–17. CELF-P Word Classes—Expressive — 261

Table 10–18. CELF-P Word Classes—Total — 261

Table 10–19. CELF Preschool Scores	261
Table 10–20. Test of Auditory Processing Skills (TAPS) Scores	262
Table 10–21. CHILD Scores by Acoustic Environment	262
Table 10–22. By the End of the Competent Communicator Stage, the Child Should:	268

Chapter 11. Advanced Communicator Stage

Table 11–1. Auditory Abilities Evidenced in the Advanced Communicator Stage	272
Table 11–2. Language and Speech Skills Evidenced in the Advanced Communicator Stage	273
Table 11–3. Auditory Goals for Understanding Sound as Meaningful in the Advanced Communicator Stage	275
Table 11–4. Auditory Feedback and Speech Production Goals in the Advanced Communicator Stage	275
Table 11–5. Auditory Goals for Language Comprehension in the Advanced Communicator Stage	275
Table 11–6. Auditory Goals for Expressive Language in the Advanced Communicator Stage	276
Table 11–7. Knowledge Areas in the Advanced Communicator Stage	277
Table 11–8. Optimal Strategies to Implement in the Advanced Communicator Stage	277
Table 11–9. Guide and Coach Parents To:	278
Table 11–10. Test of Auditory Processing Skills-3 (TAPS-3) Scores	284
Table 11–11. CELF Preschool 2 Scores by Subtest	286
Table 11–12. CELF Preschool Scores	287
Table 11–13. TACL-3 Scores	287
Table 11–14. CELF Preschool 2 Scores by Subtests at 6 Years 6 Months	289
Table 11–15. TACL-3: Age-Equivalent Test Scores at 6 Years 6 Months	290
Table 11–16. Test of Auditory Processing Skills-3 (TAPS-3) Scores at 6 Years 6 Months	290
Table 11–17. TACL-3: Age-Equivalent Test Scores at 7 Years 9 Months	291
Table 11–18. Test of Auditory Processing Skills-3 (TAPS-3) at 7 Years 9 Months	291
Table 11–19. Test of Language Development—Primary (TOLD-P:3) Scores at 7 Years 9 Months	292
Table 11–20. Test of Auditory Processing Skills-3 (TAPS-3) Scores at 9 Years 9 Months	293
Table 11–21. Test of Language Development—Intermediate (TOLD-I:4) Scores at 9 Years 9 Months	293
Table 11–22. By the End of the Advanced Communicator Stage, the Child Should:	300

Chapter 1

Speech Acoustics: The Gold at the End of the Rainbow Audiogram

Sylvia Rotfleisch

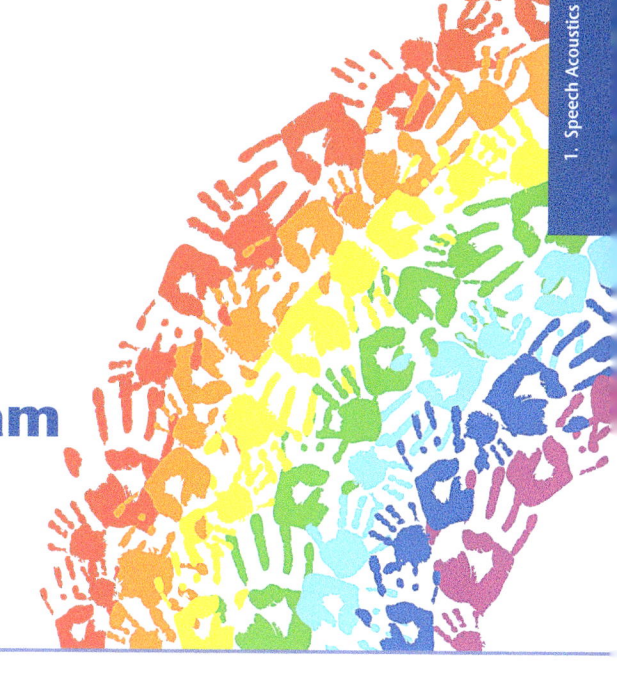

Why Do We Need to Understand Speech Acoustics?

"Of the available senses, residual audition must be regarded as potentially the most important because it is the only one directly capable of appreciating the primary characteristics of communicative speech, which are acoustic" (Ling, 2002, p. 22).

In other words, audition is the only sense capable of appreciating all aspects of speech. As professionals focused on developing listening and spoken language with children with hearing loss, we must understand that auditory access is key. Speech acoustics is the framework to understand the acoustic properties of speech phonemes and their relationship to an audiogram. By understanding speech acoustics, we can understand what sounds of speech children are hearing, better understand their perception of sounds, and use that information to plan therapy—from basic access to integration with the complexity of speech and language development. Speech acoustics is the foundation on which we consider goals and build listening and spoken language. It is also the foundation area we will look back at when there are red flags or lack of progress through stages of language acquisition.

Section I
Basics of Sound

Key Points

- The audiogram can indicate potential access or deficits related to the speech signal.
- Duration, intensity, and pitch are three dimensions of sound of significant importance in our work with children with hearing loss.
- Understanding speech acoustics principles allows us to understand factors that enhance or diminish the auditory signal for children with hearing loss.

Basics of Sound

Discussion of the perception of sound is based on three dimensions that are relevant and have applications to our work: duration, intensity, and pitch. Duration is the perceived length of the acoustic event. Loudness is the perception of intensity. Frequency is perceived as pitch. A given sound will be perceived as louder if the source of the sound is closer, and quieter if it is farther away. Loudness is the perception of how strong a sound is and can be measured objectively in units of decibels (dB) and represented on an audiogram. The larger the units for measurement of a sound, the louder it will be perceived. The audiogram is explained in more detail later. The decibel scale is complex to understand as it is a logarithmic scale, not a linear scale. Essentially, if a sound increases by 10 times, there will be a 10-dB increase in intensity, but if a sound increases by 20 decibels, there will be a 10×10 increase in intensity. This means that when a sound is 10 dB louder than another sound, it has an intensity that is 10 times greater in loudness. If the sound is 20 dB louder, then it is 100 times the intensity, and 30 dB would indicate an intensity greater by 1,000 times (Ling, 1989).

Pitch is the perception of a sound as being high or low frequency and can be measured objectively in units of hertz (Hz). A low-pitch or bass sound would have a smaller measurement in hertz in comparison to a high-pitch sound. Duration of a sound, or the length of a sound, provides information that differentiates speech sounds such as vowels versus consonants (e.g., the vowel /a/ is a longer sound and it can be made to have a longer duration, whereas the consonant /b/ is a short sound with a short duration).

Audiogram

A detection audiogram is a line graph of the dimensions of sound that indicates what a person hears. It represents the intensity level where a threshold is measured for a designated frequency. Sounds are indicated based on the graph's horizontal and vertical axes. Sounds below or louder than the indicated line can be heard, while those above cannot be heard.

The frequency of the sound is represented on an audiogram graph from low to high on the horizontal axis. It is similar to a piano keyboard from low on the left to high on the right. Continuing with the analogy of a piano which has 88 keys —the note at the middle of the keyboard, middle C, is about 250 Hz—where audiograms typically begin. An octave, or octave band, is represented by eight notes on a keyboard. An octave represents a measured doubling of the Hz (e.g., 250 Hz, 500 Hz, 1000 Hz). An octave band includes frequencies lower and higher than the named center frequency. For example, the octave band for 250 Hz, with 250 Hz as the center point, ranges from 177 to 355 Hz. The next octave band of 500 Hz is from 355 to 710 Hz. The frequencies in hertz are written across the top of the audiogram. An audiogram includes the frequencies that are most critical for hearing speech sounds, but represents less than half of the keys on a piano.

The intensity of sounds is indicated from quiet to loud in decibels (dB) as one goes down the vertical axis of the audiogram. A quiet sound, such as the wind rustling leaves in a tree, would be between 10 and 20 dB (www.sengpielaudio.com). A jet airplane taking off overhead would be about 140 to 150 dB, which is the threshold of pain for a listener with typical hearing (www.sengpielaudio.com and www.chchearing.org). Conversational speech has quiet and louder components, as well as low- and high-frequency components. Normal conversational speech ranges from about 30 to 60 dB, and from 250 to 6000 Hz, when at a distance of about 6 feet (about 2 meters.) The area on the audiogram that includes the acoustic range speech elements is most commonly referred to as the *speech banana* (Northern & Downs, 1984) or the *long-term acoustic speech spectrum* (LTASS) (Stevens et al., 1947; Niemoller et al., 1974). The goal is to achieve detection thresholds at the top of the speech banana, but perception must be assessed beyond merely detection abilities.

In audiology, noise level is compared to the signal or message being provided to the listener. The signal to noise ratio (SNR) is the comparative level of the signal in relation to ambient or background noise. If the signal is 65 dB and the noise level is 50 dB, then the signal is 15 dB louder than the noise. The SNR would be considered +15 dB. An SNR of +6 would mean the signal is 6 dB louder than the noise. A 0 SNR would be when the signal is equal to the noise. If the noise is louder than the signal, the SNR would be a negative number. For example, if the noise was 80 dB and the signal was 70 dB, we would have a −10 SNR.

A Sound Basis: The Applications

Hearing Loss and Detection

The analogy of a submarine is effective when considering an audiogram and hearing loss (Rotfleisch, 2000). To help the reader understand hearing loss, Figure 1–1 compares an audiogram and hearing levels and speech to the water level and a submarine. The audiogram, the threshold levels of the hearing, can be indicated by the water level (Ling, 2002). It is useful to understand that we do not actually improve the child's hearing loss when

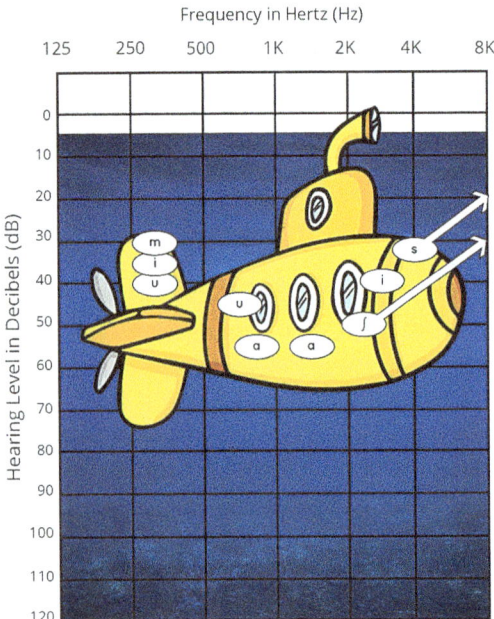

Figure 1–1. Audiogram representing normal hearing levels.

while those sounds that are above water can't be heard. An increase in decibels of the signal means an increase in the depth at which the submarine is submerged and an increase in the signal accessible.

Thresholds can be difficult to assess in children who have hearing loss. Threshold, for an audiogram, is defined as sound that we hear 50% of the time. It requires concentration on the part of the listener. Consider the threshold line on an audiogram like the water of the ocean at the beach. Threshold is like your toes being in and out of the water as the waves roll in and recede. That is how fine the line is for threshold. However, we don't listen to speech and language at threshold level. We must sink the submarine, and we do that by increasing the intensity of the signal, allowing more of the sound to reach the brain. Remember, sounds above the threshold line represented by the water (Figure 1–2) are not accessible with a hearing loss.

Modifying the Signal

How can we modify the signal to improve the outcomes in sessions and the long-term outcomes? With understanding of the dimensions of sounds and principles related to the audiogram, we can look at practical ways to apply this information to improve the auditory signal. Without question, the first way to improve the signal for a child with hearing loss is through the consistent use of technology. However, having technology does not always mean the child has the necessary access to sound. Some children with hearing loss will derive little or no benefit from hearing aids and conventional forms of hearing technology. Children may experience a delay in obtaining technology, such as

we provide technology. This is not the typical way of thinking of hearing loss. The current technologies actually increase the intensity or accessibility of the signal presented to the child at the eardrum or the cochlea. We are used to seeing an aided audiogram, which seems to indicate improvement of the thresholds. Consider the submarine represents the signal or speech and language input. Submarines belong below the water; in this analogy, below the audiogram line. We make the signal more accessible to compensate for the hearing loss. The submarine is submerged on the audiogram, and the increasing depth represents the increase in decibels. One can conceptualize sinking the submarine by increasing the auditory intensity of the speech signal (see section on modifying auditory signal). The analogy continues in that anything under water (i.e., the thresholds) can be heard,

1. Speech Acoustics: The Gold at the End of the Rainbow Audiogram 5

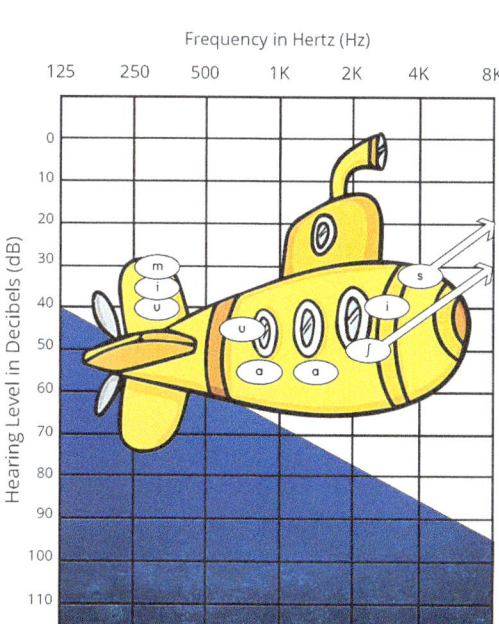

Figure 1–2. Audiogram representing a hearing loss.

cochlear implants, until they are older, if at all. Technology must be set properly, and we cannot automatically assume that because a child has technology, it is set to provide the necessary access. We must gather our own data as professionals to help figure out if the child has properly set, functioning technology that is being used to provide the auditory input required to develop listening and spoken language.

Access to sound and auditory input can be changed by multiple factors. Hearing loss is the primary factor we are addressing. Additional factors such as intensity of the sound, noise and the SNR, reverberation, distance, and imbalance of sounds in different frequency ranges can interfere with the auditory access.

The following are practical, simple ways to modify the signal, or sink the submarine, by understanding the dimensions of sound and applying principles of speech acoustics.

Ear Shot/Speech Bubble

We listen to sounds from a distance. When closer, the sounds are louder and clearer than when the distance is greater. The distance range that we can hear within is referred to as *earshot* (Ling, 1980) or the *speech bubble* (Anderson, 2002). Earshot is impacted by the child's hearing loss, speaker's clarity, and intensity of speech and ambient noise conditions. As professionals, we must determine the child's speech bubble during therapy sessions and with input from parents. We teach the parents how to monitor their child's reactions to sounds and collect further information to understand earshot in various hearing situations. Once we know the child's earshot/hearing bubble, we can be vigilant about providing the child with auditory access in a variety of situations. Effective use of a remote mic system can help us to be sure that the child is within hearing range as much as possible.

Background Noise and Noise Clutter

Let us consider the impact of noise and loudness in decibels as related to the logarithmic scale. A sound that is measured at 10 dB stronger in intensity would be perceived as a sound that is 10 times louder. An 80-dB noise or sound such as a piano or vacuum cleaner would be 10 times louder than 70-dB sounds such as a dog barking or phone ringing, and 100 times louder than a 60-dB normal conversational level (John Tracy Audiogram of Familiar Sounds, 2012; Ling, 1989).

The SNR is a critical factor when we consider the child's speech discrimination abilities. This is the relationship of the signal that we are listening to and the competing noise. Research has shown that a good SNR for typical children without hearing loss or children with hearing loss would be +15 dB to +20 dB (Nelson et al., 2002). That is, if a signal is 65 or 70 dB and the noise is 50 dB, then the signal is 15 to 20 dB louder than the noise. SNR has been examined in depth (Dubno et al., 1984). Using the data from this research, we can look at two SNR conditions: a +6 SNR and a 0 SNR. At +6 dB SNR, typically hearing individuals can score 90% correct for discrimination while individuals with hearing loss score 30% correct. At a 0 SNR, typically hearing individuals score 60% correct while individuals with hearing loss score less than 10% correct. For a child with hearing loss, improving the SNR to +12 can improve the child's score to 50% and to more than 70% with a SNR at +18. Reducing noise clutter helps to establish an environment conducive to auditory learning and significantly improves the possible speech perception for a child with hearing loss.

Consider the noise a child is exposed to in the routines of daily life and in their various listening environments. We want to explain the impact of noise and help the family address the noise factor across all of the acoustic environments. For example, for the child with hearing loss, we must consider the acoustic environment of the school (Gremp & Easterbrooks, 2018; Dockrell & Shield, 2012). An excellent acoustic environment would be 30 dB. Consider that the average ambient noise of a typical quiet room in a home can be about 50 dB. This is due to ambient noise from traffic and items in the house (e.g., a refrigerator), according to the Center for Hearing Communication (www.chchearing.org). A quiet library will have an ambient noise of about 40 dB, or 10 dB quieter than a home. Typical ambient noise in a classroom is 60 dB, or 10 dB noisier than a home. Using sound level meter apps for mobile phones, we can easily measure the noise level in a given environment. This is an excellent way to understand or demonstrate the level of noise and share it with parents.

In addition to addressing the noise in the environment, we need to consider the physical properties of the room. When appropriate, we can consider acoustic treatments in some rooms to address reverberation in the room. Acoustic treatments for walls, windows, and floors can help to diminish the echo and to establish a better auditory environment.

Audible Versus Intelligible

An audiogram is a graph of detection of the sounds that can be heard by a person. Thus, an audiogram indicates what is audible. However, just hearing the sound is not an indication of the quality of the sound or whether it can be discriminated and identified. The sound might not be adequately loud to provide for the needed perception for intelligibility of the word. Therefore, hearing (that is, detecting) words and discriminating them as different by number of syllables (e.g., sneak versus sneaking) might be possible. That would be an indication of audibility. We must determine if the child has enough auditory signal to allow for access to sounds that are critical to understand the differences of the sounds and words. Intelligibility means the listener is able to understand the important difference between *sneak, sneaker, sneaking, sneaky,* and *sneaks* (see the section on the 90/10 dilemma in this chapter). In therapy sessions we can monitor and assess if the child is able to go beyond simple detection and audibility and facilitate *listening for discrimination and identification* of sounds and words.

The 6-dB Significance

Six dB is the intensity related to a variety of listening situations. It is the level determined to be attributed to binaural summation. Binaural summation, when listening with both ears, is considered to be 6 dB louder for sounds that are at least 30 dB above detection threshold (Avan et al., 2015). Head shadow, the decreased level of a sound when it has to pass through the head to reach the other ear, is measured at approximately 6 dB. So, how much is 6 dB? Is it significant? A change in a sound of 3 dB is easily heard by most listeners, and a change of 6 dB is considered a significant difference in the level of the speech signal. In fact, an increase of 6 dB in the intensity of speech sound for a listener will be perceived as twice as loud (Ling, 1988; Boothroyd, 2019). Six dB has a significant impact. The binaural effect, listening through both ears, can be appreciated if you try this simple experiment. Listen to an auditory signal (e.g., speech, music) through one earbud and then continue to listen after putting the second earbud on. You will experience the doubling of the perception. The sound is significantly increased when listening binaurally. Keeping this in mind, when a child has a drop in their hearing of 5 or 10 dB, we should understand that this is a significant change in perception for the child and needs to be considered.

The 6-dB Rule

Dr. Daniel Ling always said, "Come closer to me, add 6 dB." The mathematics of sounds can be applied to help modify the auditory signal that reaches the listener. The rule of the inverse square law teaches us that for every doubling of the distance from the sound source, the sound intensity will be diminished by 6 dB, according to JL Audio. The reverse is true as well. By decreasing the distance, we increase the signal strength. Consider the dB scale. When working with a child, you can apply the 6-dB rule by increasing or decreasing the distance. We consider normal conversational speech to be from a distance of about 6 feet (2 meters), as previously discussed. Figures 1–2 and 1–3A illustrate the limited access to the submarine, the speech sounds, with a hearing loss from 6 feet, which is considered normal conversational distance. The 6-dB rule allows us to sink the submarine so that it submerges below the water level or thresholds (see Figure 1–3 A–E). By approaching the child and decreasing the distance from 6 feet to 3 feet, we will halve the distance, increase the sound by 6 dB, and double the perceived loudness (Figure 1–3B). We have begun to sink the submarine. We add an additional 6 dB each time we decrease the distance by half; e.g., as we move from 3 feet to 1½ feet (Figure 1–3C), from 1½ feet to 9 inches (Figure 1–3D), and then to 4½ inches (Figure 1–3E). This figure indicates the addition of another 6 dB each time we halve the distance and sink the submarine more. Consider in Figures 1–3B to 1–3E how we sink the submarine

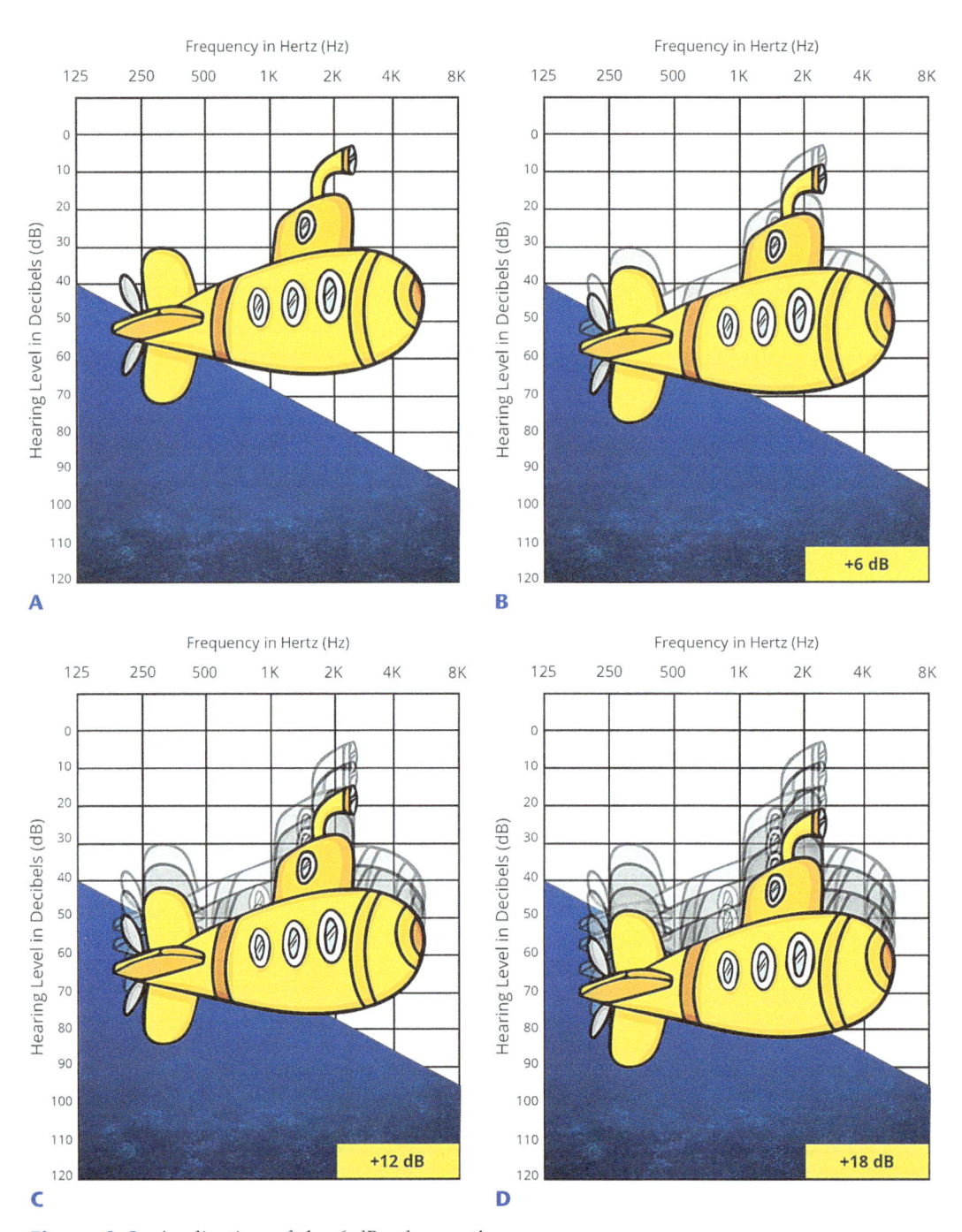

Figure 1–3. Application of the 6-dB rule. *continues*

below the water line or hearing loss and increase the access. When we are next to the child's ear, we have halved the distance four times. When we are about 4½ inches away from the child (Figure 1–3E), we have increased the signal

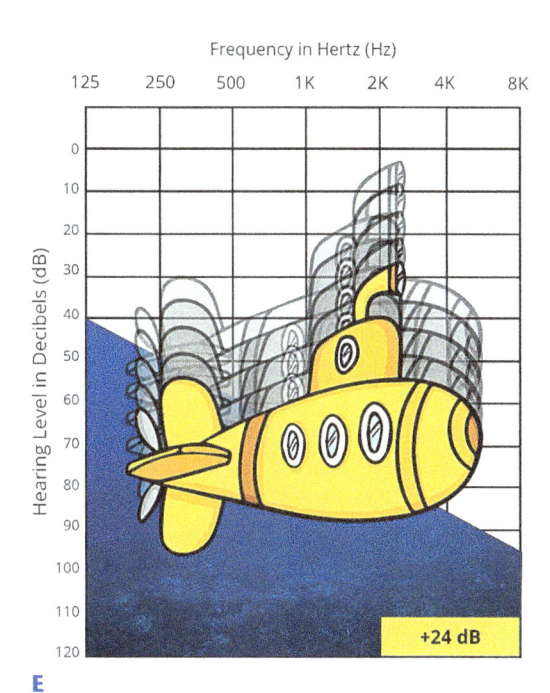

Figure 1–3. *continued*

by a total of 24 dB. This is a very significant increase in the loudness of the signal being presented to the child. As mentioned earlier, an increase of 20 dB in the signal intensity will be perceived as more than 100 times louder.

Sounds of Speech

The Basics

Speech sounds or phonemes are created by the complex speech mechanism, which includes four systems in our bodies: the respiratory, phonating, resonating, and articulatory systems. We create sounds by modifying the airflow through these systems. (Pickett, 1999; Ladefoged & Johnson, 2015). Speech patterns have a variety of features, which are defined and classified later. In addition to those speech patterns, there are some concepts that need to be understood. Discussion of this material and the acoustic correlates are based on Pickett (1999), Ladefoged and Johnson (2015), Ling (1976, 2002), and Boothroyd (2019).

Speech sounds have frequency and intensity elements that are important to understand. Phonemes can vary in frequency from 250 to 6000 Hz and above. The lowest-frequency speech sounds are phonemes such as /m/ and low components of /u/. The highest-frequency sounds are phonemes such as /s/ and /f/. However, sounds are complex. Some sounds have multiple components or formants in different frequency ranges. We will discuss sounds such as /i/ and /z/, which have both low- and high-frequency components. Phonemes in the English language have a range of intensity of about 30 decibels between the quietest and the loudest. The quietest sounds are /θ/ as in **th**in and /f/ as in **f**un, while the loudest sound is the vowel /ɑ/ as in **hot**. We will discuss the variable energy levels and the impact. When a frequency is identified for a phoneme, it is within the octave band centered in the range and not at a unique single frequency.

A spectrogram is a visual representation of speech sounds that shows the energy at specific frequencies. It is obtained by passing sounds through filters and creating a graph of time versus frequency. This allows us to understand speech sounds in relation to the frequencies. Terms for some of these visible features of speech sounds on a spectrograph are of significance to our discussion.

Speech sounds have many features that contribute to unique character of a phoneme. Fortunately, these features can also provide redundancy (Ling, 2002).

This allows a child to determine what is being said even if some elements of the sound are not heard. Details of the acoustic correlates and some of those redundancies are discussed and identified in Section II on speech features.

Resonances are clusters of energy in sounds centered at specific frequencies. They are referred to as *formants*. Formants provide a basic understanding of the correlation between speech features and the audiogram. Formants are referred to from lowest to higher frequency as the first formant (F_1), second formant (F_2), and so on. Formants and their frequencies allow us to consider the impact of hearing loss on the sounds of speech and elements of language as related to an audiogram and auditory access.

We also consider how some of the energy of the sounds can change (or not) when produced. *Invariant energy* means that by nature of the production, it does not change for the specific sound type (Pickett, 1999). This means that each specific speech feature has a property that our auditory system is able to interpret as that feature and doesn't change (Pickett, 1999). These invariant properties are a result of the way the vocal tract is shaped or constricted during the production of the phoneme and exist in the short term when we speak and produce sounds. For example, the invariant acoustic information for nasal murmur is present and doesn't vary. *Variant energy* is the energy that that can be changed and can vary. Variant energy is a result of coarticulation and the adjacent phoneme's properties.

Transitions are the variant energy components of the speech sounds. They are how a sound transitions from one phoneme to the next in typical speech production. Rapid production of strings of phonemes produces natural coarticulation as we speak in words and string words together in phrases. Transitions are named from lowest to higher frequency as the first transition (T_1), second transition (T_2), and so on. Ling (1989) explains transitions by comparing them to filling a bottle with water. As the water slowly runs into the bottle, the amount of air left decreases. This causes the air to resonate at a higher pitch, and you can hear the change in the pitch of the resonance. As the water quantity increases and the air decreases, the pitch increases. This is similar to the formant transition that occurs when you say "hot" and move your tongue to make the /t/ consonant sound.

For our purposes and applications, when you know some aspects of the acoustic energy can be varied, you can use that as a strategy. Consider that, when saying words, we move our articulators to combine strings of phonemes. This coarticulation creates transitions, or movement either up or down depending on the frequency differences between the adjacent sounds. As vowels and consonants connect to each other in running speech, they create transitions identified based on the order of the vowels and consonants. Therefore, we identity a vowel-to-consonant transition as a V-C transition. Of course, we have various combinations such as V-C-V or C-V-C and so forth. Key features of speech and their acoustic correlates, including formants and transitions, are discussed and identified in Section II on speech features.

Applications

Basic Principles

When considering access to speech sounds, we can look at general expectations or principles to have an overall view of issues for the child with hearing loss. When we consider access related to frequency areas on the audiogram, low-frequency and high-frequency information have some very different properties. Low-frequency information is typically easier to hear, more accessible, and carries more acoustic energy. High-frequency information is typically more difficult to hear, less accessible, and carries less acoustic energy. Table 1–1, *General Principles Related to Low and High Frequencies*, summarizes the key concepts related to low- and high-frequency information. Listening and spoken language therapy relies on this foundational knowledge to allow for the constant thinking and analysis back and forth between speech acoustics and the development of spoken language. We use this information to determine if all the pieces fit together properly or if something doesn't quite seem logical based on these principles. This understanding provides a foundation for selecting goals.

Table 1–1. General Principles Related to Low and High Frequencies

Low Frequency	High Frequency
Easier to hear	More difficult to hear
More accessible	Less accessible
More acoustic energy	Less acoustic energy

The 90/10 Dilemma

General principles related to low- and high-frequency speech features (Table 1–2) are the basis for what we consider the 90/10 dilemma. An estimated 90% of acoustic energy of sound (Mueller & Killion, 1990) is in the low frequencies and carries about 10% of information related to spoken language (Figure 1–4). The information in those low frequencies is less important to the perception of speech sounds and the meaning of the message. The remaining 10% of the acoustic energy is in the high frequencies and carries the 90% of information that is critical to the perception of speech sounds and the meaning of the message (Mueller & Killion, 1990; see Figure 1–4). The different properties related to low- and high-frequency speech elements (see Table 1–2) relate directly to the issue of 90% and 10% of acoustic energy. As an illustration, this means that vowels are significantly louder than consonants such as /s/, /f/, /t/, and /k/. It is easier to discriminate morphemes that have lower-frequency components such as a vowel. A vowel will add a syllable, such as the difference in *run* versus *running* or *runner* or *runny*, and take advantage of the 90% of acoustic energy. When we add the morpheme /s/ in *runs* or change the word to *runt* by adding /t/, the final consonant car-

Table 1–2. Speech Features Related to Low and High Frequencies

Low-Frequency Information Includes	High-Frequency Information Includes
Suprasegmentals: duration, intensity, pitch	Vowels: remaining F_2
Vowels: first formants and some F_2	Consonant place cues
Nasal murmur	Consonants of the fricative and affricate manner
Most consonant manner information	
Consonant voicing cues	

90/10 Dilemma

- 90% of the acoustic energy carries 10% of the meaning/intelligibility
- 10% acoustic energy carries 90% of the meaning/intelligibility

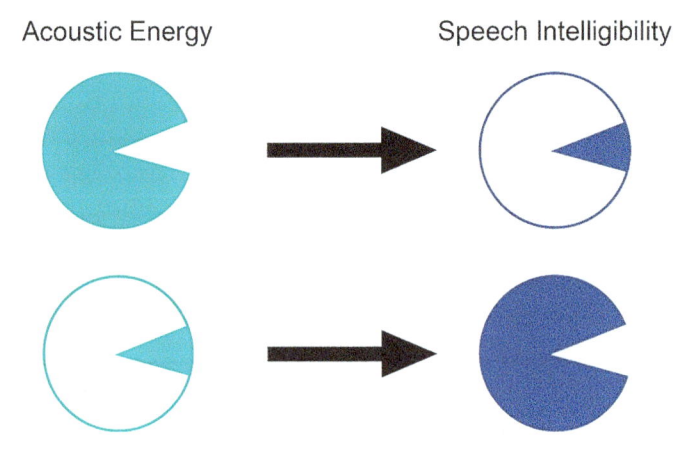

Figure 1–4. 90/10 dilemma. Rotfleisch, S. (2018). Speech perception 90/10 dilemma. *Speech acoustics detective work.* Hearing First. Used with permission.

ries acoustic information from the 10%. It is more difficult to access but impacts the meaning.

Upward Spread of Masking

A child with hearing loss might have variable access to the different elements "of speech phonemes based on their specific frequency and the intensity. We can use a variety of strategies to address the imbalance of acoustic energy that is perceived as intensity. The situation explained in the 90/10 dilemma is exacerbated when a child's hearing technology isn't set properly and the child is possibly hearing low-frequency sounds even louder than they are naturally in relation to the high-frequency sounds (explained further in the section on Ling Six Sounds).

This louder acoustic energy masks, or overpowers, the quieter acoustic information. We consider this the garbage truck syndrome. If you stand next to a loud garbage truck, it does not matter how loudly you try to produce the /s/ sound, it will not be heard above the noise of the truck. In speech, the low-frequency, loud sounds such as the vowels and the nasals would act like the garbage truck. They would drown out the important elements of the speech signal that provide the speech perception ability to understand the message. People think that speaking louder or yelling will improve the access for the person with hearing loss. However, raising our voice only makes the vowels louder, distorts the balance of sounds to a greater extent, doesn't help, and might make it more difficult to be understood. (Further discussed later in the section on suprasegmentals and vowels.) Yelling basically makes the loud sounds louder, acting like the loud garbage truck, but does nothing to increase the intensity of the quieter and high-frequency sounds. Though it seems counterintuitive when working with a child with hearing loss, whispering can sometimes help with the imbalance of speech sounds. Whispering a word will decrease the intensity of a vowel and allow the energy from the consonant to be more audible. It puts the vowel in a state more balanced with the consonant (see the section on acoustic highlighting).

Application using variant acoustic information is discussed further at a later point in the chapter with consonants.

Discussion Questions

1. Based on information in this section, how would you explain an audiogram to the parents of a child with a newly diagnosed hearing loss?
2. What topics discussed in this section would you explain to parents? Pick one and discuss how you would explain it.
3. You are working with a child who is a candidate for a cochlear implant but will not be implanted for many months or possibly longer. The family has a desired outcome of listening and spoken language. What speech acoustics applications could you explain to the parents to improve the auditory access prior to implantation?
4. Explain what information you learned in this section that you can use to help a child with hearing loss. How would you use it?

Section II
Speech Features

Key Points

- Speech elements can be classified into suprasegmental and segmental features.
- Suprasegmentals are duration, intensity, and pitch.
- Segmentals include vowels, diphthongs, and consonants.
- Consonants are classified by manner, place, and voicing.
- Speech elements have specific acoustic correlates and can be identified on an audiogram and applied to our work with children with hearing loss

Speech Features and Acoustic Correlates

The Basics

Speech patterns are composed of and classified into two main patterns: suprasegmentals (also known as nonsegmentals) and segmentals. The suprasegmental aspect has to do with the prosody of the production as perceived by the rate, rhythm, and intonation. These features are described using the dimensions of sound: duration, intensity, and pitch. Segmentals are the consonants and vowels. Each of these patterns can be classified into additional features (Table 1–3) and are discussed in more detail later. Speech elements will be related to specific areas on the audiogram. These are referred to as their *acoustic correlates* and are discussed in the following text.

Vocalization

When we produce speech sounds, the air travels through our speech-production system and vibrates within the system at a given rate or natural resonance. This is referred to as the *fundamental frequency* (F_0). Our voice has a perceived pitch based on the natural size and resonance of our vocal system. We perceive a person's voice as low or higher frequency because of the F_0 of their person's voice. The natural pitch is primarily dependent on the size of the larynx. The larger the larynx, the lower the fundamental frequency that is produced. Male voices have a lower fundamental frequency, female voices have a higher F_0, and children have the highest F_0. All fundamental frequencies are below 750 Hz, but a vocalization produces harmonics at multiples of the F_0 (Pickett, 1999; Ladefoged & Johnson, 2015; Ling, 1989, 2002).

Acoustic Correlates of Vocalizations

The fundamental frequencies for men, women, and children are all below 750 Hz.

Table 1–3. Speech Features

Suprasegmentals (nonsegmentals)	Segmentals
Duration • Long • Short • Interrupted **Intensity** • Loud • Normal • Quiet • Whispered **Pitch** • High • Normal • Low • Variable	**Vowels and Diphthongs** • Front/back • Tense/lax **Consonants** **Manners of Production:** The way the sound is produced • Nasals: resonating of the air in nasal cavity with the mouth typically closed and velopharyngeal port opens the nasal passage • Plosive: exploding sound created with buildup of pressure and burst when released. Can be produced with the pressure not released. • Fricatives: blowing sounds with friction between articulators producing an oral breath stream • Affricates: a combination of stop plosives and fricatives • Semivowels: the sound made by the movement between vowels • Liquids (laterals): two articulators in close approximation preventing breath stream release **Place of Production:** The anatomical place where the sound is produced • Bilabial: both lips • Labiodental: lower lip and upper front teeth • Linguadental: tongue tip and teeth • Alveolar: tongue tip and ridge behind upper front teeth • Palatal: front of tongue and hard palate • Velar: back of tongue and hard palate • Glottal: originating at the vocal cords **Voicing** • Voiced: vocal folds vibrating • Unvoiced: vocal folds not vibrating

Suprasegmentals (Nonsegmentals)

The suprasegmental elements of speech are duration, intensity, and pitch (DIP). These features of speech production are superimposed on all of our vocalizations. The suprasegmentals allow us to control and modify rate, rhythm, stress, and intonation (Ladefoged & Johnson, 2015; Ling, 1988, 2002). We do this by changing the vowel to be longer or louder. This is discussed further later in the text.

Vowels and Diphthongs

Vowels are produced as the airflow passes through the vocal system, and their characteristic sound is created by varying the size of the throat and mouth cavities. The shape and size create specific resonances. These resonances produce the formants at specific frequencies. Throat resonance, referred to as the *first formant* (F_1), has limited variability. The resonance that results from the mouth cavity, which is primarily shaped by tongue position, is the *second formant* (F_2) and has wider variability (Pickett, 1999). There are more than two formants for vowel sounds, but the first two are the most critical for creating the unique sound. Diphthongs are created when two vowels are produced in succession and blended together as one sound. The diphthong in b**oy** is produced by rapidly blending /o/ (as in b**oa**t) and /i/ (as in tr**ee**) (Ladefoged & Johnson; 2015; Ling, 2002). Vowels can be classified as front or back, and tense or lax (see Table 1–3). The front or back classification is based on the placement of the blade of the tongue. Tense or lax refers to how they can be used in English in different syllables. For purposes of our discussion, we will focus on the resonance of the sounds or formants as this aspect relates directly to their acoustic properties.

Acoustic Correlates of Suprasegmentals and Vowels

The suprasegmental features, which are carried by the vowels, are auditorily accessible if there is access to F_1 of all vowels. Vowels of the English language are represented with their first and second formants and are arranged in an ascending order of frequencies for their F_2 in Figure 1–5. This formant chart allows us to consider auditory access based on the frequency components of the vowels. Access

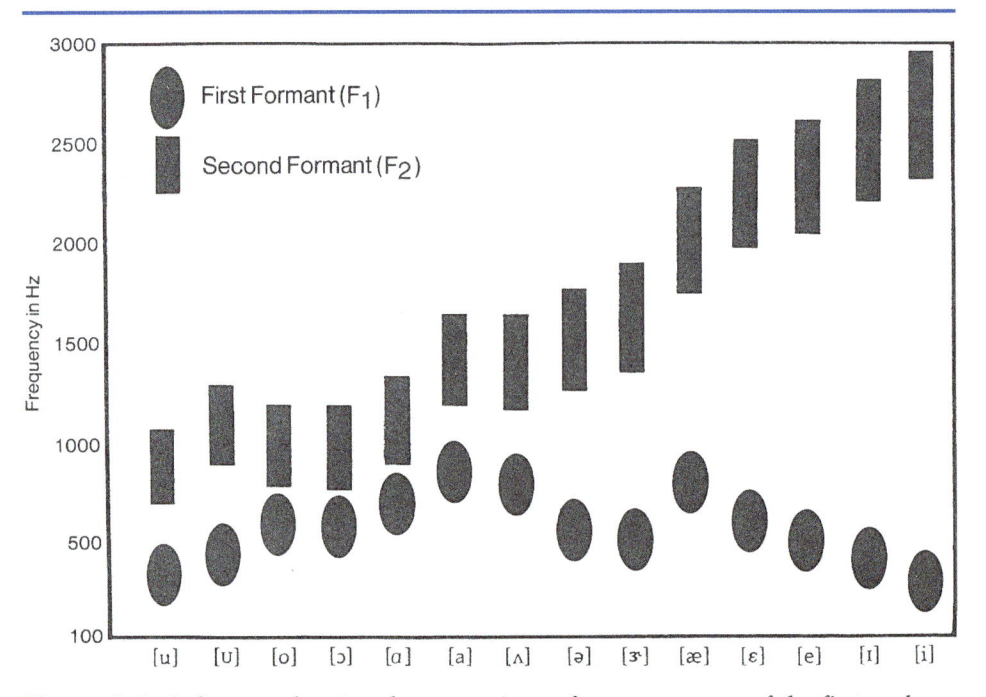

Figure 1–5. A diagram showing the approximate frequency range of the first and second formants of the English vowels as spoken by adult males. From Ling, D., & Ling, A. (1978). *Aural habilitation: Foundations of verbal learning in hearing-impaired children.* Reprinted with permission from AG Bell.

to all of the first formants provides detection of all vowels, but access to F_2 is needed to be able to discriminate the vowels (Ling & Ling, 1978; Ling, 2002). All vowels will be detected if there is auditory access up to 1000 Hz. However, the ability to discriminate the vowels is dependent on access to the second formants. Vowels with higher-frequency second formants are examples of sounds that have low- and high-frequency acoustic information. Some vowels have first formants at similar frequencies and are different by the higher-frequency second formant. Auditory access to 3000 Hz will allow for identification of all vowels. Limited auditory access at different frequencies will limit the ability to discriminate some of the vowels.

Consonants

Consonants features are created by the airflow being altered as it moves through the four systems of the speech mechanism (Pickett, 1999; Ladefoged & Johnson, 2015). This airflow creates formants, or clusters of energy, as discussed previously. Consonants are described using three dimensions: manner, place, and voicing (see Table 1–3).

The manner is how the sound is produced. Air can be diverted to the nasal cavity or the oral cavity, where it then resonates to produce an oral or nasal sound. The nasal manner of sounds is produced when air is diverted through the nasal cavity. Other manners of consonants such as plosives and fricatives are produced when air is diverted through the oral cavity. Plosives can be produced with the release of a burst of air, or be classified as a stop plosive when the air is unreleased or stopped. The plosive /b/ would be released in the word *ball* and unreleased in the word *cab* (Pickett, 1999; Ladefoged & Johnson, 2015).

The place is the location where the sound is produced. The mouth, teeth, tongue, and jaw are the components of the articulatory system that control the place of production (Ladefoged & Johnson, 2015; Ling, 2002). For example, a phoneme produced using both lips is bilabial, and a phoneme produced using the tongue tip and teeth is linguadental.

The phonation created by modulating air in the pharynx and larynx determines if the sound is voiced or voiceless, depending on if the vocal cords are vibrating or not. Voicing is if the vocal cords are vibrating when the sound is produced (see Table 1–3). An unvoiced sound indicates the vocal cords are not vibrating (Ladefoged & Johnson, 2015; Ling, 1988, 2002). One might think that we are always using our voice when we speak, but that is different than this feature of voicing. This can be demonstrated and understood by placing your hand on your throat while saying /s/ and /z/ phonemes. You will feel no vibrations for the unvoiced /s/ and vibrations for the voiced /z/. Sound pairs such as /s/ and /z/, which are of the same manner and place but only differ by the vibration of the vocal cords, are cognate pairs. The various elements within these dimensions are included and defined in Table 1–2. A completed chart (Table 1–4) classifies the consonants by manners of production and places of articulation and voicing using the International Phonetic Alphabet (IPA) symbols (Table 1–5).

Acoustic Correlates of Consonants

Acoustic correlates for consonants' manner, place, and voicing features are basic information for understanding the relationship of consonants and the audiogram. Manner information is primarily low- and mid-frequency information. For example, the nasal resonance, referred to

Table 1-4. Consonant Classification Chart

	Voicing	Bilabial	Labiodental	Linguadental	Linguaalveolar	Linguapalatal	Linguavelar	Glottal
Plosives	Voiced	b			d		g	
	Unvoiced	p			t		k	h
Fricatives	Voiced		v	ð	z	ʒ		
	Unvoiced		f	θ	s	ʃ		
Nasals	Voiced	m			n		ŋ	
	Unvoiced							
Affricates	Voiced					dʒ		
	Unvoiced					tʃ		
Semivowels	Voiced	w				j		
	Unvoiced							
Liquids	Voiced				l, r			
	Unvoiced							

Table 1–5. International Phonetic Alphabet Key

Symbol	Key Word
/b/	**b**at
/d/	**d**o
/f/	**f**ill
/g/	**g**o
/h/	**h**ow
/j/	**y**es
/k/	**k**ey
/l/	**l**ow
/m/	**m**e
/n/	**n**o
/ŋ/	si**ng**
/p/	**p**at
/r/	**r**ed
/s/	**s**o
/t/	**t**o
/v/	**v**ery
/w/	**w**e
/z/	**z**oo
/θ/	**th**in
/ð/	**th**at
/tʃ/	**ch**ild
/dʒ/	**j**am
/ʃ/	**sh**oe
/ʒ/	ca**s**ual

Source: http://www.internationalphoneticassociation.org/content/ipa-chart

as the *nasal murmur*, is centered at 300 Hz. Fricative and affricate energy is higher at 4000 Hz. Frequency information on voicing, the vocal cord vibration, is found at 500 Hz and below. Place cue information is primarily found from frequency information, including bursts of energy from 1500 to 4000 Hz and also from the energy of formant transitions. Details of acoustic cues for the speech features are in Table 1–6 and are organized as discussed earlier.

The Applications Related to Speech Features

Suprasegmentals, Vowels, and Diphthongs

Suprasegmentals and vowels are foundational related to both the ability to produce speech that others can easily understand and nuances of the linguistic message. Suprasegmentals are dependent on vowels and diphthongs. Vowels and diphthongs provide the opportunity for modulating the duration, intensity, and pitch (DIP), which carry the melody of speech and much underlying meaning. We do this by changing the way we say the vowel. In that way, vowels carry or allow us to create suprasegmentals in running speech. We can change the vowel duration to make it longer or shorter. We can change the intensity by making it louder or quieter. The perceived pitch can be modified to be lower or higher (Pickett, 1999). Control of the production of suprasegmental aspects is critical to production of speech that is intelligible to others. Poor control of these elements, such as elongating sounds or using a pitch that is not our natural resonance (i.e., too high or too low), will cause poor breath control and support of the systems used for speech production. Such inappropriate use of the underlying foundations of speech production cause poor intelligibility and error patterns, resulting in poor voice quality.

Table 1–6. Acoustic Cues for Speech Features

Vocalization		Consonants: Manners of Production	
125 Hz	Male fundamental frequency (F_0)	1000 Hz	Noise burst of most plosives
			F_2 of nasal consonants
250 Hz	Low harmonics of adult male voices		T_2 of the semivowels
			Additional cues for most consonants
	Fundamental frequency (F_0) of female and child voices	1500 Hz	F_1 of lateral liquids /r/, /l/
750 Hz	Minimum level to hear all fundamental frequencies	2000 Hz	Additional cues
			Noise burst of most plosives and affricates
1000 Hz	Harmonics of most voices		
2000 Hz	Harmonics of most voices		Unvoiced plosives: /p/, /k/, /t/
4000 Hz	Upper range of harmonics of most voices		Turbulent noise of fricatives /ʃ/, /f/, /θ/ (unvoiced)
			T_2 and T_3 of /l/ and /r/
Suprasegmentals, Vowels, and Diphthongs		4000 Hz	Turbulent noise of voiced and unvoiced fricatives
250 Hz	F_1 of high back and front vowels		Fricatives and affricates
			Noise burst of most plosives and affricates
500 Hz	F_1 of most vowels		
1000 Hz	To detect all vowels		Turbulent noise of all fricatives and affricates
	F_2 and T_1 of back and central vowels	**Consonants: Place of Production**	
2000 Hz	F_2 and T_2 of front vowels	1500+ Hz	F_2 and T_2 and burst frequency
3000 Hz	To discriminate among vowels	1500 Hz	Primary cues
4000 Hz	F_3 and T_3 of most vowels	4000 Hz	Secondary cues
Consonants: Manners of Production		**Consonants: Voicing**	
300 Hz	Nasal murmur F_1 for /m/, /n/, /ŋ/	250 Hz	Voicing cues
		500 Hz	And below for duration and intensity differences
500 Hz	Primary cues for most consonants	750 Hz	For vocal cord vibration
	T_1 of the semivowels		Voiced: at least one formant present at or below
750 Hz	Allows for ability to discriminate nasals from plosives	3000 Hz	For unvoiced: has no energy below 1000 Hz

Source: Adapted from Ling (1989), Figure 3–7, p. 69.

Adult variations of DIP are the basis for infant- or child-directed speech (IDS, CDS), which is important in early facilitation of listening and spoken language development. By controlling the suprasegmentals, we express vocal emotions, questions, statements, and other, subtler underlying messages such as sarcasm. A rising intonation by increasing the pitch of the final words in a sentence will create a question. By making a word stressed within a sentence, we can have the listener understand that it is a more significant part of the message.

As with all elements of speech and language, we must develop the auditory skills related to the elements before they can be used. These elements are lower frequency and easier to access. This is the foundation where we begin with children or new listeners. Singing and nursery rhymes, exclamations (e.g., "uh oh," "oh no!"), vocal play, and child-directed speech all take advantage of the brain's early listening ability to attend to low-frequency, stronger intensity sounds. First, children listen to these elements and discriminate them, and then produce and control them.

Even with limited auditory access, many beginning listeners will have access to this information. Auditory skills can begin with vowels and suprasegmentals. These elements are the foundations and should be initial goals for every child learning to listen. Children who do not have access to the high-frequency sounds or will be getting different technology can still begin with these elements. Sound-object associations take advantage of speech acoustics. These sounds (also referred to as the *learning to listen sounds*) should be strategically used to facilitate and monitor detection of the suprasegmentals and vowels (Vaughan, 1976). This is done by contrasting a low pitch, low-frequency vowel in *moo* for the cow with the high pitch *ch, ch, ooooo* for the train. The beginning listener attends to and learns to discriminate and identify the sounds based on their elements and develops some early comprehension (see Chapter 5).

Babies begin here with controlling their initial speech productions. By learning to control their DIP, they master the skills that are needed to support their development of intelligible speech. As children learn how to speak and use their suprasegmentals, they learn to maintain critical aspects of their speech such as prosody, rate, nasal and pharyngeal resonance, pitch, air expenditure, and other elements. These skills will allow their speech production to be intelligible to listeners. They learn to control their suprasegmental aspects of speech to express pragmatic functions to convey emotions such as happy, content, hungry, or angry (Damm et al., 2019).

Our control of intonation and stress patterns can completely alter the meaning of a sentence. In English, to ask a question, we use a rising intonation in the final word or words of the phrase. Stressing a word within a phrase by making it louder or longer or giving it an intonation curve allows the listener to know the most important part of a message. If we say the same sentence but stress a different key word, we can answer different questions. Consider the sentence "Betsy bought the lamp at the flea market." We would stress BETSY if asked who bought the lamp, but we would stress LAMP if the inquiry was what was purchased. Stressing the words FLEA MARKET would indicate the question was asking where the lamp was bought.

Vowels have two critical formants that combine to provide their characteristic sound. One is the formant created by the resonance from the throat, and the other formant is created by the resonance of the mouth or oral cavity. It is like blowing across the tops of two bottles of different volumes to create a sound, one for each of the formants. Combining the formants simultaneously creates a resonance that we hear as a pitch.

Acoustically similar vowels have the same first formant but different second formants. If the first formant is the same, one of the two bottles would be the same and the second would be different. There are several pairs of acoustically similar vowels. The vowel formant chart illustrates this issue. Looking at the vowel formant chart (see Figure 1–5), place a piece of paper horizontally at 1000 Hz, covering the top of the chart and obscuring the symbols for formants above that frequency. This provides a visual representation of how some vowels pairs such as /u/ and /i/ are acoustically similar. This vowel confusion is very common for children who do not have access to the higher-frequency second formant of /i/. Children with this difficulty will confuse the vowels and words such as *blue* and *green*, or *two* and *three*. One can move the paper to block the view, for example, at 2000 Hz, to help visualize access or lack of access to vowels due to hearing loss. Note which vowels have similar first formants.

Vowels have low-frequency energy and can mask elements of quieter, high-frequency speech phonemes. When you whisper a vowel, you are no longer vibrating your vocal cords, which is a low-frequency component of the sound. This can allow other phonemes to be more easily heard. This is one of the principles of acoustic highlighting.

Central vowels such as /ɑ/ and /a/ in the 1000-Hz octave band have more intensity than other vowels as they are produced with the mouth wide open. Vowels produced with the mouth and tongue obstructing the airflow, such as /u/ and /i/, are lower intensity.

Vowels can provide information about the consonants. The duration of a vowel will be different if the consonant that follows it is voiced or unvoiced. If the consonant is voiced, the vowel before it will be longer, but a vowel will be shorter if the consonant following it is unvoiced. This is illustrated when you say C-V-C word pairs with voiced and unvoiced consonants. If you say the words *mop* and *mob* but stop before you vocalize the word's final consonant, you will notice the difference in the length of the vowel. The duration of the vowel provides information about the consonant. It can be used to facilitate the discrimination skills related to voicing.

Important factors and applications for the suprasegmentals and vowels are summarized in Tables 1–7 and 1–8.

Consonants

When we have an understanding that the child with hearing loss has access to sounds in specific frequency ranges from their audiogram, we can select appropriate detection, discrimination, and identification tasks predicted to be within the child's range of audibility. Manner and voicing information are primarily found in the lower and mid frequencies. Such information will have more acoustic energy and be perceived as a louder intensity. These features are typically easier to hear and then easier to access, and are typically foundational skills to be developed. However, sometimes we must look at the areas of difficulty to determine beyond the detection and what is actually being accessed by the brain.

Table 1–7. Suprasegmentals: Important Factors and Applications

- Identified through duration, intensity, pitch (DIP)
- Carry the melody of speech
- Carry pragmatic meaning/coding, e.g., question, sarcasm, mood of speaker
- Are the foundation of child- and infant-directed speech
- Information is not available through vision and must be accessed through audition
- Can be accessed if child has audition up to 1000 Hz
- Babies begin to discriminate the different features of DIP with auditory access
- Babies control their early vocal productions using these elements
- Babies will learn to express different vocal emotions by controlling these elements
- Control of suprasegmentals is a preliminary skill developed during stages of babbling and control is learned and practiced
- Control and correct production of suprasegmentals are critical foundational skills for production of intelligible speech

Table 1–8. Vowels: Important Factors and Applications

- Vowels allow for modulation of the suprasegmental aspects of speech
- Auditory information is critical to detect and discriminate vowels
- First two formants are critical to making vowels distinct and identifiable
- Possible to detect but not discriminate or identify vowels
- Discrimination and identification of specific vowels requires access to both F_1 and F_2
- Access to F_1 permits detection of a vowel
- All vowel F_1 are below 1000 Hz
- Vowel F_2 range from low to high frequency
- The sentence "Who would know more of art must again learn and then take his ease" (Ling & Ling, 1978) lists vowels such that F_2 is in ascending order
- Vowel's F_2 carry information about the adjacent consonants found in the 750 to 2500 Hz range
- Acoustically similar vowels have similar F_1 and differ by F_2 and therefore can be confused (e.g., /u/ versus /i/)
- All vowels are voiced
- Vowels cannot be identified though speechreading since they are dependent on tongue position
- Cannot discriminate a vowel based on lip positions
- Lip rounding and lip spread distort the vowel and can create pitch-dependent vowels
- Duration of a vowel will be decreased when preceding a word final unvoiced stop (e.g., /p/, /t/, /k/) and longer duration when preceding a voiced stop (e.g., /b/, /d/, /g/)
- Vowels can contribute to the garbage truck syndrome
- Whispering lowers the acoustic energy for vowels—this is one of the principles of acoustic highlighting

Sources: Adapted from: Ling & Ling, 1978; Ling, 2002; Ladefoged, 2015; Tiwari, 2012

Perception errors can help to determine issues with auditory access, discrimination, or identification. When errors are found to show consistent patterns, we can look at specific areas on the audiogram as possible red flags. A child having difficulty hearing /b/ as different from /p/, and /d/ as different from /t/, is demonstrating issues with the difference between voiced and voiceless sounds. We know that voicing is in the 500-Hz range and below on the audiogram. Error analysis and the rainbow audiogram are useful to help determine frequency areas that could be potential problems and are discussed later in the text. Discrimination error patterns will impact the development of speech and language.

A child who has difficulty hearing manner differences will have difficulty with past-tense verbs where consonants of different manner cues are adjacent to each other. Examples would be the nasal adjacent the plosive in *comb* versus *combed*, or the fricative /s/ adjacent to the plosive /t/ in *cross* versus *crossed*. A child who has difficulty hearing differences in place cues will have difficulty with past-tense verbs where consonants of different place cues are adjacent to each other. This would be seen in verbs with the bilabial /p/ followed by the alveolar /t/ as in *jump* versus *jumped*, or the velar /g/ followed by the alveolar /d/ as in *bag* versus *bagged*. These issues are discussed further in the section on language development.

In normal speech production, consonants and vowels are coarticulated and have an effect on each other. Vowel information, as discussed earlier, can provide information about the nature of consonants. Duration of a vowel provides information indicating if the following consonant is voiced or unvoiced. Consonants can change based on the sound that comes before them. The /s/ phoneme will often change to a /z/ when the sound before it is voiced. For example, in the word *scissors*, the initial /s/ is unvoiced but the medial and final ones are voiced, as are the sounds before them. We see this rule in the /s/ plural and possessive functions. The word *bat* finishes with an unvoiced /t/ and the plural form, *bats*, is spoken with the unvoiced /s/. The word *bag* finishes with a voiced /g/ and the plural form, *bags*, is said with the voiced /z/. The word *mommy* ends in a vowel, always voiced, therefore the possessive form, *mommy's*, is said with the voiced /z/. Similar rule follows for the pronunciation of the *-ed* morpheme indicating past tense. When the verb ends with a voiced phoneme such as *comb*, the *-ed* is pronounced as a voiced /d/. However, when the verb finishes with an unvoiced phoneme such as *push*, then the *-ed* is pronounced as an unvoiced /t/.

All vowels and many consonants are voiced and therefore have a low-frequency component. This can bring into play the garbage truck syndrome. If the voiced sounds are too loud (for any of a number of reasons) compared to the quieter speech sounds, we may need to help the child with hearing loss to improve their access and enable them to attend to the quieter sounds. Whispering a voiced consonant or vowel can provide access to quieter consonants within the word or phrase, as whispering gets rid of the garbage truck noise. Whispering eliminates the sound of the vibration of the vocal cords. This is effective when voiced consonants might be masking the unvoiced consonants in the word. This strategy allows for a balancing of sounds and their quieter formants of the unvoiced phoneme to be more easily heard. For acoustic highlighting, we must look at which phonemes are voiced and which are unvoiced to know if we will be providing the improved access. The formant transitions provide invariant energy with information for consonant place cues. The continued discussion by Ling on the subject of transitions illustrates this (Ling, 1989). If you say the words *hop* and *hot*, and move the tongue (create the transition) to the appropriate place in your mouth, but stop before you say the final consonant, you will notice the distinct difference in the words.

Additional speech acoustics information from comparative intensities can provide cues for differentiating consonants when they overlap in the same frequency range. For example, within the same lower octave band we find both the nasal murmur and the voicing sound. However, the nasal murmur has less intensity than voicing energy. Similarly, in higher-frequency octave bands, we find that fricative turbulence produces a stronger intensity sound than the high frequency of second formants. Fricative turbulence intensity differs for different phonemes in this manner. We know that the phoneme /s/ is stronger in intensity than both the /f/ and /v/ phonemes. We find that fricatives and affricates that are unvoiced, such as /ʃ/ and /tʃ/, have louder fricative turbulence than the voiced /ʒ/ and /dʒ/ (Ling, 2002).

Though we know some sounds are within specific octave bands, and though speech features have invariant energy, they also have variant energy. Vowels can be used to take advantage of the variant energy of consonants; that is, the transitions. Vowels allow us to vary the variant energy. You can remember VVV: vowels vary variant energy.

We can take advantage of the varying nature of transitions by controlling how they vary. A high-frequency phoneme will need to connect to the adjacent one, which could be similar, higher, or lower in frequency. Think of the sounds reaching or stretching toward each other to be joined. Compare this to you reaching to grab an object. You would need stretch to get the object if it is on a high shelf, but you would bend down if it is on the floor or simply reach directly forward when it is on a counter. Consider sounds reaching for each other. If a low-frequency vowel such as /u/ is before a high-frequency consonant such as /s/, then the energy of the vowel and consonant has to connect. The vowel will make the consonant bend down to create the variant energy in the transition. If the vowel with higher-frequency energy such as /i/ is before the high-frequency consonant such as /s/, then the energy of the vowel and consonant still has to connect. However, this time there is less of a stretch.

When looking at speech perception skills, using this principle to check the child's abilities with vowels that are low frequency (e.g., /u/), mid frequency (e.g., /ɑ/), and high frequency (e.g., /i/) can be very informative. A child might be able to more clearly discriminate place cues such as /p/ versus /k/ depending on the vowel that is paired with the plosive. So, when a child has limited hearing in the higher frequencies, pairing a high-frequency consonant with a vowel that has low-frequency formants can help to enhance components of the consonants. Important factors and applications for the consonants are summarized in Table 1–9.

Table 1–9. Consonants: Important Factors and Applications

- There are three defining features for consonants: manner, place, and voicing
- These acoustic features are in low-, mid-, and high-frequency areas
- Many acoustic features overlap with features of other suprasegmentals, vowels, diphthongs, and other consonant features
- Consonants carry only 10% of acoustic energy but 90% of critical speech perception information
- Consonants are critical to understanding specifics of words and language
- Nasals, liquids, and semivowels are always voiced
- Place cue information is carried primarily by second formant transition (T_2) and burst frequency
- Voicing feature is noted by the presence or absence of the vibration of the vocal folds
- Features have specific acoustic correlates that can be related to the different frequency bands on the audiogram
- When the morphemes such as /s/ or past tense -ed are added to a word, they will take on the voicing characteristic of the previous phoneme
- A word final stop plosive will be perceived as voiceless when the preceding vowel is short in duration and perceived as voiced when the vowel is longer in duration (Lisker, 1964; Ling, 2002)
- Acoustic highlighting eliminates the low-frequency energy of voiced phonemes to help access unvoiced phonemes

Discussion Questions

1. Explain what information you learned in this section that can you use to help a child with hearing loss. How would you use it?
2. The parents of a young child with hearing loss keep asking why their child doesn't have all the sounds or any words yet. They want to know why you aren't focusing on speech sounds like /k/, /s/, and /l/. How would you explain suprasegmental aspects of speech, the acoustic correlates, and their importance to this family?
3. What topics discussed in this section would you explain to parents? Pick one and discuss how you might explain it.
4. You are working with a child who is a candidate for a cochlear implant but will not be implanted for many months or possibly longer. The family has a desired outcome of listening and spoken language. Based on speech acoustics principles and applications, how would you explain the auditory access and appropriate auditory goals for the child?

Section III
Speech Acoustics Tools and Applications

Key Points

- Ling six sounds, when appropriately administered, can provide significant information when working with children with hearing loss.
- The rainbow audiogram is a visual representation of speech acoustics and speech features on an audiogram.
- The rainbow audiogram can be used to bridge speech acoustics theory to practical applications.
- Listening and spoken language intervention is best accomplished when applying speech acoustics principles to understand the auditory access to speech for children with hearing loss.
- Understanding speech acoustics allows us to understand patterns and difficulties that children with hearing loss have in the development of speech and language skills.

Ling Six-Sound Test

Purpose and Administration

The Ling Six-Sound Test was intended as a test to quickly determine if " . . . a child's audition is at least minimally adequate for hearing speech" (Ling, 1980). The six sounds (Table 1–10) were selected to assess the range of access from low to high frequencies. Sounds are typically presented to the child by the adult/Listening and Spoken Language (LSL) professional from a distance of about 6 feet (2 meters). The six sounds are indicated on the submarine in Figures 1–1 and 1–2.

The child is taught to indicate if they hear the sound by raising or clapping their hands, responding verbally, or using a toy as in conditioned play audiometry (Ling, 1989, 2003). Additional information on the correct administration of the Ling Six-Sound Test is outlined in Table 1–11. This test can be used in different ways to assess beyond detection. The child can be asked to imitate the sounds. Identification abilities for the sounds can be determined by this imitation and can provide us with information about the entire auditory system from detection through

Table 1–10. Ling Six Sounds

Sound	Key Word
/m/	**m**e
/u/	wh**o**
/ɑ/	**o**f
/i/	**ea**se
/ʃ/	**sh**oe
/s/	**s**o

Source: Ling, 2002.

Table 1–11. Administration of the Ling Six-Sound Test

- Sounds are presented in random order
- Sounds are produced at normal conversational level
- Sounds are produced in a natural manner without exaggeration
- Sounds are presented with varying intervals between sounds to prevent responses to a perceived rhythm
- Sounds are presented from a distance of 6 feet/2 meters (or indicate the distance as additional information)
- Sounds are provided through audition only, and the child is not able to see the presenter's mouth. If the child can see the speaker's face, then an acoustically transparent screen, not a hand or other object, should be used to cover the mouth
- The child understands how to respond to hearing the sound appropriately to their skill level

technology to perception and what is getting to the brain.

Applications of the Ling Six Sounds

Detection of all the Ling six sounds from the distance of normal conversational interactions can be considered a good prognostic indication of the ability to develop speech. For additional information, we might try to determine if the child can respond to a given sound from a closer distance if they were not able to respond from the defined distance. For example, if the child does not respond to the /ʃ/ from 6 feet, we could approach to see if a response can be obtained from 3 feet or a few inches away from the child. This would indicate underamplification at that frequency range but that the child can hear that frequency.

The Ling Six-Sound Test is used to obtain basic information regarding the child's hearing access. It is not an intervention goal. It is not a substitute for an audiogram or audiological testing. However, it has a variety of applications (Table 1–12)

Table 1–12. Applications of the Ling Six-Sound Test

- To determine what the child detects
- A discrimination screening tool
- An identification screening tool
- To check if the hearing technology is working
- To be sure the FM system is connected properly
- To know what modalities are appropriate to use to teach speech
- A screening of appropriate access through cochlear implant (CI) settings/map
- To cue the child to listen

and information that can be determined based on the child's responses.

Interpretation of the Ling Six Sounds

However, when the child does not respond or identify all the sounds, patterns or errors in the response can provide useful information. For example, responses to /ʃ/

and /s/ indicate access to high-frequency speech features. The vowel /i/ can provide an abundance of information due to its formant structures and the relationship with the other sounds. These responses and errors can indicate different auditory access issues and are summarized in Table 1–13.

Consistent administration of the Ling six sounds will help to monitor for a change in any of components of the auditory chain. A child who consistently

Table 1–13. Interpretation of the Ling Six-Sound Test

Response Pattern	Indication and Concerns	Potential Outcomes
Detects all six sounds	Access to sounds across the speech range	Able to access sounds to develop speech features across the frequency range
Detects /m/, /u/, /ɑ/, /i/, and /ʃ/	Access to both formants of the vowels and access to some high-frequency sounds	Difficulty with unvoiced plosives, unvoiced fricatives, and possibly place cues
Does not detect /m/	Poor access to other low-frequency sounds	Poor prosody Errors in vowels
Does not detect /ɑ/	Poor access to mid-range sounds	Unstressed words in mid-frequency range could be missing
Does not detect /m/ and /u/ but detects /ɑ/	Underamplification of low frequency and/or overamplification of mid frequency	Detects whispered *ah* from distance (20 feet), resulting in upward spread of masking
Does not detect /i/	No access to low F_1 or high F_2	Overall limited access to high- and low-frequency speech features
Detects /i/, /m/, and /u/ but not /ʃ/	Access to low F_1 but no access to high F_2	Limited or no access to high-frequency speech features
Detects /i/ and /ʃ/ but not /m/ and /u/	Access to high F_2 but no access to low F_1	Poor prosody Errors in vowels
Detects /i/, /ʃ/, and /u/ but not /m/	Access to high F_2 but no access to nasal murmur	Issues with nasalized productions of vowels
Does not detect /s/ but detects other sounds	Access to both formants of most vowels and access to moderately high-frequency sounds but not the very high sounds	Difficulty with unvoiced plosives, unvoiced fricatives, and possibly place cues
Confusions with /u/ versus /i/	Access to low F_1 but no access to high F_2	Errors in vowel discriminations and productions when critical high-frequency access is limited
Confusions with /u/ versus /m/	Need to verify possible technology issues as possibly causing the confusion	Need for work to facilitate identification of the sound

Source: Compiled from Ling, 2003.

responded to all sounds and then has a change in their responses could indicate a new problem. It could be a dead battery in the technology or other technology problem that requires troubleshooting. The child who does not respond or discriminate low-frequency sounds, but previously responded, could have fluid in their ear or an ear infection. Changes in responses to high-frequency sounds could indicate a microphone beginning to malfunction, roll off in responses, or wax buildup in the ear canal. A persistent change could indicate the onset of a problem with technology or a change in hearing abilities that should be further investigated.

The Rainbow Audiogram

The rainbow audiogram was introduced as a concept by Rotfleisch (2000), and some of its applications are explored in this section. It is a visual representation of speech features and their acoustic correlates plotted directly on an audiogram (Figure 1–6). We refer to this visual representation as the rainbow audiogram (Rotfleisch, 2000). The rainbow audiogram is a tool used to help visualize some key acoustic correlates (Table 1–14) and bridge theoretical information with practical applications. The rainbow audiogram illustrates the connection between speech acoustics, hearing, and an audiogram. Speech acoustics and audition are considered the foundation for this therapy model for developing listening and spoken language.

Applications of the Rainbow Audiogram

We are taking this opportunity to explore five suggested applications of the rainbow audiogram in a variety of analyses related to speech acoustics. We can also use it as one of the tools when determining a functional audiogram. (See Functional Audiogram later in the text.)

1. Identifies Speech Features as Low, Mid or High Frequency

The rainbow audiogram visualizes speech features as low-, mid-, or higher-frequency areas on the audiogram. When considering speech features and the development of skills related to those features, we remember basic principles and differences in low- and high-frequency auditory information (see Table 1–2, Table 1–14, Figure 1–6). In developing auditory skills, children with hearing loss typically begin from the easiest, most accessible sounds, which are typically in the low-frequency range on the left side of the audiogram. Initial goals would include speech features on the low-frequency sounds.

Looking at the rainbow audiogram, it is easy to identify beginning skills by speech features in the lower-frequency ranges (e.g., detection of voices, nasals, voicing, nasal plosive manner discrimination, vowel detection, and suprasegmentals). Skills then proceed to develop toward the mid- and higher-frequency ranges toward the right side of the audiogram. Speech features such as the additional manners of production, vowel discrimination based on second formants, and place cues are the intermediate and advanced skills.

2. Identifies Acoustic Correlates for Errors and Error Patterns

The rainbow audiogram assists in looking at the acoustic correlates of a child's skills and difficulties. Once an error pattern is determined, the rainbow audiogram can

Rainbow Audiogram

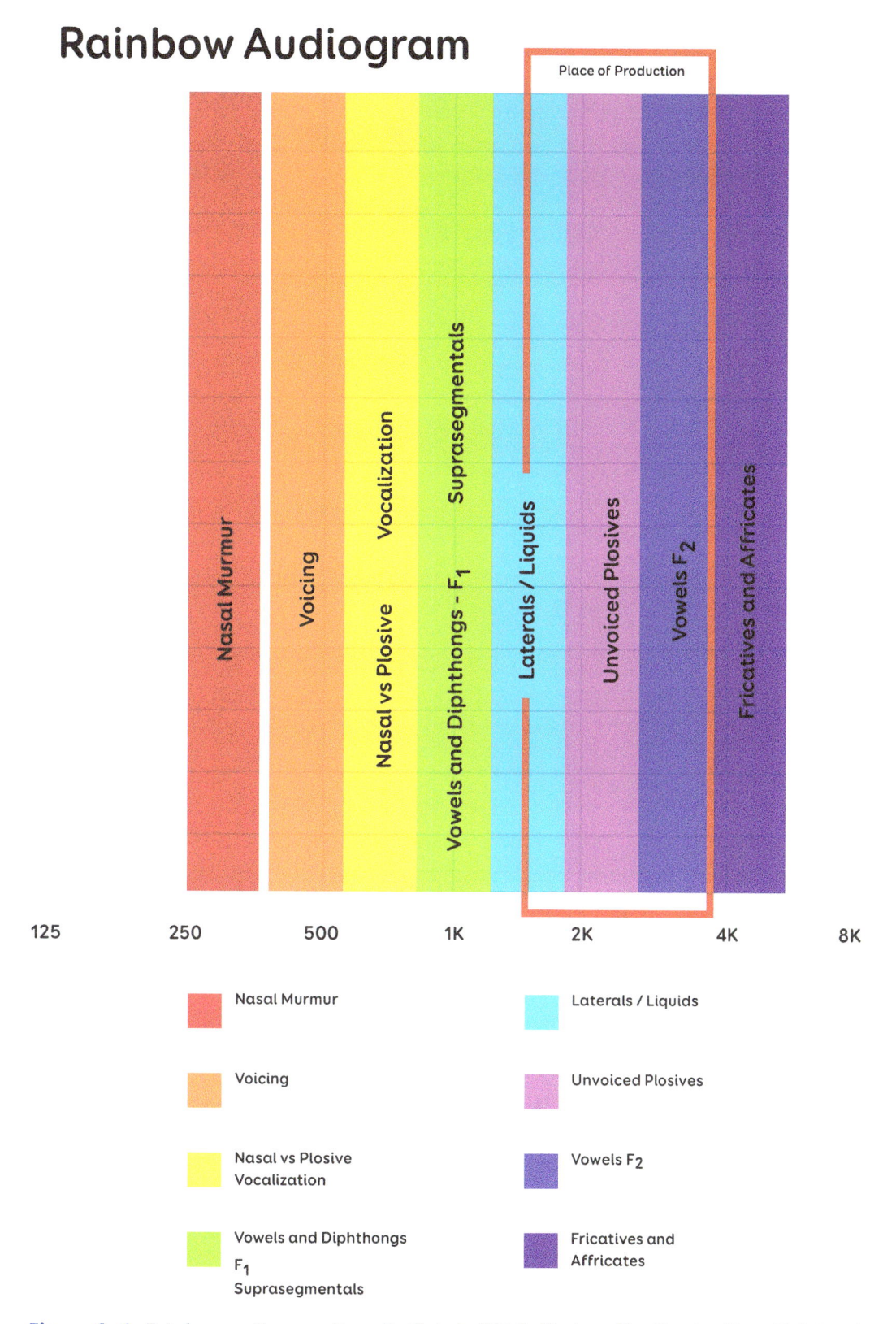

Figure 1–6. Rainbow audiogram. From Rotfleisch (2018). Designed by Hearing First, LLC. Used with permission.

Table 1–14. Rainbow Audiogram Features

Acoustic Correlates of Speech Features
Vocalizations: Fundamental frequency (F_0) of vocalizations for men, women, children: minimum of 750 Hz
Suprasegmentals: Acoustic information at and below 1000 Hz
Vowels: Detection of vowels by first formants which are below and up to 1000 Hz Discrimination of vowels by second formants are up to 3000 Hz
Consonants **Manner information:** • Nasal murmur: 300 Hz • Nasals versus plosives: 750 Hz • Laterals: 1500 Hz • Fricatives and affricates: 4000 Hz • Unvoiced plosives: 2000 Hz
Consonants **Place Information:** Place features are from burst frequency at 1500 to 4000 Hz
Consonants **Voicing Information:** 500 Hz and below

be used to identify areas on the audiogram that would be required for the specific speech perception ability. If the child is able to perform a skill such as discrimination and identification for all the vowels, the rainbow audiogram would indicate that the child has reasonable access to first and second formants with hearing up to the area of 3000 Hz. A child with hearing loss who has difficulty with the perception of nasal sounds and discriminating or identifying a nasal from a plosive is identified as having low frequency difficulties on the rainbow audiogram, with the vertical bars 300 and 750 Hz. As previously discussed, this information shown on the rainbow audiogram can assist in determining a functional audiogram.

3. Helps Identify Availability of Other Speech Features

Knowing that a child is making specific errors, we can use speech acoustics, an error analysis, and the rainbow audiogram to determine the frequency band that could be causing the error. The rainbow audiogram provides a quick visual representation of the features found in a similar acoustic range. This can allow us to predict and assess for other errors that might be probable. Once we have determined the frequency area, we are aware of what other features might be difficult for the child. If a child is demonstrating difficulties with voicing features for consonants, we can look at the rainbow audiogram and see that the orange band is the low-frequency range. We could then determine if other low-frequency speech features such as nasal murmur or plosive versus nasal manner are showing any error patterns. If we know that a child with hearing loss has the ability to discriminate all the vowels, that indicates they have access to the vowels' F_2. Looking at the vertical band for vowels' F_2 on the rainbow audiogram, we can see that place cue information and unvoiced plosives are in similar frequency ranges.

Knowing the child has access to sounds up to 3000 Hz, we can expect the child to be able to develop those discrimination abilities. We can assess for those features and appropriately set auditory goals. However, if the child demonstrates difficulty with the ability to discriminate all the vowels, that indicates they have potential issues with the access to the vowels' F_2. Therefore, based on the rainbow audiogram, we would be concerned about auditory abilities related to place cues and unvoiced plosives. If another child had difficulty discriminating /p/ and /k/, analysis would determine the difference is place cues for unvoiced plosives. On the rainbow audiogram, we see the frequency range would be between 1500 and 4000 Hz. Features such as unvoiced plosives, laterals, and second formants of vowels would be speech features to assess and monitor. All of these error patterns could indicate issues to be addressed in therapy with appropriate goals or could indicate problems with the setting of the technology.

4. Auditory Abilities and Difficulties to Verify or Predict Auditory Access

The rainbow audiogram provides a way to compare diagnostic information gathered while working with the child with hearing loss and to use it to verify audiological information provided by the audiologist. This helps the professional in determining what is getting to the brain and what goals are appropriate to be targeted. The starting point for this would likely be a detection audiogram using technology. The goal is to look for agreement between the detection audiogram and the abilities and difficulties that indicate the functional audiogram for a child with hearing loss. We would look at skills and difficulties and match them with speech features as indicated on the rainbow audiogram with thresholds from the audiology testing. If the skill such as discriminating a nasal from a plosive is demonstrated, then, looking at the rainbow audiogram, we know the child is able to use the auditory information in the 750-Hz range. We expect that the detection audiogram would show access to that frequency range.

5. Auditory Access to Predict Auditory Abilities and Difficulties

Speech is a complex signal, and sounds can be changed based on their acoustic surroundings. With this information in mind, we must realize that predicting what a person can hear based on an audiogram is not accurate. Ling (1989) writes, "Predictions based on audiograms rather than evaluation in the course of training are likely . . . to be neither accurate nor reliable" (p. 62). He goes on and explains, "Audiograms are much more useful as indicators of what children cannot hear than as predictors of what auditory skills they will be able to acquire" (p. 62). We must evaluate children's abilities during intervention to be certain of areas of abilities and areas of difficulties rather than relying on detection audiograms. As suggested by Ling (1989), when provided with a child's aided detection audiogram, we can use the rainbow audiogram as a framework to predict possible limitations in specific frequency ranges but not as definitive.

We can plot a child's audiogram on the rainbow audiogram. For example, if a child does not have hearing in the frequency ranges past 2000 Hz, or only has access at high intensity, the rainbow audiogram would point to potential difficulties for skills related to the speech features of laterals, unvoiced plosives, vowel discriminations dependent on F_2, consonants differing by place cues, and the fricative and affricate manners. This allows us to follow Ling's words of caution to look at which speech features might be difficult to perceive or will be most accessible. Though we can apply the rainbow audiogram directly to a child's audiogram or to a hearing loss configuration, we must also remember Ling's recommendation to evaluate the child's abilities. (See Hearing Loss Configurations later in the text.)

Functional Audiogram

A functional audiogram is how the child functions related to hearing. It is an indication of their use of audition. It looks to answer key questions in listening and spoken language therapy: What does the child hear? What is getting to the child's brain? (Flexer, 2017). It should be thought of as the hypothesis of the auditory input that is getting to the child's brain. By gathering data related to speech acoustics, professionals can hypothesize a child's functional audiogram. When there is not a completed audiological assessment, or when red flags point to issues of auditory access, a functional audiogram provides valuable information to support the child's audiological management.

Professionals are charged with facilitating and monitoring the child's listening and spoken language abilities through hearing. We <u>always</u> go back to the hearing. Speech features and acoustics are the fundamental building blocks of hearing for the child to acquire listening and spoken language. We assess and analyze abilities and difficulties in listening, speech perception, speech production, and language error patterns. Using the variety of speech acoustics tools available (e.g., vowel formant chart, rainbow audiogram, consonant speech features, acoustic correlate and formant tables, audiograms with sounds), we find the relationship between skills, errors, speech acoustics, and the audiogram. This allows us to assess for optimal access and to determine goals.

An analysis of the errors related to the rainbow audiogram can contribute information for the functional audiogram. The use of a task analysis to look at errors and error patterns is an effective way to gather information to determine the functional audiogram. Analyze the abilities or difficulties. Look for specific speech feature patterns. Identify the acoustic correlates on the audiogram. This information could provide cross-validation or refute existing assumptions related to the child's hearing loss. In addition, data obtained by the professional can be useful to the audiologist in relation to technology settings.

Error Analysis to Determine Perception and Error Patterns

Perception and production of speech phonemes are closely tied. Children will produce what they hear (Ling, 1976). Many professionals refer to this as "garbage in, garbage out" or "muddy in, muddy out." With the understanding that the child's speech production is a reflection of their perception, it follows that a child's error patterns indicate areas of poor perception or poor discrimination. Professionals must be aware of appropriate abilities for a child based on their hearing experience with hearing technology and the appropriate sequence of development of the segmental aspects of speech, particularly the consonants. We know that consonants have a typical developmental sequence (see Chapter 3) and a typical time span for their development. Lack of production of consonants at given times in a child's development is therefore developmentally appropriate. Some specific consonants are not expected to be present or emerging at a given stage of development. Additionally, certain error patterns are developmentally appropriate.

Analysis of the error pattern is important, followed by relating it to the acoustic correlates. The following task analysis procedure (Table 1–15) can be used to look at specific speech features, a specific phoneme, an error pattern, and/or contrasts between two or more phonemes. These patterns can be identified when anyone working with the child notes speech perception errors, speech production issues, or a language morpheme error. When looking at errors, we look for evidence of a pattern. If there is only one example of an error, it could be that the child has an old habit or it is just an isolated error.

If a child has difficulties with /b/ and /m/ perception and instead of "mama" says "baba" or says "my, my" for "bye, bye" we can look at the identifying speech features to do an error analysis (Table 1–16). We can identify the sounds as a voiced bilabial plosive and a voice bilabial nasal. This allows us to understand that the sounds are different by manner: a nasal and a plosive. From viewing the rainbow audiogram, we can see that the information necessary to hear a nasal murmur is centered around 300 Hz and the frequency information needed to differentiate a nasal from a plosive is centered around 750 Hz. This information can help us determine if the child has access to the necessary balance of low-frequency information to hear the nasal murmur and to differentiate between a nasal and a plosive. We should keep in mind that low-frequency information for a nasal resonance carries strong acoustic energy and is typically an easier discrimination.

Table 1–15. The Steps for a Systematic Task Analysis

1. Define the phoneme or phonemes by manner, place, and voicing.
2. Compare two phonemes to identify features that differ.
3. Identify the features and the acoustic correlates using the rainbow audiogram, vowel chart and consonant chart, or other resources.
4. Identify other issues that could be causing the error.
5. Assess for agreement between the detection audiogram and the access to the feature.

Table 1–16. Task Analysis: Consonant Manner of Production

Step 1. Define the phoneme or phonemes by manner, place, and voicing	
/b/	/m/
• Manner: plosive	• Manner: nasal
• Place: bilabial	• Place: bilabial
• Voicing: voiced	• Voicing: voiced
Voiced bilabial plosive	Voiced bilabial nasal
Step 2. Compare two phonemes to identify features that differ	
Error by manner	Plosive versus nasal
Step 3. Identify the features and the acoustic correlates using the rainbow audiogram, vowel chart, and/or consonant chart	
Features	**Acoustic Correlates**
Nasal murmur	300 Hz (red on rainbow audiogram in Figure 1–6)
Plosive versus nasal	750 Hz (yellow on rainbow audiogram in Figure 1–6)
Step 4. Identify other issues that could be causing the error	
Nasal murmur and voicing (both low frequency)	
Visually same, as they are both the same place of production (bilabial)	
Step 5. Assess for agreement between the detection audiogram and the access to the feature	
Possible access issues in low-frequency range, as illustrated in red and yellow on the rainbow audiogram (Figure 1–6)	

An additional factor to consider for this phoneme pair would be that these sounds are produced in the same place. That means they look the same when produced and could be visually confused if the child is relying on the visual information available from lipreading rather than on auditory input. This error pattern would indicate possible access issues in low-frequency areas and would be information to discuss with the audiologist.

Error analysis for a pair of phonemes that differ by voicing is illustrated in Table 1–17. We can see that /b/ and /p/ are the same by manner and place and vary only by the voicing feature. Using the rainbow audiogram, we can quickly identify voicing as low-frequency information. As in the previous example, this pair of phonemes are produced in the same place. The same place of production would mean that the sounds can be visually confusing if the child is relying on lipreading rather than on auditory input. We should keep in mind that low-frequency information for voicing carries strong acoustic energy and is typically an easier discrimination. This error pattern would indicate possible access issues in low-frequency areas and would be information to discuss with the audiologist.

Error analysis for a pair of phonemes that differ by place cue is illustrated in Table 1–18. We can see that /m/ and /n/ are the same by manner and voicing and vary

Table 1–17. Task Analysis: Consonant Voicing

Step 1. Define the phoneme or phonemes by manner, place, and voicing	
/b/ • Manner: plosive • Place: bilabial • Voicing: voiced **Voiced bilabial plosive**	/p/ • Manner: plosive • Place: bilabial • Voicing: unvoiced **Unvoiced bilabial plosive**
Step 2. Compare two phonemes to identify features that differ	
Error by voicing	Voiced and voiceless
Step 3. Identify the features and the acoustic correlates on the rainbow audiogram, vowel chart, and/or consonant chart	
Features Voiced versus unvoiced	Acoustic Correlates 500 Hz and below (orange and red on rainbow audiogram in Figure 1–6)
Step 4. Identify other issues that could be causing the error	
Visually same, as they are both in the same place of production (bilabial)	
Step 5. Assess for agreement between the detection audiogram and the access to the feature	
Would indicate possible access issues in low-frequency range at 500 Hz and below	

Table 1–18. Task Analysis: Consonant Place of Production

Step 1. Define the phoneme or phonemes by manner, place, and voicing	
/m/ • Manner: nasal • Place: bilabial • Voicing: voiced **Voiced bilabial nasal**	/n/ • Manner: nasal • Place: alveolar • Voicing: voiced **Voiced alveolar nasal**
Step 2. Compare two phonemes to identify features that differ	
Error by place	Bilabial, alveolar
Step 3. Identify the features and the acoustic correlates on the rainbow audiogram, vowel chart, and/or consonant chart	
Features Place cues	Acoustic Correlates 1500 to 4000 Hz (red on rainbow audiogram in Figure 1–6)
Step 4. Identify other issues that could be causing the error	
None	
Step 5. Assess for agreement between the detection audiogram and the access to the feature	
Would indicate possible access issues in higher-frequency range	

only by the place cue feature. Using the rainbow audiogram, we can quickly identify place cue as mid- to high-frequency information. In contrast to the previous examples, this pair of phonemes is produced in different places. The place of production is visually available and can be used if the child is relying on lipreading rather than on auditory input. It is critical that we always assess the discrimination for phonemes through audition only and do not use or provide visual information. Place cue information, due to the nature of this feature and acoustic correlates, is a more difficult discrimination. This error pattern would indicate possible access issues in mid- and higher-frequency areas and would be information to share with the audiologist to collaborate for the child's benefit.

Case Study Application of Speech Acoustics Tools

We must gather our own data as professionals to help figure out if the child has properly set, functioning technology that is being used to provide the auditory input required to develop listening and spoken language. Knowing that a child is not able to detect some phonemes or has specific abilities, we can look at where those speech features are on the audiogram, determine a functional audiogram, and determine other phonemes or speech features that are likely to be accessed or not. Consider a child that is able to say "ma, ma, ma" in a babble and can change the production to "ba, ba, ba" when they hear an adult say the different sound. However, the child doesn't change to "pa, pa, pa" when that sound is modeled. The ability to change from the /m/ phoneme to the /b/ indicates that the child is able discriminate a nasal from a plosive at the 750-Hz range, as indicated on the rainbow audiogram. Knowing this, we can look at what other features should be accessible in that range. This could include first formants for many other vowels, some second formants, and the suprasegmentals.

There is evidence that supports this as the child detects /ɑ/ but doesn't respond or indicate detection to /ʃ/. It hasn't been determined if the child can detect /s/. We can look at the rainbow audiogram or tables, which indicate frequencies for speech features. The formants for the /ɑ/ are around 500 Hz and about 1000 to 1500 Hz. Detecting and discriminating this vowel would only require hearing up to that range and doesn't confirm that the child has access to the second formants. Looking at the vowel formant chart and placement of the /ʃ/ on an audiogram, that would allow us to conclude that the child will have limited access to some of the higher-frequency second formants. Lack of response to the higher-frequency fricative /ʃ/ might indicate the child would be able to hear some of the second formants of vowels and might not have access to place cue features. This would indicate possible problems in the mid- and high-frequency range.

If a child has difficulty with discrimination of voiced and unvoiced sounds, this indicates possible difficulty with the voicing feature at 500 Hz and below. This information, or specific bits of data points, can be compiled as a functional audiogram. In this case, we might hypothesize that the child has poor access to the low- and mid-frequency sounds and has better access to the higher-frequency ranges. We are not able to say if the child has access to /s/, but suspect the inability to identify and produce the higher-frequency unvoiced plosive /p/ in "pa, pa, pa."

Our functional audiogram would have responses in the low frequencies, decreasing to the mid and the lower ranges of high-frequency sounds. It is possible that the child's audiogram or auditory access goes up in the higher ranges. In this case, the functional audiogram is a partial answer to what is getting to the child's brain. It provides valuable information to share with the audiologist and other professionals. If this child has hearing aids, it indicates that either they are not optimally set or the child might require different technology—different hearing aids or cochlear implants. If the child is using cochlear implants, the lack of response to /ʃ/ indicates mapping is not optimal.

Speech Acoustics and Hearing Loss Configurations

Defined audiogram configurations such as a corner audiogram, a reverse slope, a downward slope, or a cookie bite result in different auditory access for the child with the hearing loss. As mentioned above, predictions based on hearing loss are not accurate for each individual. However, it is useful to understand potential limitations of different hearing loss configurations. The audiograms (Figures 1–7 to 1–10) are used to indicate audiogram configurations that are useful to consider in relation to speech acoustics and speech features. They are not actual aided or unaided audiograms. In some instances, we would consider an unaided audiogram. In other cases, an audiogram obtained with technology might show patterns similar to some unaided hearing loss configurations. We stress that, as we look at the audiogram configurations, we are looking at patterns of access or limited access. Remember that just because a child has technology does not guarantee they have full access. Technology could be poorly set or mapped or not appropriate.

Applying information from the rainbow audiogram to these audiograms allows us to anticipate and assess possible limitations in specific frequency ranges. Additionally, it allows us to look at possible areas of abilities for each individual child with hearing loss. We must realize that a child with a corner audiogram hearing loss with responses only up to 500 Hz will have different abilities than the child who has a similar configuration but who has access to up to 1500 Hz. A cookie bite audiogram can vary in access in low and high frequencies for the individual. One child might have more access in the high frequencies as a result of quieter thresholds beginning at 1000 Hz, while another might have more access beginning at 2000 Hz or higher. Audiogram configurations are illustrated (see Figures 1–7 to 1–10) with prognostic indications (Tables 1–19 to 1–22). The examples are merely a framework as a starting point for assessing each individual child.

Speech Acoustics and the Impact on Speech Production

Speech acoustics can be applied to the development of speech sounds. The babbling stages are where speech production and control of suprasegmentals begins. Access to sound is critical as the infant or young child with hearing loss develops babbling abilities or has difficulty moving through the differentiated babbling

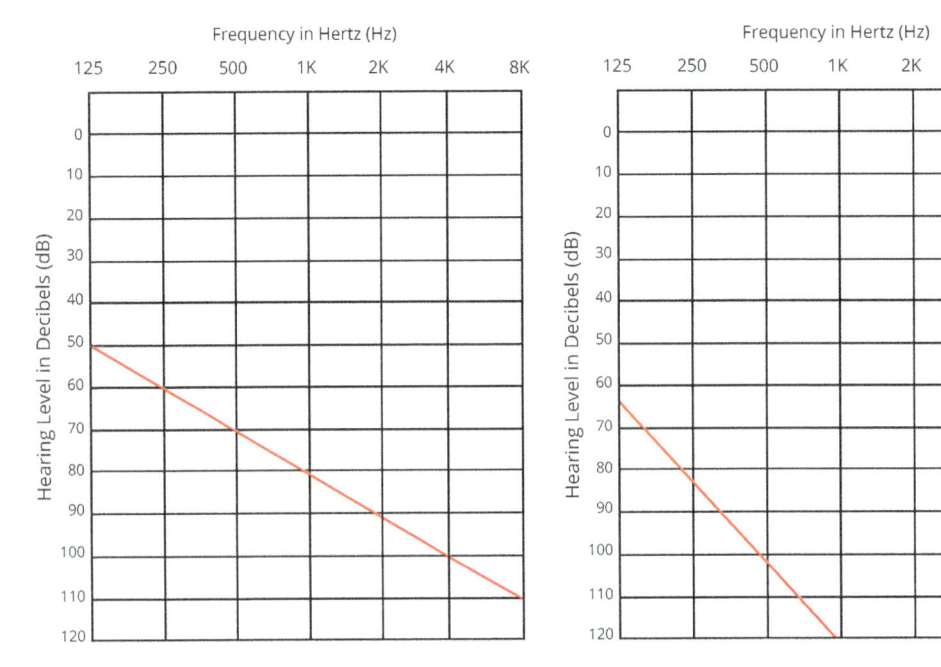

Figure 1–7. Downward sloped audiogram.

Figure 1–8. Corner audiogram.

Table 1–19. Prognostic Indications Based on Downward Sloping Audiogram Configuration

Expected Access	Expected Limitations
• Suprasegmentals: OK • Vowels: F_1 OK • Manners: nasals and plosives	• Vowels: some /u/ /i/ confusion • Manners: difficulty with fricatives • Place: problems especially with fricatives, plosives

Table 1–20. Prognostic Indications Based on Corner Audiogram Configuration

Expected Access	Expected Limitations
• Suprasegmentals: OK • Vowels: F_1 OK • Manners: nasals and plosives	• Vowels: F_2 differences limited • Manners: trouble with manners besides nasals and plosives • Voicing: could be inconsistent • Place: not expected

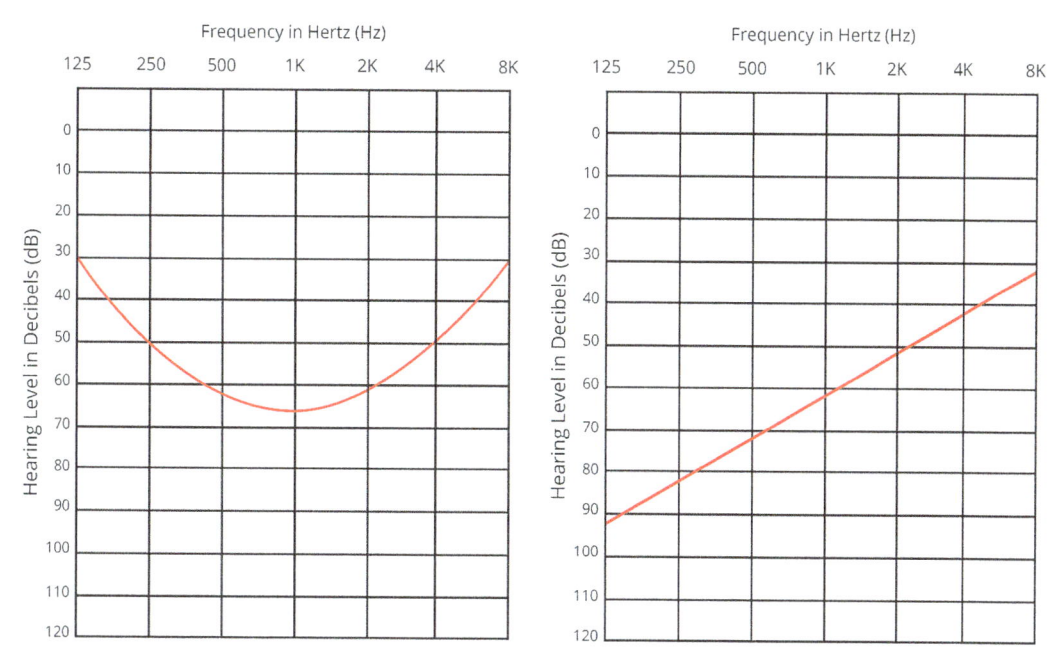

Figure 1–9. Cookie bite audiogram.

Figure 1–10. Reverse slope audiogram.

Table 1–21. Prognostic Indications Based on Cookie Bite Audiogram Configuration

Expected Access	Expected Limitations
• Low- and some high-frequency vowels • Fricatives: good development • Manners: some manners	• Vowels: limited variety in mid frequency • Nasal plosive discrimination • Nasals and laterals discrimination between /m/ and /l/ • Nasals versus plosives • Place cues: mostly good

Table 1–22. Prognostic Indications Based on Reverse Slope Audiogram Configuration

Expected Access	Expected Limitations
• Suprasegmentals: inconsistent • Vowels: F_2 • Manners: nasals and plosives • Good articulation of high-frequency sounds	• Poor control of suprasegmentals • Limited nasal phonemes • Discrimination of voicing

Table 1–23. Babbling Stages Related to Speech Features and Acoustic Correlates

Babbling Stage	Auditory Skills Needed/Speech Feature	Acoustic Correlates
Quasi-resonant sounds, reflexive vocalizations	n/a	n/a
"gooing," "cooing"	Vocalizations	750 Hz
Fully resonant sounds	Suprasegmentals Vowels: F_1 for detection Vowels: F_2 for discrimination	1000 Hz, 3000 Hz
Canonical Reduplicative	Consonants: plosives versus nasals manner emergence /b/ or /m/	750 Hz (low frequency)
Canonical Variegated	Variety of consonants and vowels	All frequencies

stages (Eiler & Oller, 1993). Primary speech features as they are related to the babbling stages are indicated in Table 1–23, which summarizes key features and their frequencies related to the stages. Limited or no access to the specific speech features required for a stage will impact or arrest progression of the production abilities developed and practiced in babbling.

Speech phoneme development will be impacted by access to sounds, as discussed previously. Knowing where speech elements are located on the audiogram can help to understand the specific issues that might be apparent in developing speech. For example, the child with hearing loss who has poor access to the low frequencies can be expected to have difficulty with voice quality issues including resonance, pitch control, prosody, vowels, and consonant voicing. These speech error patterns would significantly impact the intelligibility of her speech productions, even though she might have a good variety of consonants. This is an important point, as professionals often assume that poor speech intelligibility is due to articulation of consonants. The relationship of some speech production issues and speech acoustics as generalized by low-, mid-, and high-frequency auditory information is illustrated in Figure 1–11 and summarized in Table 1–24.

Remedial formal speech correction intervention for a child with hearing loss should consider auditory access and speech perception. Limitations of auditory access in different frequency ranges will impact the ability to use audition as the primary modality for correction and remediation. We understand that audition is the only sense able to access all aspects of speech (Ling, 2002), and therefore we use sensory correlates on the audiogram to determine feature accessibility. We must be able to determine if the feature can be taught through hearing or if other sensory modalities (e.g., vision or tactile stimulation) will be needed. When access is limited, we must select additional sensory modalities for remedial teaching of a speech phoneme. Table 1–25 summarizes

LOW-FREQUENCY SPEECH FEATURES

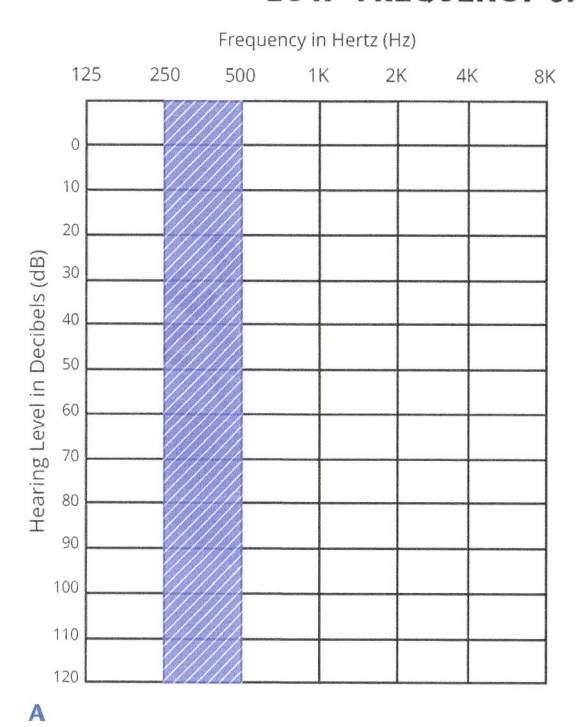

(250-500 Hz)

- Weak or breathy voice
- Falsetto voice
- Poor prosody
- Nasalization or denasalization
- Syllable deletion
- Confusions of nasals and plosives
- Confusion of voiced and unvoiced consonants

A

MID-FREQUENCY SPEECH FEATURES

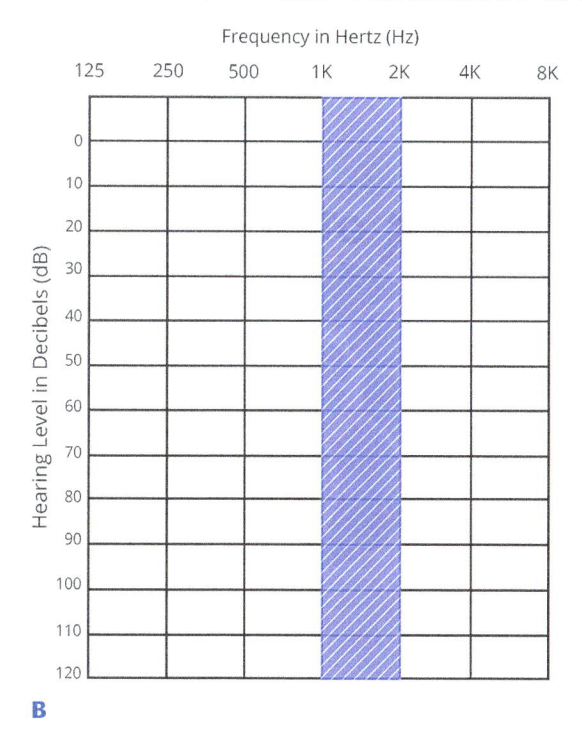

(1000-2000 Hz)

- Omission of unstressed morphemes
- Neutralization (centralization) of vowels

B

Figure 1–11. A. Low-frequency speech features. B. Mid-frequency speech features. *continues*

HIGH-FREQUENCY SPEECH FEATURES

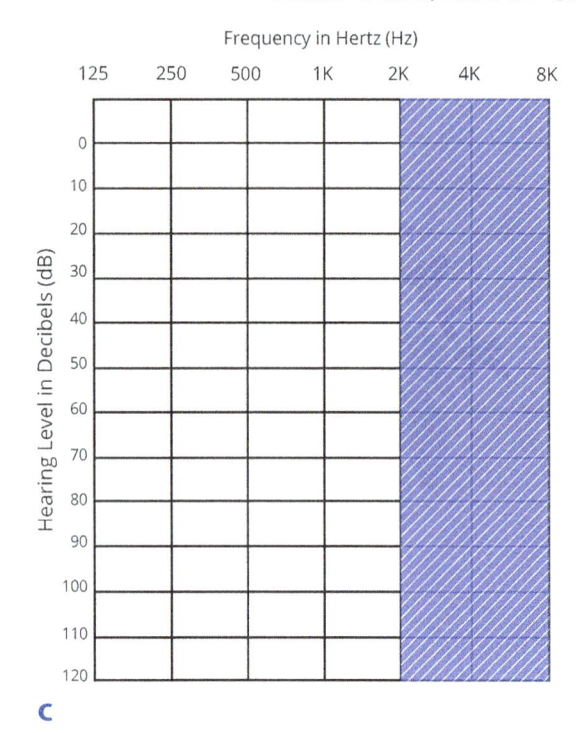

ABOVE 2000 Hz

- Omission and/or distortion of fricatives
- Omissions of final consonants
- Distortion or substitution of stops

C

Figure 1–11. *continued* C. High-frequency speech features.

Table 1–24. Speech Acoustics Applied to Speech Production Patterns

Low-Frequency Information 250 to 500 Hz	Mid-Frequency Information 1000 to 2000 Hz	High-Frequency Information Above 2000 Hz
Weak or breathy voice	Omission of unstressed morphemes	Omission and/or distortion of fricatives
Falsetto voice		
Poor prosody	Neutralization (centralization) of vowels	Omission of final consonants
Nasalization or denasalization		Distortion or substitution of stops
Confusion of nasals and plosives		
Confusion of voiced and unvoiced consonants		

Source: Compiled from Ling (2002).

expected auditory accessibility of speech features for application to structured remedial speech strategies. When we consider the patterns of availability as indicated in this table, we realize that many features are available in low- and mid-frequency ranges. This means that, for children with hearing loss who are not yet

Table 1–25. Speech Feature Availability Based on Audition

	Voice Features			Vowel Features		Consonant Features		
	Duration	*Intensity*	*F_0*	*F_1*	*F_2*	*Manner*	*Place*	*Voicing*
Audition								
Up to 750 Hz	A	A	A	A	U	P	U	P
Up to 1500 Hz	A	A	A	A	P	A	P	A
Up to 3000 Hz	A	A	A	A	A	A	A	A
Cochlear implant	A	A	A	A	A	A	A	A

Note: A = available; P = partially available; U = unavailable.
Source: Used with permission and adapted from Ling (2002).

optimally provided with access through their hearing technology, there is work to be done to help them. Children with hearing loss will have difficulties using control of the suprasegmentals to express emotions (Damm et al., 2019). However, when working with these children, we must remember that 90% of the information for understanding speech is carried by the high-frequency information such as the consonants.

Speech Acoustics and Language Development

Inadequate access has a domino effect. Initially, it is apparent that perception and auditory skills suffer, resulting in speech production issues and then issues with the emergence of language structures. A child with poor access in the mid frequencies will have difficulties with suprasegmentals. The resulting poor discrimination of durational cues will impact development of many low-intensity grammatical morphemes such as articles, pronouns, and prepositions. When the child is learning past-tense verbs, irregular verbs (e.g., *eat/ate*, *fall/fell*) typically rely on access and ability to discriminate different vowels. When learning the regular *-ed* endings, we remember that it can be produced as a /t/ or a /d/. The child who presents with difficulty with consonant discrimination will be impacted. If they are not distinguishing between some manners of production, they could have issues hearing the difference between the present- and past-tense verb. If this difficulty is discrimination between the nasals and plosives, then *comb* versus *combed* or *climb* versus *climbed* might not be perceived. Similarly, the child with place cue discrimination issues might confuse *walk* versus *walked* or *stop* versus *stopped*.

When we consider the child with poor access to the high frequencies, the expectation would be difficulties with detection of and production of an /s/. Keeping in mind that /s/ carries a significant morphemic burden in the English language, we consider the impact of poor access to /s/ on language development. During spoken language intervention, we can anticipate multiple grammatical difficulties including plurals, possessives, third-person regular present-tense verbs, and possessive pronouns (e.g., *hers*, *his*, *yours*). These different morphemic functions are expected to develop at different ages, but plurals and possessives are among the first morphemes to emerge after about age 2 years (see Chapter 3, and Table 3–7 for morphemic development). Analysis of morphemic functions related to speech acoustics is included in Table 1–26. This analysis illustrates some specific morphemic functions expected to develop as related to speech features and acoustics. Use of this table will assist in

Table 1–26. Speech Acoustics Analysis of Morphemic Functions

Language Structure Skills	Auditory Skills Needed/Speech Feature	Acoustics/ Frequency
Regular plural /s/	Unvoiced fricative /s/	4000 to 8000 Hz
Regular plural /z/	Voicing	500 Hz
	Fricative /z/	4000 to 8000 Hz
/s/ possessive	Unvoiced fricative /s/	4000 to 8000 Hz
/z/ possessive	Voicing	500 Hz
	Fricative /z/	4000 to 8000 Hz
Third-person regular, present-tense /s/	Unvoiced fricative /s/	4000 to 8000 Hz
Third-person regular, present-tense /z/	Voicing	500 Hz
	Fricative /z/	4000 to 8000 Hz
Regular past tense	Plosives: *-ed* /d/ or /t/	
	Voicing	500 Hz
	Unvoiced plosive	2500 to 3000 Hz
	Discriminate manners	500 Hz
	(e.g., *canned*)	2500 to 3000 Hz
	Manners: plosive versus nasal	750 Hz
	Discriminate manners (e.g., *washed*)	
	Unvoiced fricative versus plosive	2500 to 3000 Hz
	Discriminate plosive place cues (e.g., *walked, jumped, talked*)	2000 to 4000 Hz
Irregular past tense	Vowels	1000 Hz for detection
		3000 Hz for discrimination

selecting language goals that are appropriate based on speech acoustics and will help to understand the auditory skills required to support the development of those targets.

The relationship of some language structures to speech acoustics as generalized by low-, mid-, and high-frequency auditory information are illustrated in Figure 1–12 and summarized in Table 1–27.

Table 1–27. Speech Acoustics Analysis of Language Structures

Low-Frequency Information 250 to 500 Hz	Mid-Frequency Information 1000 to 2000 Hz	High-Frequency Information Above 2000 Hz
-ing verb ending	Articles	/t/: past-tense -ed verb ending
Irregular past tense	Conjunctions	Verbs: /s/ marker; present tense
Prepositions (found all over frequency range usually unstressed)	Pronouns	Irregular past tense
	Irregular past tense	/s/ morphemic functions
	Prepositions	Prepositions

Source: Used with permission and adapted from Ling and Ling (1978); Ling (1989).

LOW-FREQUENCY LANGUAGE STRUCTURES

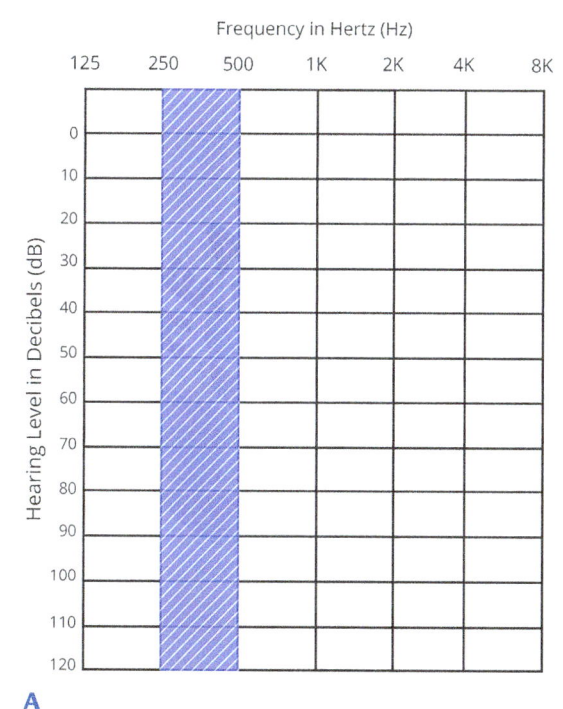

(250–500 Hz)

- Verbs "ing" at 250 Hz
- Irregular past tense
- Prepositions
  found all over whole frequency range usually unstressed

A

Figure 1–12. **A.** Low-frequency language structures. *continues*

MID-FREQUENCY LANGUAGE STRUCTURES

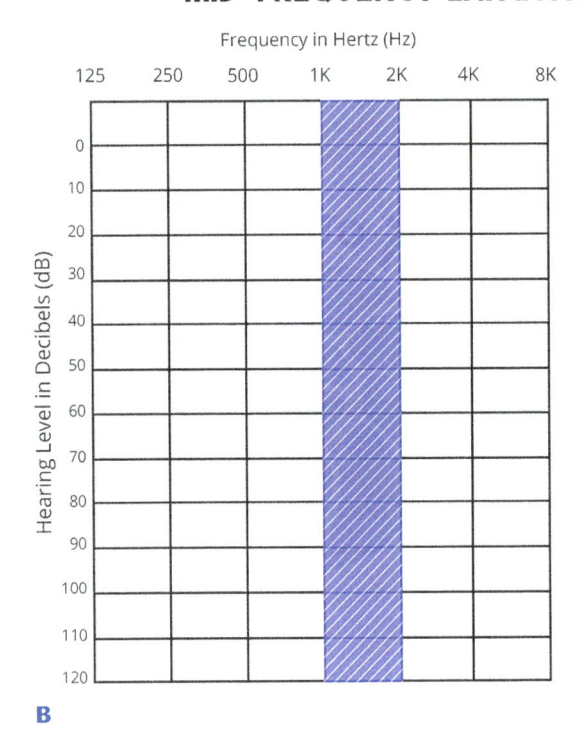

(1000-2000 Hz)

- Articles
- Conjunctions
- Pronouns
- Irregular past tense
- Prepositions

B

HIGH-FREQUENCY LANGUAGE STRUCTURES

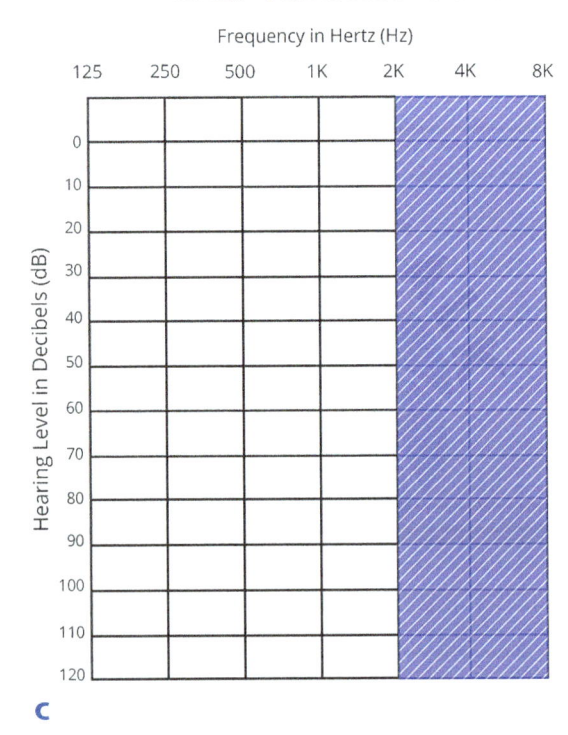

ABOVE 2000 Hz

- Verbs - [t] past tense "ed"
- Verbs - [s] marker
- Irregular past tense
- S morphemic functions
- Prepositions

C

Figure 1–12. *continued* **B.** Mid-frequency language structures. **C.** High-frequency language structures.

Case Study Application of Speech Acoustics for Speech and Language Development

Consider a child with hearing loss limiting access past 2000 Hz. When we consider the child's speech perception and production, we anticipate this child will likely have difficulty with fricatives, word-final consonants, plosives, and stops. In language, the morphemic functions /s/ and past-tense *-ed* ending produced as a /t/ and prepositions are more apparent as probable issues. However, irregular past-tense forms might be less obvious.

Let's go through an analysis to understand why this would be an issue. When we look at irregular verbs, we are most frequently looking at a change of the vowel (e.g., *eat/ate, ride/rode, sleep/slept, fall/fell*). Look at your rainbow audiogram and consider vowel detection versus discrimination. That is the clue that gives you the answer if you consider vowels and 2000 Hz. Detection requires only access for the first formants up to 1000 Hz. This child be able to detect all the vowels. Discrimination requires hearing access for the second formant up to 3000 Hz. This child will not be able to discriminate all the vowels. Remember the Ling sentence that organizes the vowels by second formant (Ling & Ling, 1978). The vowels in the key words "and then take his ease" have F_2 that are mostly above 2000 Hz.

Irregular past tense verbs do not add an *-ed* but typically change the vowel sound. If you consider <u>eat and ate</u>, the F_2 for both of these is above 2000 Hz. This child will not hear these as different. In <u>drink and drank</u>, the child might hear part of most of the second formant for /æ/ but likely will not hear that vowel as different than /ɪ/. You can go through this analysis with other irregular past-tense verbs and look at the vowels that need to be discriminated and identified. You can think about the changes in these examples: *take/took, fall/fell, read* (present tense)/*read* (past tense), *drive/drove*, and *give/gave*. Once again, examine your vowel chart to consider if the child will be able to hear these as different. If the child can't hear them as different, the child will not learn them.

The Gold at the End of the Rainbow Audiogram: Applications for Speech Acoustics

Speech acoustics is the foundation on which all therapy to achieve listening and spoken language should be based. It allows for the constant thinking and analysis back and forth between speech acoustics and the development of spoken language. We use this information to determine if all the pieces fit together properly or if something doesn't quite seem logical based on these principles and as a foundation for selecting goals.

Information regarding aspects of sounds and speech features has been examined and related to audiograms and children with hearing loss. Some preliminary and basic applications to the developing of babbling, speech production, and language development are addressed throughout the chapter.

With the understanding of the principles addressed, we have compiled a list of ways that professionals can and should apply speech acoustics to listening and spoken language intervention with children with hearing loss and their families (Table 1–28), organized by areas of application. You will notice that some applications are listed in more than one area as there is overlap.

Table 1–28. Applications of Speech Acoustics

Audiology Testing, Audiogram, and Technology

1. Prepare a child for a more accurate hearing test by starting with the most audible sound when teaching conditioned play responses.
2. Validate hearing testing/audiogram.
3. Determine discrimination and identification expectations based on an audiogram.
4. Draw probable audiogram based on abilities/predict hearing configuration.
5. Raise questions about hearing testing.
6. Determine if child is a candidate for a CI.
7. Determine if technology is adequate.
8. Determine if technology is optimal.
9. Determine if technology is appropriately set.
10. Determine if technology needs remapping.
11. Monitor for upward spread of masking.
12. Determine if the clinical results match testing results.
13. Provide information to the audiologist and team regarding access.
14. Provide information to the audiologist to assist in setting technology.
15. Assist in finding possible red flags of technology.
16. Create a functional audiogram for the child.

Listening and Spoken Language Strategies

1. Modify the auditory signal by considering distance.
2. Modify the auditory signal by using acoustic highlighting strategies.
3. Modify the auditory signal related to noisy environments.
4. Teach parents about auditory access and modifying the auditory signal related to distance.
5. Teach parents about auditory access and modifying the auditory signal by using acoustic highlighting.
6. Teach parents/child about signal to noise ratio (SNR) and noise.
7. Teach parents about speech features.
8. Teach parents about speech features on an audiogram.
9. Teach parents about speech development related to an audiogram.
10. Teach parents about language development related to an audiogram.
11. Determine/define appropriate acoustic strategies for acoustic highlighting.
12. Make sounds more audible by bringing sounds into an audible range.
13. Help enhance the child's perception of speech sounds by the acoustic environment and variant energy.
14. Relate to the Ling six sounds to understand potential issues.
15. Match strategies with individual's abilities based on speech acoustic principles.
16. Determine most effective strategies and modalities for specific speech targets.
17. Guide and coach parents about speech acoustics and walk them through their child's development based on speech acoustics.

Table 1–28. *continued*

18. Basis for speech production and development and the use of modalities.
19. Analyze articulation errors and determine which feature of any speech sound the child is missing.
20. Provide an awareness of possible skills and difficulties based on an audiogram.
21. Select auditory goals to facilitate specific speech targets.
22. Select auditory goals to facilitate specific language targets.

Diagnostic Work

1. Predict skills or difficulties based on an audiogram.
2. Determine what is getting to the child's brain.
3. Monitor for errors that indicate a pattern of auditory difficulties.
4. Monitor development of auditory discrimination abilities.
5. Monitor initial access and development for babies.
6. Monitor initial access and development for new CI users based on speech acoustics.
7. Analyze voice errors such as pitch control, resonance, nasal quality, and ability of breath control to support vocalizations.
8. Analyze speech feature errors through task analysis as an indication of auditory access and perception.
9. Determine if speech errors are appropriate based on auditory access or other possible problems.
10. Provide information to determine if errors are auditory perception based.
11. Analyze articulation errors and determine which feature of any speech sound the child is missing.
12. Determine if child has enough hearing access to learn spoken language.
13. Determine if child is a candidate for a CI.
14. Determine if a child might have additional difficulties that are causing speech errors.
15. Determine if language errors are appropriate based on auditory access or other possible problems.
16. Analyze language errors and determine if there is a pattern indicating the child has issues with auditory access.
17. Select auditory goals to facilitate specific speech targets.
18. Determine how child is functioning with their current amplification on a daily basis to monitor if they hearing as well today as they were yesterday.

Goals

1. Set auditory goals based on access and limited access.
2. Know when to appropriately select modalities other than audition if needed.
3. Select auditory goals to facilitate specific speech targets.
4. Select auditory goals to facilitate specific language targets.
5. Set auditory perception goals.

Discussion Questions

1. What topics discussed in this section would you explain to parents? Pick one and discuss how you would explain it.
2. Using speech acoustics information, how would you explain the importance of using technology to the family of a child with hearing loss? Their desired outcome is listening and spoken language. What tools or figures would you use to help in the explanation and how?
3. How would you explain possible access issues to the parents of a newly diagnosed child with a corner audiogram?
4. A child is a candidate for a cochlear implant but will not be implanted for a period of time. Based on speech acoustics, predict what auditory access this child might have. What would be possible auditory goals based on the child's access?
5. Select a hearing loss configuration (i.e., corner audiogram, sloping audiogram, cookie bite, reverse slope). Using speech acoustics information, how would you explain to a family if their child is or is not a candidate for a cochlear implant? What tools or figures from this chapter might you use?

References

Anderson, K. (2002). Early listening function (ELF). Parent involvement: The magic ingredient in successful child outcomes: Improving parent participation using the ELF and the CHILD. *Hearing Review, 9*(11), 24–27, 56.

Avan, P., Giraudet, F., & Buki, B. (2015). Audiology and neurotology proceedings. Importance of binaural hearing. *Audiology Neurotology, 20*(Suppl. 1), 3–6.

Boothroyd, A. (2019). The acoustic speech signal. In J. R. Madell, C. Flexer, J. Wolfe, & E. Shafer (Eds.), *Pediatric audiology: Diagnosis, technology, and management* (3rd ed., pp. 203–213). Thieme.

Center for Hearing and Communication. (n.d.). *Common environmental noise levels*. https://chchearing.org/noise/common-environmental-noise-levels/

Damm, S. J., Kulkarni, A., & Chatterjee, M. (2019). How vocal emotions produced by children with cochlear implants are perceived by their hearing peers. *Journal of Speech, Language, and Hearing Research, 62,* 3728–3740.

Dockrell, J., & Shield, B. (2012). The impact of sound-field systems on learning and attention in elementary school classrooms. *Journal of Speech, Language, and Hearing Research, 55*(4), 1163–1176.

Dubno, J. R., Dirks, D. D., & Morgan, D. E. (1984). Effects of age and mild hearing loss on speech recognition in noise. *Journal of the Acoustic Society of America, 76*(1), 87–96.

Eiler, R. E., & Oller, D. K. (1993). Infant vocalizations and the early diagnosis of severe hearing impairment. *Journal of Pediatrics, 124*(2), 199–203.

Engineering ToolBox. (2010). *Octave band frequencies*. https://www.engineeringtoolbox.com/octave-bands-frequency-limits-d_1602.html

Flexer, C. (2017). How to grow a young child's listening brain. *Hearing First* https://www.continued.com/early-childhood-education/articles/to-grow-young-child-listening-22841

Gremp, M. A., & Easterbrooks, M. A. (2018). A descriptive analysis of noise in classrooms across the U.S. and Canada for children who are deaf and hard of hearing. *Volta Review, 117,* 5–31.

JL Audio. (2019). *Doubling power vs. doubling output*. https://jlaudio.zendesk.com/hc/en-us/articles/217201737

John Tracy Clinic. (2012). *Audiogram of familiar sounds*. https://www.jtc.org/wp-content/uploads/2015/11/Audiogram_What_Does_Child_Hear.pdf

Ladefoged, P., & Johnson, K. (2015). *A course in phonetics* (7th ed.). Cengage Learning.

Ling, D. (1976, 2002). *Speech and the hearing-impaired child*. Alexander Graham Bell Association for the Deaf.

Ling, D. (1980). Keep your hearing-impaired child within earshot. *Newsounds, 6*, 5–6.

Ling, D. (1989). *Foundations of spoken language for hearing-impaired children*. Alexander Graham Bell Association for the Deaf.

Ling, D. (2003). The Ling Six-Sound Test. *The Listener*, 52–53.

Ling, D., & Ling, A. (1978). *Aural habilitation: Foundations of verbal learning in hearing-impaired children*. Alexander Graham Bell Association for the Deaf.

Lisker, L., & Baer, T. (1984). Laryngeal management at utterance-internal word boundary in American English. *Language and Speech, 27*, 163–171.

Mueller, H. G., & Killion, M. C. (1990). An easy method for calculating the articulation index. *Hearing Journal, 43*(9), 14–17.

Nelson, P. B., Soli, S. D., & Seltz, A. (2002). *Acoustic barriers to learning*. Technical Committee on Speech Communication of the Acoustical Society of America.

Niemoller, A. F., McCormick, I., & Miller, G. A. (1974). On the spectrum of spoken English. *Journal of the Acoustical Society of America, 55*, 461.

Northern, J. L., & Downs, M. P. (1984). *Hearing in children*. Lippincott Williams & Wilkins.

Pickett, J. M. (1999). *The acoustics of speech communication: Fundamentals, speech perception theory, and technology*. Allyn & Bacon.

Rotfleisch, S. (2000). Soda bottles & submarines: Essential speech acoustics. *The Listener*, (Summer), 51–56.

Rotfleisch, S., & Martindale, M. Why do most children in auditory-verbal therapy and education acquire highly intelligible speech but some do not? In W. Estabrooks (Ed.), *101 frequently asked questions about auditory-verbal practice*. Alexander Graham Bell Association for the Deaf.

Stevens, S. S., Egan, J. P., & Miller, G. A. (1947). Methods of measuring speech spectra. *Journal of the Acoustical Society of America, 19*, 771–781.

Studio and Audio Calculations: Audio and Acoustic Conversions 1. (n.d.). www.sengpielaudio.com

Tiwari, M. (2012). Speech acoustics: How much science? *Journal of Natural Science: Biology and Medicine, 3*(1), 24–31.

Vaughan, P. (1976). *Learning to listen: A book by mothers for mothers of hearing-impaired children*. Scribner.

Chapter 2

Guiding and Supporting Parents/Caregivers

Maura Martindale

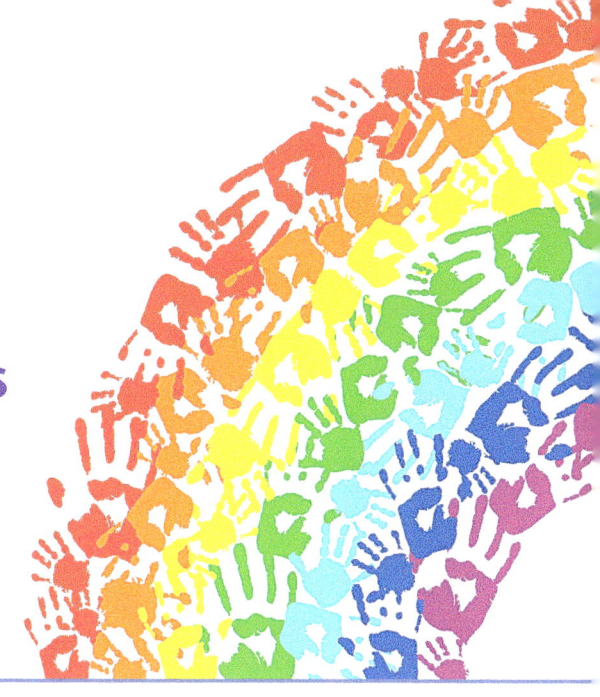

Key Points

- Parents spend more time with their child than anyone, so they need to be partners in spoken language learning, thus increasing the quantity and quality of intervention.
- Professionals need to learn as much as possible about the family's daily life.
- Parents are adult learners whose acquisition of knowledge differs from that of children.
- Parents engage in language interactions with their child all day, during activities for daily living, where listening and spoken language take place as part of natural routines and activities.
- Following the identification of a hearing loss in their child, parents will experience a range of emotions, which is to be expected. The professional's role is to avoid judgment and to be a good listener.
- There are numerous tools to help professionals actively engage parents, but incidental, teachable moments occur naturally and can be used to achieve desired goals.

Why Are Parents Included in Auditory Sessions?

If you have decided to become a professional who provides listening and spoken language support to children with hearing loss, you will be guiding and supporting families, not just teaching a child who has hearing loss (see Auditory-Verbal Principles on companion website). As you see in the 10 auditory-verbal (AV) principles, guiding and coaching parents are over half of them. Parents are key members of the team, more so than simply attending parent-teacher conferences or meetings to decide on annual goals. Each individual session should include the parents, who are with their child more than we ever will be. They hold the dreams and goals for their child and they are the constant, as there will always be changes in teachers, doctors, therapists, audiologists, and other professionals. They are partners in this and they have a greater amount of investment in the outcomes. Parental involvement is a significant predictor of the learning language (Moeller, 2000).

Getting Started: Planning

Before your first sessions, review typical and atypical child development. Not all children's behaviors are related to the hearing loss, and parents often need to be reminded of this. Have takeaways at the ready in the form of single sheets that can be affixed to the refrigerator. Do avoid giving these in any specific order, but follow the needs of the family. Overplan your sessions. In this way, if you were going to sort laundry (using clothing language), and the parent shares that the child dislikes doing this, you have plan B ready to go, such as dressing a doll or stuffed animal. Plan to model as opposed to long lectures or explanations, narrating and providing short reasons and intended goals as you work together. Turn control of the activity over to the parents. Look for ways to praise the parents! Their sense of child-rearing confidence may have been shaken by the identification of the hearing loss.

Emotional Supports for Families

You will need to *become comfortable dealing with strong, varied, and difficult feelings* that many hearing parents experience when they learn that their child has a disability. The feelings may be readily apparent or not. This is particularly true immediately after an identification of hearing loss is established via audiological, medical, and other assessments. In our experience, strong feelings of distress and worry can also emerge again during times of transitions, such as when the child changes schooling or is about to graduate from high school (Lederberg & Golbach, 2002). As Luterman (1979, 2010) points out, it is not our job to make parents feel better, make their feelings go away, or minimize these feelings. Their feelings are their own. It is our job to listen and to be aware that much of the early advice and information that we provide to families may not be remembered or even register depending upon where they are emotionally. This may be the first time they have even thought about having a child who is deaf or hard of hearing in their family.

In the Discussion Questions for this chapter, think about: When it comes to talking about and responding to others' difficult feelings, how comfortable are you? As you read more about working with parents, think about your own responses to others' difficult feelings and be ready to discuss!

Why? Responding to the strong feelings of guilt, worry, grief, anger, loss, fear, sadness, pain, and denial will be a part of your interactions with parents and caregivers whose child has a disability. It is unavoidable. These feelings are not good or bad, right or wrong. They just are. You do not need to be a psychologist or counselor to provide support to parents. Each emotion has a purpose and is not to be ignored or dismissed. Moses (1994) created a valuable framework to help professionals engage with families at the emotional level, called ENUF. Remember, this takes practice!

- **E**mpathizing. Truly sensing what the other person is feeling at that

moment. Not sure? Try rephrasing what you think was shared with you.
- **N**onjudgmental. Authentically staying neutral and not deciding/believing whether these feelings are good or bad.
- **U**nconditional. Feelings are permitted because we are human. They are to be expected.
- **F**eeling focused. While it is tempting to stay in territory that you are most comfortable with, parents and caregivers who are dealing with powerful emotions may want to share them with someone like you.

There were many times when the session we had planned had to be put aside so that the parents could talk to a trusted professional who allowed them to feel whatever they are feeling. Knowing that this is OK can be comforting to you. Other tips and thoughts:

- Introduce and connect families to other families who have children with hearing loss. Parents often say that meeting other families who are dealing with similar feelings is helpful.
- Arrange to have older children, teens, and adults with hearing loss talk to families. If you do not know any of these groups right now, there are a number of books, videos, organizations, websites, and webinars that can be shared with families.
- If a parent is upset and does not want to share, let them know that if they want to at a future time, you are open to it.
- Have your own resources available by collecting websites, service providers, emails, and phone contacts should parents have specific issues and request them.
- Many parents go through a period of shopping for information, communication approaches, schools, programs, and other supports. This is not an insult to you, but a journey they are taking. It's a good time to practice ENUF!
- Remember that life happens! Families face crises in the course of their lives, such as a job loss, death of a family member, or other tragic events. A broken hearing aid or the need for new earmolds may not be at the top of their list of primary concerns when that happens.
- Even parents who seem to have it together may experience strong feelings that are triggered by what seems like a minor event, such as a birthday.
- Always keep the family's culture or cultures in mind when talking about feelings. The good news is that regardless of the cultural gaps you may be experiencing, your efforts at compassion will be appreciated. For example, if you are planning food preparation activities, use foods that the family actually eats.
- It will be important to consider how different cultures typically handle communication breakdowns, and what sounds are associated with children's toys and activities, to show respect and avoid offense.

Teaching Parents and Caregivers: Why Are They Part of Every Session?

Parents are critical team members who can keep the learning going 24/7, particularly if they are included in weekly sessions. Thus, these sessions will assist them via modeling, guiding, and coaching, thus building toward spoken language. Numerous studies have shown that the quality and amount of parental language input to young children with typically hearing children (Hart & Risley, 1995) and for children with hearing loss are significant factors in the quality and quantity of spoken language outcomes (Nittrouer et al., 2019). Keep in mind that parents may come to your sessions with a preconceived idea about what therapy ought to look, sound, and feel like to them, based on their own life experiences such as their culture, school and therapy experiences, education level, and role of a parent.

Even if you are helping children with hearing loss in settings where parents cannot or do not participate, regular communications with the family about their child's progress, and ideas to promote listening and spoken language in the home, can still be shared. Over the past decade, children with hearing loss and their families have been successfully taught using telepractice (Daczewitz et al., 2020).

In situations where caregivers cannot be physically present during listening and spoken language (LSL) sessions, telepractice may work for their situation by connecting virtually over the internet. If you are in a school setting with a caseload of children with hearing loss and minimal access at all to caregivers, you may want to consider adding to the number of sessions each week for practice and carryover. Regardless of how you schedule your sessions, parents are a member of the team!

Since parents are essential to their child's listening and spoken language development, what are ways to think about teaching, supporting, and guiding adults?

In a qualitative study by Neuss (2006), the term *ecological transition* was introduced. It is the journey many families take, changing from their expected role for a child to one that will assume many additional important duties that are needed for parents whose child has a hearing loss. These include teacher, advocate, equipment manager, data gatherer, and social skills facilitator. This transition does not occur overnight for most parents. Regardless of how and when these other roles are assumed, professionals can facilitate this by knowing more about how adults learn.

Because the parents will be assuming additional roles in intervention, we need to think about how adults learn. The term *andragogy* was coined by Knowles (1980) to explain how adults learn differently than children. He theorized that adults come to a novel experience with a lifetime of knowledge and learning. They are typically self-directed, internally motivated, and oriented to problem solving. For these reasons, your student is an adult who is interested in practical solutions and specific actions relevant to their daily lives. Your guiding and coaching needs to demonstrate success and focus on how the parents can best incorporate what you are modeling into their family situation. The adult learner needs to know what you are doing, why you are doing it, and how it will be useful to them.

As a first step and first session, gather as much information about the family as possible, along with their feelings. Remember that not everyone will be comfortable sharing feelings with you until trust is built over time. We also want to know what the parents' desired outcomes are for therapy and education. Abundant research has shown us that certain key variables will impact a child's progress and parents' expectations. These include age of identification of the hearing loss, age of acquiring hearing aids and/or cochlear implant(s), usage of hearing technologies, all audiological data, educational programming, additional disabilities, language(s) of the home, maternal education, and developmental milestones (Ching et al., 2018). If possible, secure all assessment data that has already been conducted and ask about the child's daily schedule, siblings, other family members who interact frequently with this child, and playmates. This information is vital to all professionals on the team.

Ask how their environment at home can become more conducive to listening to natural conversations by reducing background noise such as from appliances (Caldwell & Nittrouer, 2013). Provide some suggestions on how to improve the auditory environment in the home, such as keeping the television off during mealtime conversations, and emphasize turn taking at family gatherings. Use open-ended questions to gain an understanding about each family!

A word about level of parental education is needed here. As our population becomes more diverse, a therapy caseload will probably include some families where parents' educational experiences are more limited. Being aware of your own biases and assumptions is a good idea. Compensation for this is achievable, given the time to build trust and with attention to approaches which encourage parents. Ask yourself, does the family have access to the internet? Do you need to use take-aways that are translated into the home language? Would diagrams be a better way to explain something or answer a question? Is there a better school situation that can be determined at meetings with other professionals providing services? Any family may experience job loss, persistent poverty, crises with other family members, and other events that impact the ability to follow through on appointments or care. You may need to take time during sessions to guide parents in gaining access to needed services and audiological follow-up visits. The professional can help anyone realize that they bring many strengths to their child's learning.

It is not uncommon for parents to have expectations based on the hope that once a child has access to sound, talking will follow immediately. They might assume that as soon the sensory device is appropriately set for the child that the child will begin to behave as other children of the same chronological age, to point to their ears when they hear a sound, localize sounds, and to begin to immediately babble or respond to their name or say words. As previously discussed, a critical element of intervention is working with the parents and providing them with the knowledge base and appropriate expectations. This is a good time to have the parents talk with other parents whose beginnings were similar.

As you meet with parents initially, be aware that they are likely new to dealing with technology or might be adjusting to different technology for their child with hearing loss. The need to monitor responses to sound is among one of the first goals for the professional and therefore for the parent as well. With newly emerging auditory abilities, we must observe the sometimes-subtle responses to sound and other behaviors that are evidence of auditory access. We expect parents might have limited experience and understanding of what initial responses might look like in their young infant or child or how verbal productions would indicate auditory access and emerging perception (see Chapter 6, Tables 6–1, 6–10, 6–11).

To be effective in coaching parents, the professional needs to spend more time and effort directed at the parent than at the child. This involves more than collaborating on goals or reviewing assessments. It means modeling, observing parent-child interactions in a variety of contexts, providing useful feedback and suggestions in the moment, and fostering reflections about these interactions (Fey et al., 2006; Brown, 2012). Parents are active participants in coaching, and the professional feedback needs to be strength based and positive. Parents often enter sessions seeking solutions to problems, which may or may not be related to listening and spoken language. A parent could be concerned about eating, sleeping, academics, homework, general development, or other professionals. Professionals can share resources, provide suggestions, and always encourage the parents to enhance their own problem-solving skills.

Does all this guiding and coaching of parents via modeling work in promoting a child's language acquisition? What can we tell parents about the benefits of parental involvement in sessions? We know from the Hart and Risley study (1995) that there is a relationship between the amount and quality of parent/child talking and typical children's language development over time. Ramirez et al. (2019) studied how intervention with one group of parents made a significant difference in children's language growth compared with children who were in a no-intervention parent group. Spoken language growth was higher in the intervention group, as measured within the home settings of both groups of children at 6, 10, 14, and 18 months of age. For children with hearing loss, the quality and quantity of parental language input are significant factors in the quality and quantity of spoken language outcomes (Nittrouer et al., 2019; Rufsvold et al., 2018).

Family Life: Activities of Daily Living (ADL) as the Foundation of Every Session

To ensure parents are critical partners in the intervention, we must engage and empower them. An excellent starting point is to consider: what do all parents and children do on a daily basis? At a basic level, parents care for their children by feeding, clothing, washing, and comforting them. Every parent/child interaction from changing diapers, dressing, washing their hands, and running errands to food shopping, preparing meals, and engaging in countless other events are part and parcel of daily living and can include listening and language. These are activities of daily living (ADL). ADL should be considered the blueprint, and are activities with which parents feel competent and comfortable already, building their sense of confidence and "I can do this" (Spagnola & Fiese, 2007).

It is important to learn about the family's day-to-day life and their living situation to be able to model language within ADL (Bloom & Lahey, 1978). ADL uses the family's daily life, not just toys or flash cards, to bathe the child in language. Keep in mind that many families may not have the resources or desire to purchase expensive toys and games. Moreover, these are not essential to learning spoken language, as a simple walk around the block can provide a rich and interesting source of conversation. Furthermore, there is an increasing number of families from diverse cultures whom you will undoubtedly meet in any educational setting today. Learn what you can about the culture of each family and home language. Incorporate the family's holidays, celebrations, music, clothing, traditions, and foods into your sessions as appropriate.

Structured therapy sessions can be intimidating for parents who are probably overwhelmed. Professionals can assist and guide parents in carefully selecting materials for play in sessions in a way that mirrors the family's culture, goals, and life situation. Otherwise, this may unintentionally give the message that only professionals can teach a child with hearing loss or that there are specific materials that need to be used. Mentor parents in material selection for activities so that they can do the same in their home.

Parents are dealing with the hearing loss, technology, and possibly a child who is very delayed in their development while still trying to learn their many new roles. Parents wonder if their child with hearing loss can reach the desired outcome of listening and spoken language. In natural situations, parents are always teaching their child, and children are always learning from their parents. We need to guide, coach, and empower parents to take advantage of what they are already doing in all things and talk about changing diapers, making lunch, taking a walk, and so on.

ADL should be seen as a springboard for examining opportunities to facilitate the skills of the child with hearing loss. The professional can guide the parents to the realization that everyday life is a listening and spoken language process with a wealth of language that awaits their discovery. As professionals guiding and coaching parents to support the successful development of a child with hearing loss into a competent spoken language communicator, we must understand that auditory access is the primary building block necessary for developing an auditory brain.

Through guiding and coaching caregivers, parents understand that they can teach through the course of everyday activities and that language learning situations are part of the entire day. ADL naturally incorporates meaningful, everyday language along with repetitions needed to facilitate the development of competent young communicators. Parents will feed their children, but they are less likely to sit down at a table to complete a structured activity that the professional modeled in the child's therapy session (Snow & Beals, 2006). In sessions, we can explain the natural advantage of using everyday scenarios for improving the desired outcomes.

Parents will use stereotypic phrases during the ADL activities that will allow children to develop a sense of routine and to predict what is going to happen when provided with a verbal message that is routinely used by the adults in the environment as they begin to hear and learn language. Young children with hearing loss and limited language will look to make sense of their lives, particularly with older children who have limited or no receptive language. Verbal routines paired with ADL routines provide a collection of phrases, many of which are unique to that family, that help a child with hearing loss make sense of the language and vocal pattern of stereotypic phrases. When it is time to eat, one family may be called with a sing-song chorus of "Dinner time!" while others could say, "Soup's on," "Everyone to the table," or "Last one here is a rotten egg!" Regardless what the expression is, we can expect the expression to be consistent and to have a specific intonation pattern that is not confused with "Wave bye-bye to Daddy" or "Uh oh, it fell down?" or "What a mess!" or a clean-up song.

Stereotypic phrases might be different at Grandma's home, in daycare, or in preschool.

Why focus so much attention on ADL? For typically developing children, language is caught through daily life and meaningful communicative interactions. This is the process we facilitate with the child with hearing loss. Always sitting at a therapy table is not an efficient way compared to the natural way the brain learns language (Beals, 2001). This basic premise needs to be established or re-established in every interaction during sessions and ADL; i.e., that we use our voice and our language for interacting and communicating with others. The underlying message that must be made clear to the child is that "You want to communicate something to me, and I really want to understand you."

Consider the abundant opportunities to use spoken language during ADL with a child with hearing loss. The following **ADL Formula** illustrates the amount of repetitions of meaningful language that can be embedded into daily routines and activities:

R = Repetitions per day

N = Number of days activity performed

P = Potential language repetition within ADL

X = Exposure to language structure

$$R \times N \times P = X$$

For example, mealtimes:

Activity—meals R = 3

Number of days per year N = 365

Language repetition P = 10

$$3 \times 365 \times 10 = 10{,}950!$$

This formula provides professionals and parents a clear picture of the essential part that Activities of Daily Living play in promoting listening and language (Rotfleisch, 2001)!

Engaging Families in Sessions

Having read about the strong feelings that parents may have at various points during your time with them, how can professionals engage with parents so that the child with hearing loss will develop a listening brain and spoken language? Table 2–1 contains a few suggestions for engaging parents.

Cultural Considerations

You will be providing intervention to families who belong to cultural group(s) that are different from your own. This is a certainty. Their views and perceptions of hearing loss will be influenced by their own experiences, norms, values, and cultural lens, which may be in conflict with goals and your own expectations. Even if you are supporting a family who states that their cultural experiences are very similar to your own, we do know that no group is homogeneous. For example, it can be tempting to assume that a family whose home language is Spanish is similar to all other Spanish-speaking families. In addition to cultural norms, values, and experiences, issues of race, class, ethnicity, language, gender, financial status, and geographic region will have an impact on how disability is viewed, ideas on parenting and child rearing, family roles and relationships, medical models, and perceptions of the role of professionals.

Table 2–1. Increasing Engagement With Families

Creating High Levels of Engagement	Tools for You to Share With Parents	Tools for You
Provide takeaway items for everyday use and to share with others	Information about how the amount of talking at home impacts language learning	Hart and Risley (1995) charts
Model what to talk about during ADL	Lists of stereotypic phrases to use throughout the day	Talk Around the Clock curriculum (Rossi, 2006)
Relate speech acoustics to diagnostic/error analysis	Use the charts in Chapter 1 to meet their child's needs	Speech acoustics chapter charts
Explain hearing loss to families; make communication choices	Numerous materials to share with parents	https://successforkidswithhearingloss.com/for-professionals/early-childhood-infants-toddlers-preschool/
SPICE auditory curriculum Spice for Life	Comes with toys, songs and picture cards, a video, YouTube videos, etc. Useful for remedial children	Central Institute for the Deaf (Moog et al., 1995) West and Manley (2012)
Children's books with characters with hearing loss	Books to share with the family and peers	*Gracie's Ears* (Blackington, 2011)
Pragmatics in natural environments	*It Takes Two to Talk*, Hanen Center	Weitzman, E., & Cupples, P. (2017). *It takes two to talk: A practical guide for parents of children with language delays.* The Hanen Center.

We have also observed that families from diverse cultural backgrounds have varying ideas of what therapy looks like and their role in it. Pragmatics, or social conversational norms such as communication repair strategies, may not be the ones you use, so ask the parents how their culture typically addresses this. The sounds that we often associate with specific toys, such as farm animals, may be distinctly different in a family's heritage language. As an example, many people say "peep-peep" for a baby chick, but someone from another culture may say "peopeo." Those of us for whom English is a first language may not be able to hear phonemes from other languages.

Given the essential role and importance of language and speech development for children with hearing loss, consideration of potential cultural challenges and strategies are presented in Table 2–2. Remember to avoid stereotyping a family based on their cultural background!

Wang and Lam (2017) recommend that professionals seek out a cultural interpreter who can assist in shaping therapy and intervention in a way that is culturally

Table 2–2. Connecting With Families and Their Cultures

Challenges			
Family life and roles	**Goals of education**	**Language of home**	**Audiology/implants/ diagnosis/aids**
Strategies			
Fold all objectives and activities into existing cultural family roles. For example, if mom sees her role as family caregiver and not as a teacher, avoid giving her flash cards and worksheets. Instead of using phrases such as "You need to work with your child," find ways to maximize natural parent-child interactions (e.g., food preparation) to promote linguistic outcomes; emphasis on language stimulation.	Ask the parents what they would like to see as an eventual outcome for the school year. Instead of imposing goals and objectives stated in education-speak such as "Child will produce all step-one English vowels and diphthongs," restate it as "Child will learn to use vowel sounds that are shared in both English and the home language in words and phrases." Be aware that family relationships may be viewed as equally important to individual achievement, as evidenced by behaviors such as extended visits to home countries to see family.	Identify the home language on the school documents without judgment. Utilize informal assessment techniques such as *evidence gaining* to gain knowledge of the child's known spoken language; acquire and analyze a *language sample* in the home language if the child can express himself spontaneously; encourage parents who do not speak English to continue using the home language to keep auditory neural pathways stimulated; utilize known checklists of pragmatic/conversation skills or language rating scales and modify them as needed; stress early vocabulary words that are important and similar in both languages	Provide abundant information and resources that will result in complete access to the sounds of the home language and English for the child; target this population for early diagnosis, hearing aids, and cochlear implants. Structured auditory skills curricula may be required for children who are older but new to listening.

responsive to children with disabilities. This person is more than a language interpreter, but someone who could share possible family perspectives on cultural norms and values related to disability. Reflecting on your own knowledge about cultural diversity is a good way to start!

Screen Time

We are aware that more and more children, even infants and toddlers, are spending increasing amounts of their time with portable devices with touchscreens. In a study of children with typical hearing, ages 6 months to 3 years of age, a survey of 715 parents found that some children spent as much as 75% of every day on a touchscreen device. The researchers found that children who used these devices frequently were associated with sleep problems and delays (Cheung et al., 2017). Our overuse of touchscreen devices with very young children will send a signal that listening and language can be learned through these devices. So, we recommend that devices be used sparingly if at all.

piness for any family. Parents of children with hearing loss face additional sources of stress related to the disability (Lederberg & Golbach, 2002). The multitude of decisions and issues regarding hearing technology, schooling, language and communication, siblings, and socialization arise at different times in the child's life. Supportive, unbiased information, along with a willingness to listen to the family, is a major part of our work.

Speech Acoustics and Parents

As caregivers gain knowledge and experience, they might want additional information about their child's hearing loss, speech acoustics, and the nature of spoken language. Some topics that might be of interest to them include:

- auditory access and modifying the auditory signal—distance;
- auditory access and modifying the auditory signal—acoustic highlighting;
- signal to noise ratio (SNR) and noise clutter;
- speech features;
- speech features on an audiogram;
- speech development related to an audiogram;
- language development related to an audiogram; and
- a walk through their child's development based on speech acoustics.

Summary

Parenting can be stressful, challenging, and at the same time a great source of hap-

Discussion Questions

1. When it comes to talking about and responding to the difficult feelings of others, where are you? What aspect of ENUF might be challenging for you?
2. Practicing ENUF: What would you say to a parent who says:
   a. "Emma just doesn't want to sit down for sessions with me."
   b. "I noticed that Matthew, who sees Jenny for therapy, seems to have better speech than my child."
   c. "I couldn't find any parking," says a chronically late parent who has attended therapy for 6 months.
   d. "She will do much better without me in the room with her."
3. How can you bridge between your own cultural experiences and those who are members of a different cultural group(s)?
4. In explaining speech acoustics to parents, what resources do you need to gather for parents as takeaway items? What resources do you already have?

References

Beals, D. E. (2001). Eating and reading: Links between family conversations with preschoolers and later language and literacy. In D. K. Dickinson & P. O. Tabors (Eds.), *Beginning literacy with language: Young children at home and school* (pp. 75–92). Paul H. Brookes.

Behl, D. D., Blaiser, K., Cook, G., Barrett, T., Callow-Heusser, C., Brooks, B. M., . . .White, K. R. (2016). A multisite study evaluating the benefits of early intervention via telepractice. *Infants and Young Children, 29*(4), 147–161. https://doi.org/10.1097/iyc.0000000000000090

Bloom, L., & Lahey, M. (1978). *Language development and language disorders*. John Wiley & Sons.

Brown, J. (2012). *Exploring coaching strategies in a parent-implemented intervention for toddlers* [Unpublished doctoral dissertation]. Florida State University.

Caldwell, A., & Nittrouer, S. (2013). Speech perception in noise by children with cochlear implants. *Journal of Speech, Language, and Hearing Research, 56*(1), 13–30.

Cheung, C. M., Bedford, R., De Urahain, I. S., Karmiloff-Smith, A., & Smith, T. J. (2017). *Daily touchscreen use in infants and toddlers is associated with reduced sleep and delayed sleep onset*. https://www.nature.com/articles/srep46104

Ching, T. Y. C., Dillon, H., Leigh, G., & Cupples, L. (2018). Learning from the longitudinal outcomes of children with hearing impairment (LOCHI) study: Summary of 5-year findings and implications. *International Journal of Audiology, 57*(Suppl. 2), S105–S111.

Daczewitz, M., Meadan-Kaplansky, H. & Borders, C. (2020). Telepractice coaching for a parent of a child who is hard-of-hearing. *Deafness and Education International, 22*(2), 113–138.

Fey, M. E., Warren, S. F., Brady, N., Finestack, L. H., Bredin-Oja, S., Fairchild, M., . . . Yoder, P. J. (2006). Early effects of responsivity education/prelinguistic milieu teaching for children with developmental delays and their parents. *Journal of Speech, Language, and Hearing Research, 49*, 526–547.

Hart, B., & Risley, T. (2003). *Meaningful differences in the everyday experience of young American children* (4th ed.). Paul H. Brookes.

Knowles, M. S. (1980). *The modern practice of adult education: From pedagogy to andragogy* (revised and updated). Cambridge Adult Education.

Lederberg, A. R., & Golbach, T. (2002). Parenting stress and social support in hearing mothers of deaf and hearing children: A longitudinal study. *Journal of Deaf Studies, 7*(4), 330–345.

Luterman, D. (1979). *Counseling parents of hearing-impaired children*. Little, Brown and Company.

Luterman, D. (2010). 10 ideas for parenting a child with hearing loss. *Volta Voices, 17*(6), 34–35.

Moeller, M. P. (2000) Early intervention and language development in children who are deaf and hard of hearing. *Pediatrics, 106*(3), 1–9. http://www.pediatrics.org/cgi/content/full/106/3/e43

Moses, K . (1994) Grief groups: Rekindling hope. Voices. *The Journal of the American Academy of Psychotherapists*, (Summer). http://www.griefcounselor.org/articles/prof-article-grief-groups-Moses-1994.pdf

Neuss, D. (2006). The ecological transition to auditory-verbal therapy: Experiences of parents whose children use cochlear implants. *Volta Review, 106*(2), 195–222.

Nittrouer, S., Lowenstein, J. H., & Antonelli, J. (2019). Parental language input to children with hearing loss: Does it matter in the end? *Journal of Speech, Language, and Hearing Research, 34*, 234–238.

Ramirez, N. F., Lytle, S. R., & Kuhl, P. K. (2019). Parent coaching increases conversational turns and advances infant language development. *Proceedings of the National Academy of Sciences in the United States of America*, 1–8. www.pnas.org/cgi/doi/10.1073/pnas.1921653117

Rossi, K. (2006). *Talk around the clock: A professional's early intervention toolbox.* Alexander Graham Bell Association for the Deaf.

Rotfleisch, S. (2001). E = mc² (English equals milk and cookies too!). *The Listener,* Fall, 39–42.

Rufsvold, R., Wang, Y., Hartman, M. C., Arora, S. B., & Smolen, E. R. (2018). The impact of language input on deaf and hard of hearing preschool children who use listening and spoken language. *American Annals of the Deaf, 163*(1), 35–60.

Snow, C. E., & Beals, D. E. (2006). Mealtime talk that supports literacy development. In R. W. Larson, A. R. Wiley, & K. R. Branscomb (Eds.), *New directions for child and adolescent development. Family mealtime as a context of development and socialization* (pp. 51–66). Jossey-Bass.

Spagnola, M., & Fiese, B. H. (2007). Family routines and rituals: A context for development in the lives of young children. *Infants and Young Children, 20*(4), 284–299.

Wang, M., & Lam, L. (2017). Evidence-based practice in special education and cultural adaptations: Challenges and implications for research. *Research and Practice for Persons with Severe Disabilities, 42*(1), 53–61.

Chapter 3

Stages Not Ages Model

Sylvia Rotfleisch and Maura Martindale

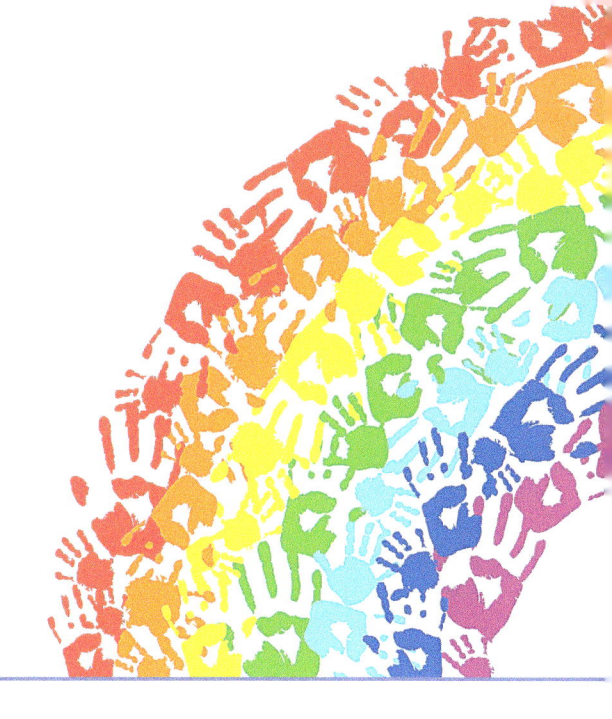

Key Points

- Children develop complex skills in a developmental sequence whereby they acquire foundational skills that supports the next step toward mastery.
- The habilitation stages model is an orderly process facilitating the abilities of children to follow the normal sequence of development.
- Clear and realistic expectations are important to the habilitation process.
- Development of listening and spoken language competence is dependent on the facilitation and emergence of the auditory skill development.
- Professionals working with children to develop listening and spoken language mastery must understand the normal sequence of development of listening, speech, language, and the cognitive and social components of communication.
- Development of listening and spoken language competence is dependent on and scaffolded by the facilitation and emergence of the auditory skill development.

This chapter and the following chapters present a model for habilitation that is developmental and sequential. We are not presenting a remedial approach, but rather a sequence of stages that is applicable to a child with either delayed skills or typical development. This habilitation model is an auditory-based therapy that follows typical child development in each domain: listening, speech, language, and the cognitive and social components of communication. Information on the stages model for habilitation is summarized along with information to help determine which stage of habilitation is most appropriate for an individual child. The intervention chapters are designed to assist and support professionals in the development of goals based on thorough assessments in a variety of domains, using both formal and informal approaches. A number of detailed developmental tables are included here for your reference and to help focus on where and how the child should be progressing over time. Tables provided can be used to assist in determining each child's individual level of performance, and as the foundation for treatment planning of long-term goals and short-term learning outcomes for instruction.

When lesson planning for therapy sessions based on goals, consider that individual learning outcomes during therapy sessions may include a number of the goals within a single activity, such as food preparation. Sharing the intended outcomes of any activity with parents prior to beginning each session will help them see progress, areas of need, and what strategies worked (and which did not). At times, a spontaneous action or reaction may touch on a learning outcome that was not planned, such as the child wanting to know what an article of clothing or utensil is called. Careful note taking in sessions is essential to keep track of whether or not learning outcomes were achieved.

Stages/Sequence of Development (Flow Chart)

Newborns have limited abilities but will master many complex skills as they mature and as their brains develop. This is evidenced from the time they are born as they master skills such as walking and talking that have predictable, known sequences for typically developing children. Infants do not just walk or run without developing through the necessary foundational skills such as head control, trunk and leg control, balance, weight transfer, and reciprocal leg movement. Just as other complex skills develop in a known sequence, so too do listening and spoken language abilities. In this book we address habilitation based on that premise. We must begin with the foundation abilities and in particular the auditory access. Given appropriate and sufficient auditory input, we provide habilitation, facilitating progress through developmentally sequential stages of listening and spoken language development. Language begins significantly before the child utters their first word approximation and has a definite progression, just as other complex developed skills. We must begin at the beginning. We start at the foundational skills and proceed in a systematic developmental sequence. This is the way the brain wants to develop.

The premise of the intervention chapters is based on determination of the child's stage in the development of listening and spoken language and progressing through to the more advanced stages. With that in mind, this habilitation model follows six defined intervention stages (Table 3–1). Chapters 6–11 represent each stage and consist of detailed information on skills in audition, listening and spoken language skills, recommended goals, activities to illustrate implementation of goals, and a comprehensive case history accompanied by a sample intervention session.

As you begin to apply the stages to intervention, you first decide at what stage the child is functioning. Once the child's level is determined, you begin habilitation from that stage and allow

Table 3–1. Model for Intervention

Stages Model for Intervention
1. prelinguistic
2. single word
3. emerging word combinations
4. communication with childlike errors
5. competent communicator
6. advanced communicator

the listening and spoken language levels to build as skills are mastered. In this way, habilitation begins at the appropriate skill level and progresses developmentally and sequentially from the early language stages to the advanced ones. Formal assessments and informal evaluations of the child will assist in determining the starting point for the child's habilitation program (see Chapter 4), but we can use some primary characteristics to determine the stage. The most important criteria for understanding the stage to begin with in the intervention model are listed in Table 3–2. There will be differences within the stages of what individual children are able to do. A newly identified child in the prelinguistic stage might have some of the skills or none depending on previous auditory access. If the child experienced some auditory access prior to being fit with technology, they might be vocalizing and turn taking, and may have one or more receptive words. Another child might have had no auditory access at all prior to receiving their technology and could have no auditory attention to sounds, could not yet understand that sounds have meaning, and could be nonvocal. Another example could be with children in the communication with errors stage. One child in this stage might have ongoing errors that are limited to /s/ morphemic functions such as plurals and possessives due to continued limited access to the high frequencies. Another child also in this stage might be using telegraphic phrases with only key words (e.g., "daddy go bye-bye car") and have limited use of grammatical structures while learning to attend to quieter sounds and unstressed words within complete sentences.

Following this intervention model means that a 2-month-old or late-identified 2-, 3-, or 4-year-old child could all be in the same stage of listening and spoken language development, working toward the same goals. The selected activities and

Table 3–2. Indication for Placement Into Stage

Expressive Language Indication	Stage/Chapter
Does not have a word approximation or protoword	prelinguistic stage Chapter 6
Uses a word approximation or protoword	single-word stage Chapter 7
Has combined two words together to create an original phrase	emerging word combinations stage Chapter 8
Combines three to four words	communication with childlike errors stage Chapter 9
Speaks with complex, grammatically correct language	competent communicator stage Chapter 10
Fully competent language communicator with an ever-growing vocabulary	advanced communicator stage Chapter 11

interaction style would need to be individualized appropriately for a 2-month-old compared to the 2-year-old or the 4-year-old based on their developmental and cognitive levels. Considering this example, we realize that the newly identified older child should not begin intervention working on skills that are typical for a child of their chronological age. As professionals, we must guide the family to understand that we do not begin with language skills based on the chronologic age level. We begin with the foundation skills, understanding that spoken language has meaning and expresses communicative intent.

Parents and some professionals working with such cases will be concerned about the lack of expressive language and want the child to be talking. However, that would be like expecting a 2-month-old to walk. It would be building the house by starting on the second floor without the foundations of auditory access and understanding premise of audition, listening, and spoken language. Habilitation needs to be approached systematically and developmentally. The child must begin with auditory attention, learn to use their voice for communication, and then start to develop receptive and expressive words. Word combinations cannot begin until there is adequate listening and some basic expressive and receptive vocabulary, just as the child cannot take a first step before they can stand up and balance. The 2-year-old in this example is not ready to be doing what their peers are doing—combining two words together or using plurals and possessives. Similarly, the 4-year-old with new auditory access cannot have goals for the skills expected in typically developing 4-year-old peers. This child is not able to understand or answer "wh-" questions because he does not have the receptive language and cannot be expected to combine three and four words together when he does not have expressive words.

There is not a defined period of time that a child might be in a given stage; it is dependent on the skills being facilitated and mastered. It is important to monitor and evaluate the child for progress in development of listening and spoken language, and the mastery of skills targeted in the goals. Skill development can also be used to help determine transition to the next stage. Skills that are indicative of transition to the next habilitation stage are included briefly in Table 3–2 and in tables in the therapy chapters.

Determining Child's Level

Skills to be developed during the various stages are included in detail in each of the tables of each intervention chapters. Expected listening, speech, and language skills from the stages are indicated in Table 3–3 to illustrate the progression of habilitation stages.

Each intervention chapter includes multiple tables. These tables are provided for ease of use, for continuity across the chapters, and to summarize the content for each stage of intervention. They are intended to be used for reference. For these reasons, the tables are used to address important content areas for each specific stage, and are presented in the same format and with consistent numbering across the intervention chapters. For example, the auditory abilities will consistently be in Table 1 in the therapy chapters, whether at the prelinguistic level or the word combination stage. The content areas covered in the tables in the intervention chapters are summarized in Table 3–4.

Expectations for Growth

What are realistic expectations of spoken language growth in children using an auditory-based approach? In addition to monitoring the child's growth over time in many domains, the **parents' growth** in the intervention process would also be important to document. Cole and Flexer (2007) created an excellent and easy to use checklist with 21 specific parent/caregiver behaviors that promote listening and spoken language in young children. You may need to start with the importance of full-time device wearing and model how to respond to communicative intents that maximize language development.

For **children's growth** over time, desired outcomes are a focus at the onset of therapy at any stage to determine if the expectations are realistic, depending on multiple factors involved for the family and the child with hearing loss (Macaulay & Ford, 2013). If the child is older and the parents are dealing with the identification of hearing loss, they might need to look at the research indications for the outcomes for older children with hearing loss who are delayed or have late access to audition.

The desired outcome of auditory-based therapy is for the child with hearing loss to develop age-appropriate spoken language for full participation in society. With advances in the early identification of hearing loss and access to high-quality hearing technologies, there is ample research to document excellent outcomes for children whose hearing loss is detected at less than 1 year of age and who receive access to high-quality auditory-based intervention (Rotfleisch & Martindale, 2012).

The best way to know if a child is making adequate progress toward this goal is through a well-designed and comprehensive assessment plan in which data is systematically collected, analyzed, and evaluated at defined intervals. This plan paints an overall picture of the child's maximum performance and typical performance. Data collected from standardized assessments can be compared to that of peers who are developing typically. These assessments are the best instruments to provide ongoing information regarding adequate progress, help professionals obtain objective measures, allow for accountability of service delivery, and identify areas of concern (Geers et al., 2017).

Best practices and standards of care indicate that a child in an appropriate intervention service should make at least *1 year of growth in 1 year's time*, keeping pace with their peers across multiple domains. These domains include auditory skills, prelinguistic communication, receptive and expressive language, speech perception and production, pragmatic skills, literacy, inclusion, cognition, social skills, and academic abilities.

Skills are expected to emerge as a result of auditory access in an expected sequence over periods of time and must be facilitated and monitored. The lack of progress in acquiring auditory abilities will indicate that auditory access may not be appropriate. Based on the auditory information the child with hearing loss is accessing through the hearing technology, we should expect to monitor skills emerging in the appropriate sequence and time frame. We collect data on initial auditory access through observed behaviors of the emerging auditory skills. Numerous informal checklists and formal assessments can assist in tracking emerging skills and are discussed in Chapter 4 on assessments. As we gather details on auditory abilities, we must be certain that responses are

Table 3–3. Basic Indications of Progression Through Stages of Intervention

Indications of Prelinguistic Stage

Demonstrates inconsistent or no responses to variety of sounds

Shows limited or no comprehension of words

May or may not use their voice with any communicative intent

Does not have a word approximation or protoword

⬇

Indication of Progression to Single-Word Stage

Demonstrates access to and responds to variety of speech sounds and features

Shows comprehension of a few different words

Uses voice in babbling with communicative intent

Uses a word approximation or protoword

⬇

Indication of Progression to Emerging Word Combinations Stage

Demonstrates a two- to three-item auditory memory

Follows two-part related commands

Has consistently emerging receptive and expressive vocabulary on a weekly basis

Has combined two words together to create an original phrase (e.g., "more juice")

Uses variety of consonants in words and word approximations

⬇

Indication of Progression to Communication With Childlike Errors Stage

Combines three to four words

Shows comprehension of a variety of grammatical structures including pronouns, negatives, prepositions

Uses some grammatical morphemes typically; e.g., -ing verb endings, prepositions (in, on), plural and possessive /s/ functions

Rapid increase in receptive and expressive vocabulary with early concepts emerging

⬇

Indication of Progression to Competent Communicator Stage

Speaks with complex, grammatically correct language

Uses language consistently to converse and express themselves

Follows a conversation of an appropriate subject/language, maintains the topic

Uses discourse format to tell a story or explain something.

Knows a variety of words of multiple meanings (e.g., too/to/two, trunk, hare/hair, fly [noun and verb])

Uses irregular plurals and past tenses

Understands passive voice sentences, subordinate and coordinate clauses

Limited or no grammatical errors

Table 3–3. *continued*

⬇

Indication of Progression to Advanced Communicator Stage
Has conversations using most conversational norms
Fully competent language communicator with an ever-growing vocabulary emerging in Tiers 2 and 3
Consistently discriminate:

Initial consonants different by manner	Final consonants different by manner
Initial consonants different by voicing	Final consonants different by voicing
Initial consonants different by place	Final consonants different by place

⬇

Indication of Progression to Successful Language Communicator With Advanced Competence Stage
Uses listening and spoken language comparable to an adult
Learns new vocabulary regularly from both Tier 2 and 3 in academic and daily life settings
Competent conversationalist and emerging skills for public oral presentations
Understands social language and cues including jokes, idioms, sarcasm, and inferences

Table 3–4. Organization of Table Content in Intervention Chapters

Table Number	Content Area
1	Auditory abilities
2	Language and speech skills
3	Auditory goals for understanding sound as meaningful
4	Auditory goals for development of the speech production system
5	Auditory goals for language comprehension
6	Auditory goals for developing expressive language
7	Knowledge areas for professionals and to guide parents
8	Optimal strategies to be implemented
9	Guide and coach parents to do with child
Summary table	Skills that are expected by the end of the stage and indicate progression to next stage

through audition only and not a response to visual input (e.g., lipreading, mouth movements, visual awareness of physical movement of objects or person).

If a child enters therapy and is already behind in language, speech, and listening skills, based on assessments, then the rate of progress will need to be increased with the idea of catching up. In other words, more than a year's growth in 1 year of time will be needed to make this happen. The older the child and the greater the delay, the more urgent it is to identify causes. This is not an easy task and may require adjustments in the child's educational situation/placement, amount and type of other therapies, parental knowledge, audiology and hearing technologies, and consideration of other disabilities. It is not an easy conversation to have with families, but the sooner an identification of potential barriers to progress is made, the better. McConkey-Robbins (2005) used the term *red flags* to signal an issue with progress in children who use cochlear implants and do not meet expectations for growth in spoken language.

Brain Functions of Audition

Audition is the foundation of speech, language, and literacy. Communication begins from the simple, yet critical ability to detect and access the spoken word through audition and use the different auditory processes of the brain. These processes take sound and allow us to make it linguistically meaningful through discriminating certain sounds as unique from other sounds, remembering and identifying them, and comprehending and retrieving the words. Thus, given access to sound and spoken language, our brain is wired and ready with the functions and processes to develop speech and language.

As discussed in Chapter 1 on speech acoustics, the professional will need to know a child's hearing levels with and without hearing technologies in the right and left ears for the frequencies across the speech spectrum. Only recent evaluations are useful. If the evaluation of a young child is more than 3 months old, a trip to the audiologist needs to be planned as soon as possible. Based on the child's hearing levels with hearing technology, we can gain a good idea (not a perfect one) of what and how the sounds of speech are detectable to that child. Does the family understand the audiogram in terms of what speech and environmental sounds are available to their child? It is very possible that this was explained to the family, but they may not have understood it at the time or remember the information at this time. There are several publicly available visuals of audiograms and simulations of levels of hearing loss that can bring this information home (see resources on the companion website).

Lack of auditory access results in limitation of the foundational materials required for the child with hearing loss to begin the process. Once children with hearing loss are appropriately fitted with technology, we can expect progress in the different skill areas needed for listening and spoken language development. The goal is to aggressively aim for full-time use of technology, which provides optimal auditory access (McConkey-Robbins, 2005).

The model often used for auditory abilities is based on Erber (1982) and the levels of auditory training: detection, discrimination, identification, and comprehension. Since that time, auditory learning, rather than training, is a more common way to think of the role of audition in habilitation. Mischook and Cole (1986) looked at Erber's model of auditory learning and proposed a new model in which the defined levels were developing and overlapping as they progressed, and that comprehension occurred at the center of the process of the development. The American Speech-Language-Hearing Association (ASHA) further defined auditory processes (Table 3–5) to look more closely at children's abilities or deficits

Table 3–5. Brain Functions for Listening and Spoken Language

Auditory Processes for Using Sound Meaningfully

Auditory Attention: Focusing one's selective attention on sound. Hearing becomes an active listening sense and a passive source of information. Advanced stages of attention include hearing at a distance, listening in the presence of background noise, and understanding over the telephone.

Auditory Memory: Remembering what one heard to perform cognitive functions in the working memory. Both short-term and long-term memory are needed to attach meaning to sound. Auditory memory span must also be developed in order to remember sequences of sounds for understanding words, phrases, sentences, and stories.

Auditory Discrimination: Judging two sounds as different: This is necessary so meaning can be assigned to each sound. It leads to the recognition of environmental sounds and the use of speech.

Auditory Integration: Experiencing sound in all activities; for sound to be useful, it must be associated, or integrated, with other sensory experiences.

Auditory Processes for Learning to Talk

Auditory Feedback: Hearing the sounds produced by one's own speech muscles when talking. Hearing is the sense through which normal-hearing infants learn to speak. It is also used to monitor and correct the pitch, loudness, vocal rhythm, and articulation as one speaks.

Auditory Processes for Learning Language

Auditory Recognition: Associating a sound with its referent; that is, the symbolic function of sound.

Auditory Sequencing: Remembering the order of sounds heard. We must learn to retain sounds in their correct order to understand the word, phrase, or sentence spoken.

Auditory Comprehension: Understanding the linguistic structures of the language; these include the semantic, syntactic, morphologic, and pragmatic aspects of the language.

Auditory Retrieval: Using words that are stored in our memory. With this skill, we can use spoken language to express our thoughts and use spontaneous, expressive communication.

Auditory Application: Applying all of the above auditory functions when using arbitrary symbols such as letters for reading and writing and numbers for mathematics. This allows for learning in school, at work, and in daily life.

Sources: ASHA (1996); Daniel et al. (1999). Used with permission.

(American Speech-Language-Hearing Association Task Force on Central Auditory Processing Consensus Development, 1996). The different skills develop from simple to more complex within each defined process. Therapy goals for the habilitation process, in this chapter and the intervention chapters, are organized in tables to follow these ASHA-defined processes and the Mischook and Cole's comprehension-focused model when looking more closely at the stages of the habilitation process.

Auditory Processing

There are several auditory processes or skill areas that the brain uses to understand and learn that sound is linguistically meaningful. The professional needs to be knowledgeable about how the brain is accessing, processing, and organizing incoming auditory signals and set goals for these different areas. Goals in the intervention chapters are organized based on the use of audition to use sound meaningfully for learning to speak and for developing language. See Table 3–5 for a description of the auditory processes that will be addressed in the intervention goals related to developing listening and spoken language.

Typical Development

Language

Language is a complex, learned behavior. It is critical that professionals are well versed in its development to set expectations that are realistic and focused on maintaining progress toward typical milestones. Better to habilitate than rehabilitate! Typical milestones for receptive and expressive skills in typical language development, morpheme development, and vocabulary milestones are summarized in Tables 3–6 to 3–8.

The initial auditory processes involve access to the information to allow us to use sound meaningfully through discriminating the sounds as unique from other sounds, remembering the sounds and identifying which sounds they are, and comprehending and retrieving the words. Relevant research in the field of speech perception in infants has revealed many elements that are linked to the emerging comprehension of language. Typically developing babies of 9 months have determined appropriate sound sequences that are and are not representative within words of their native language (Friederici & Wessels, 1993).

Typically developing infants show comprehension of first words by age 4 to 5 months after normal auditory exposure for that period of time, allowing the brain appropriate time to go through the needed steps to begin to respond to their name and understand other highly repeated words. All children will understand many words receptively before their first expressive word. Facilitating and monitoring comprehension will assist in knowing if the child is making progress and when it might be appropriate or inappropriate to expect the child to be progressing to the next stage of spoken language development.

Skill development in the areas of sound awareness and in phoneme, discourse, sentence, and word levels are outlined in progressive sequence steps from simpler to more complex in the Auditory Learning Guide by Simser (1993).

Table 3–6. Language Development Milestones

Receptive Language	Expressive Language
Birth	
Listens to sounds around them	Cries or coos for pleasure/pain/discomfort
Startles to loud sounds	Nonspeech sounds produced
0 to 3 months	
Responds to voices by turning toward them	Smiles when content
Is comforted by familiar voices	Coos when happy
	Differentiated crying when hungry or in discomfort
4 to 6 months	
Responds to tone of voice in words such as *no*	Vocalizations: beginning babbling with gestures
Enjoys music, singing, and voice variations	Enjoys playing with voice, generally on vowels
Interested in sounds in the environment	Indicates emotions with voice variations and crying
7 to 12 months	
Responds to name	Emergence of canonical and variegated babbling
Begins to understand familiar words and phrases	Gesturing and pointing are specific, along with babbling
Responds to requests such "where is your nose" and other body parts	First words produced with varied intonation and babbling to indicate meaning
	MLU 1.0
12 to 24 months	
Follows simple commands	Begins to produce intelligible single words
Points to known people and picks up known objects	Begins to create two-word utterances (e.g., "where doggie?")
Understand 50 to 75 common words and phrases (e.g., *mommy*, *milk*, *cookie*)	Expands language functions (e.g., questions, comments, negation)
Enjoys songs and rhymes	MLU 2.0 to 2.5
2 to 3 years	
Responds to two commands	Expansion of vocabulary is rapid and illustrates cognitive growth such as adjectives (e.g., *big*, *little*), possessives (e.g., *mine*, *yours*), and pronouns (e.g., *I*, *you*)
Receptive vocabulary grows to 200+ words	
Understands varied functions of language such as storytelling	
Understands opposites	Uses culturally based expressions (e.g., "wow")
	MLU 2.5 to 3.5

continues

Table 3–6. *continued*

Receptive Language	Expressive Language
3 to 4 years	
Understands question words easily (e.g., *who, what, where, when*)	Longer sentences of 4+ words
	Talks about experiences away from home
Vocabulary grows rapidly, needing fewer repetitions	Intelligible to all listeners
	MLU 3.5 to 4.5+
Understands complex verb tenses (e.g., infinitives, past progressive)	
4 to 5 years	
Comprehends complex directions	Uses irregular plurals
Memorizes songs and nursery rhymes	Uses complex prepositions and pronouns (e.g., *ours, their, until, anything*)
Understands reversible plurals (e.g., "The dog was chased by the cat")	Uses infinitives
5 to 6 years	
Understands indirect discourse	Can tell a word that rhymes with a given word
Understands "what is ___ made of"	
Follows directions with "ask" and "tell"	Uses present and future progressive verb forms
Understands reflexive pronouns and adverbs of time	Uses clauses (e.g., *as soon as, while, before, after*)
	Can tell the days of the week in order
6 to 8 years	
Knows which one in a set of words does not belong	Can summarize a story upon hearing it
	Gives multistep directions
Responds appropriately to compliments	Uses indefinite pronouns
Understands absurdities and jokes	Uses irregular comparatives

Sources: Wilkes (2001); Brown (1972); Bowen (1998).

Vocabulary

A word here about the importance of setting high expectations for children' vocabulary growth, both in number of words and a wide variety of semantic categories and monitoring as a measure of growth. These categories include nouns, verbs, adjectives, conjunctions, modifiers, interrogatives, stereotypic phrases, and so on. There are a number of both criterion-referenced and norm-referenced assessment instruments to assist professionals in gauging vocabulary growth in both number of words understood and expressed, but also in the variety of categories.

There is abundant research to support an association between a child's vocabulary and academic achievement and behavioral functioning by kindergarten. Keep in mind that receptive word knowledge typically exceeds spontaneous expression of words and that children will

Table 3–7. Mastery of Morphemes

Morpheme	Age for Mastery (in months)
Present progressive -ing	19 to 28
Preposition in	27 to 30
Preposition on	27 to 33
Regular plural –/s/, /z/, /ɪz/	27 to 33
Irregular past tense	25 to 46
Possessive 's 'z	26 to 40
Uncontractible copula Verb "to be"	28 to 46
Articles	28 to 46
Regular past tense -ed	26 to 48
Third-person regular, present-tense /s/, /z/, /ɪz/	28 to 50
Third-person irregular	28 to 50
Uncontractible auxiliary	29 to 48
Contractible copula	29 to 49
Contractible auxiliary	30 to 50

Sources: Bowen (1998); Wilkes (2001); Brown (1973); http://www.speechtherapyct.com/whats_new/Early%20Morphological%20Development.pdf

Table 3–8. Number of Receptive Words to Expect at Different Ages

Age in Years	Expected Receptive Words
1	6 to 50
1½	50 to 260
2	150 to 300
3	900 to 1,000
4	1,500 to 2,500
5	5,000 to 10,000

Source: https://www.stanfordchildrens.org/en/topic/default?id=age-appropriate-speech-and-language-milestones-90-P02170

vary in the rate of acquisition of vocabulary words. An ever-expanding vocabulary is to be expected and learned directly and indirectly. It is important that children listen to new words in conversations directed toward them, and equally important that they overhear vocabulary in conversations all around them. There are many strategies to promote vocabulary acquisition by the children themselves as it is not possible to teach every single word in a language such as English, which has the highest number of vocabulary words of any language in the world.

Specific goals and strategies for vocabulary development over time can be found in Chapters 6 through 11. It is important to note that with the Common Core State Standards (used in the public school system in the United States), there is an increased emphasis on acquiring academic vocabulary, as well as every day, basic vocabulary words. Beck et al. (2013) developed a framework to illustrate three tiers of vocabulary words specifically aimed at instruction for school-age children in content areas. Tier 1 words are commonly known words used by family and peers. Tier 2 words are high-frequency or high-utility words, also known as academic vocabulary. Professionals working with school-age children need to focus their vocabulary efforts on Tier 2 words to maximize success in reading comprehension, writing, and speaking. Tier 3 words are higher level in nature than Tier 2 but are subject and domain specific. Table 3–9 is an example of tiered vocabulary in teaching a unit about plants.

Since typically hearing children's first words are highly functional (e.g., foods,

Table 3–9. Tiers Framework of Vocabulary Acquisition

Tier	Relevant Information	Examples
One	Commonly known words used by family and peers Learned during activities of daily living	flower, seed, water, green, grow, plant
Two	Academic vocabulary High-frequency or high-utility words Not subject or domain specific Mature and connected to higher-level concepts	agree, compare, contrast, perform, required, emerge, admit, maintain
Three	Domain-specific words that are only used within a certain, limited area, such as science	pollination, filament, germination, photosynthesis, chlorophyll

actions, clothing, toys, places, family members' names), planning activities for the earliest stages of vocabulary development ought to focus on those words. Our goal is to follow the development of typically hearing peers, so we need to take advantage of our knowledge of that development. Plans for children at the prelinguistic stage would not focus unnaturally on words such as colors, numbers, and shapes.

Speech

Speech is another complex learned behavior with typical stages and sequences of development, including babble stages. Stages of children's vocalizations and sounds prior to spoken language are not random. The babbling stages that have been defined by researchers and analyzed to consider the necessary speech features for the stage are summarized in Table 3–10 for quick reference. These are predictable, specific stages that children move through and should be understood by professionals and caregivers. These stages can be monitored to see if the child is making progress in an appropriate sequence and time frame. Babbling development can be useful to help parents to know and listen for the next steps in speech development. The late onset of canonical babbling is a predictor of later speech and language disabilities, and infants with severe hearing impairment are at risk for not developing canonical babbling (Eiler & Oller, 1993; Oller et al., 1999).

Spoken languages consist of rapid consonant-to-vowel transitions, which are essential for typical speech development and for the required automaticity to communicate naturally with spoken words. Early language learners will understand several words before they speak their first one. Young language learners use their speech system and develop control of their suprasegmentals and vowels in vocal play and babbling stages. Control of the suprasegmental aspects of speech allows for mastery of control and appropriate use of the respiration, phonation, resonation, and articulation systems that are physiologically responsible for the production of speech. The control of the

Table 3–10. Babble Skills Typically Evidenced at the Prelinguistic Stage

Stage	Age Emergence	Description/Features
Quasi-resonant sounds, reflexive vocalizations	0 to 3 months	• Infant has mouth partially open and produces an utterance
"Gooing," "cooing"	2 to 5 months	• Lots of back articulations • Crying is very tense and usually nonspeechlike at this age
Fully resonant sounds	4 to 8 months	• Uses full resonant sounds with mouth wide open • Will add raspberries, squeals, growling, yells • Practices and plays with the suprasegmentals • Sounds like singing when happy (/ɑ/) • Some marginal babbling (i.e., alternation of full opening and closure of vocal tract) starts at end of this stage

Reduplicated babbling/canonical babble	6 to 10 months	• Canonical stage: beginning of reduplicated babbling
		• Canonized
		  ○ CV, VC (Consonant, Vowel)
		  ○ full resonant nucleus
		  ○ consonant
		  ○ rapid and unbroken
		• Child combines their vowels with other sounds they can make with other articulators; e.g., /bababa/ (C-V-C-V-C-V)
		• Children with hearing loss often stop here—need to get them to go beyond this stage or to begin babbling again if stopped completely

Variegated babbling/canonical babble	9 to 12 months	• More like gibberish or jargoning • Using syllables and nonsyllables that sound like stress categories in long trains

Source: Oller et al. (1999).

suprasegmentals within the speech allows for the production of intelligible speech. Emergence of consonants is usually evidenced in babbling.

Babies appear to use speech sounds mastered in babbling preferentially within their early meaningful speech. Limited babbling might be characteristic of poor access across all the frequencies or might be specific to some frequency bands, although some have noted a period when babbling decreases or stops prior to true speech production. Professionals who provide intervention for infants who are deaf and hard of hearing must encourage and promote canonical babbling to promote mastery of sounds. Social and vocal reinforcement increases the quantity of the babbling but not the consonants used.

There are universal tendencies for infants and young children in that certain sound classes need to be mastered before other sounds can expect to be produced and mastered. The babbling stages and vocal play allow for the mastery of these systems to produce controlled and varied vocalizations with suprasegmentals and segmental speech features. The child with hearing loss will initially use limited vocalizations with typically just one or two neutral mid-frequency vowels. They will learn to control the intensity of their voice and produce extremes of loud or very quiet sounds. Initially pitch will be limited and a reflection primarily of their psychological state or feelings, where high-pitch sounds are indicative of the child feeling tense and low-pitch sounds are indicative of relaxed or content demeanor.

Additional vowels, diphthongs, and the initial consonants /b/, /m/, /p/, /h/, /n/, and /w/ will emerge as the child begins to increase vocalizations. Some of these vocalizations will be directed at others in a communicative intent or to initiate an interaction. Suprasegmental aspects of speech emerge and become controlled with the development of more segmental speech features. Vocal play allows for durational control, which will be demonstrated by longer vocal productions, and the control of intensity and pitch will be evident in the use of a sing-song-y voice. Progression of duration control will also be evidenced by two syllables and then longer strings of babbling. Vowels are expected to be developed by the age of 3. Children continue to develop in their intelligibility past the age of 47 months, and phonemes emerge until the age of 8 and some beyond (Hustad et al., 2020). The developmental sequence of consonant mastery is indicated in Table 3–11. The age indicated is when the phoneme is customarily produced by 90% of children.

Table 3–11. Sequence of Development of Consonants in Children

Age	Consonants Showing Mastery
3	/p/, /m/, /h/, /n/, /w/
4	/b/, /g/, /k/, /d/, /f/, /j/
6	/t/, /ŋ/, /r/, /l/
7	/tʃ/, /ʃ/, /θ/, /dʒ/
8	/s/, /z/, /ð/, /v/, /ʒ/

Source: Templin (1957).

Theory of Mind

What is Theory of Mind and how can it be used in therapy sessions to promote positive socialization skills for children with hearing loss?

Parents of children with hearing loss often have similar goals: that their child will be included in general education, be successful academically, and make and sustain friendships with peers and family members. Theory of Mind (ToM) is the ability of a person to empathize and put oneself in the mind of another. ToM starts and is evident to some degree in children as young as 1 year in a typically developing child (Peterson et al., 2012). The child begins to understand that people can have thoughts, preferences, and emotional reactions that differ from those in their own minds. Research in this area has been tied directly to language development in children with hearing loss (Courtin & Melot, 2005). It is an important component in the child achieving goals listed earlier, specifically socialization and developing authentic friendships (Paffhouse, 2018).

Many children with hearing loss who are integrated into general education settings report difficulties in making friends and relationships with hearing peers (Bat-Chava et al., 2005). When integrating ToM into therapy sessions, it will be important for children who are deaf or hard of hearing to think about how their behavior might impact others and how to deal with their own emotions, thus promoting successful social interactions. Help the child to think about how other children might feel in given situations. Ask the child with hearing loss open-ended questions, even as young as preschool age, about typical social situations, particularly those related to peers, and have them think about what the other child is thinking and feeling. An example would be, "If you are always first in line, how would that make your friends feel?" For children who have difficulty putting themselves in the mind of another, ask how they would feel if a friend was always first in line or always won every board game. To promote ToM, use questions that begin with "What would happen if . . . " or "If you feel this way, how could you show it?"

The sequence of development of these important early skills is summarized in Table 3–12.

Table 3–12. Theory of Mind Developmental Timeline

2 to 3 Years	3 to 4 Years	4 to 5 Years
• Announces intentions • Uses language to express own preferences (e.g., like/don't like) • Uses words to express emotion • Begins using state of mind vocabulary (e.g., *mad*, *scared*, *sad*) • Attempts to control situations verbally • Begins to understand the distinction between thinking and knowing • Begins to tell about a past event • Imaginatively role-plays with peers	• Engages in longer conversations (four to five turns) • Explains how they know something by using *because* • Uses polite language (e.g., please, thank you) • Increases perspective taking in role-play • Assumes the role of another person in play • Has long, detailed conversations • Uses variety of thinking words in conversation (e.g., *think*, *know*, *forgot*, *wonder*, *remember*) when talking about others • Retells a short sequence of past events to a listener	• Can understand that others can make decisions on what they believe to be true and not what is visually apparent (i.e., false belief) • Attends to understanding of conversation partner (e.g., adjusts information, asks questions, offers clarification) • Explains how they know the perspectives of others • Develops sense of humor • Understands and tells jokes or riddles

Sources: Walker et al. (2017); Hearing First website.

Self-Advocacy

Another area of importance to emphasize with parents is the development of self-advocacy skills in their child with hearing loss. It is considered one area within the overall domain of self-determination. Self-advocacy is the ability of a child to actively promote and communicate one's own self-interest and needs to others in a specific and positive manner. An example would be asking a teacher for preferential seating or requesting that family members not cover their mouths when speaking. In self-determination, a child reflects on, is aware of, and takes responsibility for their own choices, such as reflecting on why they chose to stay up late at night texting friends and the consequences (Anderson & Arnoldi, 2011; English, 2012).

There are numerous resources that have been developed by professionals in the listening and spoken language field, providing us with a wealth of information on assessment, goal setting, and progress monitoring of individual skills, organized by developmental levels. These skills support children, particularly those included in general education, with the tools to be successful and happy at home and at school with their parents, teachers, family members, and peers. It is often thought that children only need these skills when they transition to college or careers. However, it is best to begin developing them as young as possible for practice and integration into daily life (Anderson, K., 2021).

Once a professional and parents assess the child's self-advocacy skills and after goals are chosen, the goals can be interwoven into activities of daily living. Encourage parents to allow even preschool-age children to make their own choices, to learn to care for their own hearing technology, to problem solve when communication difficulties arise, and to learn the importance of using captions on television. Within therapy sessions, role playing can provide practice for children with skills such as asking for help from a relative or ordering food at a restaurant. Use auditory closure strategies by starting a sentence stem such as "When I can't understand someone, I can . . . "

Higher-Order Thinking

Higher-order thinking involves problem-solving skills, complex judgments, creating, and innovating. How can higher-order thinking abilities be incorporated into the session? When learning about the family's daily life and cultural heritage, it is important to plan activities that parents and family members can easily incorporate into conversations and items that exist in the child's home. For example, if we learn that a family possesses certain books, toys, games, foods, clothing, and household items, the intervention team would model how to create challenging activities applicable using the family's real possessions.

Holt's research (2019) found that a family's contribution to a child's growth in various cognitive areas is significant. We can be hopeful that by providing families with the tools the child needs to develop at a rate similar to hearing peers, much of the delays can be reduced or eliminated entirely.

It is suggested that professionals assess cognitive skills and include higher-order thinking activities during intervention and within developmental norms. Suggestions for activities are aligned here with the updated Bloom Cognitive Domain Taxonomy (Anderson & Krathwohl, 2001). In this way, a variety of outcomes can be expected via more and more complex questions.

Applications of the Bloom taxonomy are provided in Table 3–13 to assist in transitioning from the theoretical to applications. The table reads from the bottom up. Easier cognitive tasks are at the bottom, the foundation skills for the next levels. Initial levels are remembering and understanding, while the more challenging cognitive tasks such as evaluating and creating are at the top. The verbs on the left-hand side of the table can assist in goal writing and lesson planning. These verbs are observable and measurable, aligning them with the taxonomy level as well as the questions and activities that you would pose to promote higher-order thinking.

Summary

This chapter provides professionals with some resources to design complete and well-developed short- and longer-term goals for children with hearing loss in a variety of domains (e.g., speech, audition, language, cognition). These tables can also assist in planning lessons (e.g., learning outcomes, materials, questions, sequence of activities, auditory foundations) for individual children who are at various levels of performance. The intervention chapters will illustrate these levels of performance in even more detail so that for each individual child on your caseload, you will be able to place children, design the scope and sequence of your instruction, and meet the levels of expectation for growth over time.

Discussion Questions:

1. For the case studies that follow, determine the child's stage of habilitation. Are there any concerns or red flags?
2. Develop goals for audition, language, speech, and cognition using the developmental tables provided in this chapter.

Cases

Case 1

History: Rosa is 3 years 8 months old. She passed her newborn hearing screening but her mother reported that Rosa did not respond to all sounds as an infant. At 1 year of age, she failed her hearing screening at her pediatrician's office, only had one word, and was showing physical and motor delays. Further audiological testing was recommended, and she underwent an auditory brainstem response (ABR), and was aided at 1 year 5 months in the left ear. She was implanted in the right ear at 2 years 7 months. Genetic testing was completed at the age of 3 years 6 months and indicated that she has Warsaw Breakage syndrome. She attends a preschool program for children with special needs, and receives support monthly from the DHH itinerant. The focus of the classroom has been to teach classroom routines and concepts such as colors, shapes, and numbers. Adults in the

Table 3–13. Cognitive and Higher-Order Thinking Activities for Therapy: Aligned With Bloom's Taxonomy Levels—Cognitive Domain

Sample Verbs	Questions	Sample Activities
Creating		
Assemble, categorize, collect, combine, compile, compose, condense, construct, create, design, develop, expand, generate, guide	How can we improve on ____? How would you organize ____?	Plan an upcoming birthday party. Design a gift for mom. Create your own, new pizza. Reorganize the kitchen. Make up a song about numbers.
Evaluating		
Argue, assess, champion, compare and contrast, conclude, critique, debate, decide, deduce, diagnose, evaluate, forecast, improve, judge, justify, measure, prioritize, prove, rank, rate, recommend, resolve, revise, score, select, solve, support, value, verify, weigh	What's a better solution to a problem? In what ways are these items the same and different? Can you put these items in order (most important to least)?	In the event of an earthquake, what is the order of things to do? What should happen to Goldilocks for breaking and entering? Prove that *Star Wars* is the best movie of the year. Compare shapes and decide which one is the most attractive.
Analyzing		
Analyze, associate, break down, criticize, discriminate, dissect, distinguish, elect, establish, explain, inspect, question, refute, separate, simplify, subdivide, summarize, test	What is the difference between ____ and ____? Can you retell the story in your own words?	Provide problem scenarios such losing a cell phone and explain how to find it. Divide up a dozen cookies evenly among three friends. Establish a schedule of household chores for a week.
Applying		
Add, apply, calculate, change, complete, conduct, coordinate, demonstrate, direct, divide, formulate, generalize, infer, make, model, multiply, operate, perform, present, provide, schedule, show, subtract, use	Why did ____ do ____? What questions would you ask ____? How will you take care of your new pet? What would happen if ____? What's wrong here?	Tell adult how to make a peanut butter and jelly sandwich. Show pictures of a kitchen with zoo animals. Show what would happen if you don't tie the end of balloon after blowing it up. Describe an alternative ending to the *Three Little Pigs*.
Understanding		
Classify, confirm, contrast, differentiate, examine, express, generalize,	How are these things alike?	Make a list of everything that might be seen on a walk around the block.

Table 3–13. *continued*

Sample Verbs	Questions	Sample Activities
Understanding *continued*		
give examples, group, interpret, liken, order, paraphrase, predict, reorder, rephrase, rewrite, sort, specify, substitute	What does not belong here? Why not? What is an example of ____? What do you think will happen next?	Guess what is in mommy's purse. Look in the refrigerator and take out what does not belong (shoes).
Knowing/Remembering		
Define, describe, draw, duplicate, identify, label, list, locate, match, name, pick, recall, recognize, repeat, reproduce, sequence, underline	What happened? What do you see? What did you do? What does the ____ say? (animals) What is this called?	Recall what was eaten for breakfast. Label the parts of a plant. Sequence cards on how to carve a pumpkin. Draw a picture of something you like to do. Match new vocabulary words with definitions. Make a list of what is needed to make a pizza.

classroom use signs, gestures, physical prompts, and touches to elicit speech sounds. She is seen weekly by a private speech-language pathologist who focuses on eliciting speech sounds.

Auditory Detection, Attention, Discrimination: Responds consistently to three of the Ling six sounds (/m/, /u/, /ɑ/), inconsistently to /ʃ/ and /i/, and doesn't respond to /s/. Auditory abilities as assessed by the Infant-Toddler Meaningful Auditory Integration Scale (IT-MAIS) indicate the following auditory abilities: responding to her name in quiet, alerting to sounds in new environments, associating meaning to vocal tone, vocal behavior affected while wearing hearing technology, alerting to environmental sounds in the home, and discriminating between two speakers though hearing only. Other auditory skills developed include producing a nasal and a plosive, and discriminating a fricative. She comprehends five words with context provided and comprehends two stereotypic phrases. She will follow familiar simple commands with gestures and context.

Auditory Feedback: Rosa has difficulty discriminating suprasegmentals, and demonstrates some use of the suprasegmental aspects of speech. She uses some different durations (long and short) in productions. She is able to use a quiet voice. She will use some intonation and inflection in her productions. This was noted in particular when she was upset and her vocal tone was modified to reflect her mood. Rosa has limited vowels and consonants, which she will produce spontaneously. Her mother reports that most of these phonemes are inconsistent. Mother reports that Rosa only uses the vowels /o/ as in *know* and /ʌ/ as in *must*. In sessions there was some limited use of what seemed to an emerging production of /ɑ/ as in *of*. In addition to the limited variety and use of mostly neutral vowels, it was noted that there was a nasal/oral balance issue noted in words such as *noo*, which has been taught with exaggeration and visual input. Issues with nasal/oral balance were also noted in attempts to imitate other vowels modeled to her through audition only. Her mother and speech professional reported she most frequently and most consistently will produce: /b/ as in *bee*, /p/ as in *pea*, /d/ as in *do*, /g/ as in *go*, /m/ as in *my*, /n/ as in *no*, and /ʃ/ as in *she*. These sounds need to be elicited with a prompt or are inconsistently produced when imitating a known word. Only a few of these sounds were heard during the assessment sessions.

Auditory Comprehension and Auditory Retrieval: The Receptive-Expressive Emergent Language Test (REEL) assessment was administered, and results indicated an age equivalent of 15 months receptively and 14 months expressively. Mother reports that Rosa has about 10 word approximations that she will use spontaneously but they aren't intelligible to most people. When she produces them, they are mostly accurate by syllables and some but not all vowels. She will say approximations for: *hi, bye bye, mama, no, up, ouch, eat, milk,* and *down*.

Case 2

History: Jason is 2 years old and was identified at 2 weeks of age when he was seen for an ABR, which was not completed as he didn't fall asleep. At 4 weeks of age, testing was completed during natural sleep and indicated a symmetrical mild bilateral sensorineural hearing loss (SNHL). earmold impressions were taken and he was aided at 6 weeks of age. His parents and professional noticed and reported that his babbling diminished between the age of 6 and 7 months. He was producing more gruff, guttural sounds. Follow-up audiology testing was scheduled at age 8 months, which indicated a change in his hearing with responses slightly poorer in his left ear. At 14 months of age, audiological testing indicated a moderate hearing loss cookie bite configuration to severe in the mid-frequency ranges, slightly poorer in his left ear. He was fitted with new hearing aids. Jason's parents are choosing to raise him to use listening and spoken English. His family has been seen weekly for auditory-verbal therapy since he was 6 weeks of age.

Auditory Detection, Attention, Discrimination: LittlEARS (2004) indicates that he has all the auditory abilities attributed to a 2-year-old. Additional auditory abilities were assessed with his language assessment.

Auditory Feedback: As reported by his parents, Jason uses a variety of consonants spontaneously. The phonemes are of varying manners, voicing, and places of production. A phonologic evaluation noted errors with /l/ and /r/, /f/, /v/, /θ/ and /ð/. His speech is very intelligible to familiar and naïve listeners.

Auditory Comprehension and Auditory Retrieval: The REEL assessment was completed and shows Jason scoring at 36 months in receptive and expressive language. Jason has reached the ceiling on this assessment. This assessment shows above age level skills at this time and 19 months' growth in the past 12 months.

Jason's language skills were also assessed at this time using the Pre-School Language Scale (PLS) by Zimmerman et al. (2011). This evaluation assesses auditory comprehension and verbal ability of language and provides an age equivalent score compared to normal-hearing children. Jason's auditory comprehension score yielded an age equivalent of 3 years 3 months with a standard score of 123. Jason's expressive communication score yielded an age equivalent of 3 years 5 months and a standard score of 135. His total language score as assessed by this evaluation was 3 years 2 months with a standard score of 133. His standard scores of above 131 are associated with the description of "very superior."

His parents reported difficulty with the use of some pronouns; for example, he said "you," but really meant "me" or "I" and where he said "your" he meant "my." Language samples and parent reports were used to inventory his use of Brown's morphemes. Jason was consistent in his use of present progressive -ing, prepositions in and on, regular /s/ plural forms, irregular past tense, possessive form /s/, uncontractible copula articles, regular past-tense -ed endings, and uncontractible auxiliary. He was inconsistent but showed emerging abilities with his use of regular third-person singular present tense, irregular third person, contractible copula, and contractible auxiliary.

Some typical spontaneous sentences are:

> Put the batteries in there.
>
> Let's go upstairs and read books.
>
> Let's put them in.
>
> The library was closing.
>
> It's not working.

> The animals are sleeping.
>
> Put the blue cap on.
>
> Now it's working!
>
> Should we take the key?
>
> Look at this magazine.
>
> Mommy come too.
>
> Don't put that on there!
>
> We eat pizza.
>
> Going to the park right here.
>
> What should we talk about?
>
> Mommy sleep here in the corner.

Case 3

History: Calvin is 3 years 3 months old and was identified with a sloping mild to moderately severe bilateral hearing loss at birth through the newborn hearing screening. He received his hearing aids at 3 weeks of age and consistently wore them until 6 months of age. At 6 months, he began pulling his hearing aids out. He fought not to wear them by pulling them out or screaming and crying when parents attempted to insert them. His parents took him back to the audiologist, who reprogrammed the hearing aids, but he still refused to wear them. This continued until Calvin was 1 year old. At that time, his speech professional and early start professional suggested discontinuing use of the aids as he seemed to hear without them. Hearing aid use was discontinued at that time. Prior to attending preschool, he received weekly early intervention through the local school system, and private speech language therapy. He attends a local preschool with typically developing peers.

When Calvin was 3 years old, his parents were concerned about his limited ability to communicate and felt nobody could understand his speech. They reported that he was having trouble communicating in school with his peers. His parents met with an auditory-verbal professional for a second opinion. They were referred to another audiologist for a second opinion and earmolds were made so he could wear his hearing aids. His parents reported that Calvin continued to refuse to wear his hearing aids. At the insistence of the professional and as a requirement for enrolling in auditory-verbal therapy (AVT) services, Calvin was required to wear his hearing aids. His parents were able to get full-time hearing aid use within a month with the support of the AVT and his preschool classroom teacher.

Auditory Detection, Attention, Discrimination: Calvin responded to the Ling six sounds but was not able to consistently discriminate the sounds. He confused /i/, /s/, /ʃ/, /m/, and /u/. He showed some discrimination and identification for phonemes of nasal, semivowel, and plosive manners. He would inconsistently imitate a fricative by blowing.

Auditory Feedback: Calvin spoke in a very quiet voice with no use of intonation patterns. His parents report he has a variety of vowels but doesn't use /e/, /ɪ/, or /i/. The only consonants that he produces in his word approximations are /m/, /b/, /w/, and /n/.

Auditory Comprehension and Auditory Retrieval: Calvin's comprehension and expressive language skills were tested at the age of 3 years 3 months using the Clinical Evaluation of Language Fundamentals—Preschool version (CELF-P) (2020). The scores for the subtests administered are indicated in Table 3–14.

This assessment indicates that Calvin is scoring in the low average range with gaps in his language development as indicated by his error patterns for several subtests. In the sentence structure subtest, Calvin passed the first three items and then would randomly get items correct but didn't get five consecutive zero scores before reaching a ceiling on this subtest. His skills in expressive word structure development indicate gaps. He was able to pass the first five items, similar to his performance as explained for the sentence structure subtest.

Table 3–14. CELF-P Scores

Subtest	Scaled Score	Percentile	Age Equivalent
Sentence structure	10	50	3 y 5 m
Word structure	11	63	3 y 6 m
Expressive vocabulary	8	25	<3 y
Concepts and following directions	9	37	<3 y
Recalling sentences	9	37	<3 y
Basic concepts	13	84	4 y 3 m

Calvin shows areas of weakness in receptive skills in the following areas: number of critical items, adjectives, negatives, verbs, verb tense, subordinate clauses, and passive voice.

Calvin shows areas of weakness in expressive skills in the following areas: pronouns, plurals, present tense, present-tense progressive use of copula, regular and irregular past tense (*-ed* endings), verb-noun agreement, possessive forms, and derivational forms.

Calvin's scores are mostly in the average range, but his performance is indicative of gaps in his language development over time due to his limited auditory access as he was not using hearing aids. Overall, his performance indicates poor receptive and expressive abilities for the morphemes. His areas of deficit reflect his lack of auditory access and are particularly apparent in /s/ morphemic functions and speech perception errors that are interfering with development of present progressive verb tense, past tense *-ed* endings, irregular past tense, and pronouns. These test results are also reflected in his spontaneous language use. He would typically speak in two- to three-word utterances with no use of grammatical morphemes. He confused *I* and *you* in expressive sentences.

References

American Speech-Language-Hearing Association (1996). Central auditory processing: Current status of research and implications for clinical practice. *American Journal of Audiology, 5*(20), 41–52

Anderson, K., & Arnoldi, K. (2011). *Building skills for success in the fast-paced classroom: Optimizing achievement for students with hearing loss.* Butte Publications.

Anderson, K. L. (2021). *Success for kids with hearing loss.* http://successforkidswithhearingloss.com

Anderson, L. W., & Krathwohl, D. R. (2001). *A taxonomy for teaching, learning, and assessing: Vision of Bloom's taxonomy of educational objectives.* Longman.

Bat-Chava, Y., Martin, D., & Kosciw, J. G. (2005). Longitudinal improvements in communication and socialization of deaf children with cochlear implants and hearing aids: Evidence from parental reports. *Journal of Child Psychology and Psychiatry, 46*(12), 1287–1296.

Beck, I. L., McKeown, M. G., & Lucan, L. (2013). *Bringing words to life.* Guilford Press.

Bowen, C. (1998). *Ages and stages summary: Language development 0–5 years.* http://www.speech-language-therapy.com/

Brown, R. (1973). *A first language: The early stages.* George Allen & Unwin.

Cole, E. B., & Flexer, C. (2007). *Children with hearing loss: Developing listening and talking, birth to six.* Plural Publishing.

Courtin, C., & Melot, A. M. (2005). Metacognitive development of deaf children: Lessons from the appearance–reality and false belief tasks. *Developmental Science, 8*(1), 16–25.

Daniel, L., Daniloff, R., & Schuckers, G. (1999). A language rehabilitation program for children with cochlear implants. *Journal of Louisiana Applied Health Professionals, II,* 35–44.

Eiler, R. E., & Oller, D. K. (1993). Infant vocalizations and the early diagnosis of severe hearing impairment. *Journal of Pediatrics Training, 124*(2), 199–203. Alexander Graham Bell Association for the Deaf.

English, K. (2012). *Self-advocacy for students who are deaf or hard of hearing* (2nd ed.). University of Akron/NOAC.

Erber, N. P. (1982). *Auditory training.* Alexander Graham Bell Association for the Deaf.

Friederici, A. D., & Wessels, J. M. I. (1993). Phonotactic knowledge of word boundaries and its use in infant speech perception. *Perceptions and Psychophysics, 54,* 275–287.

Geers, A., Mitchell, C. M. Warner-Czyz, A., Wang, N. Y., & Eisenberg, L. S. (2017).

Early sign language exposure and cochlear implantation benefits. *Pediatrics, 140*, 1–11, https://pediatrics.aappublications.org/content/pediatrics/140/1/e20163489.full.pdf

Holt, R. F. (2019). Family environment contributions to children's neurocognitive development. *Volta Review, 119*(1), 98–114.

Hustad, K. C., Mahr, T., Natzke, P. E., & Rathouz, P. J.. (2020). Development of speech intelligibility between 30 and 47 months in typically developing children: A cross-sectional study of growth. *Journal of Speech, Language, and Hearing Research, 63*, 1675–1687.

Ling, D. (2003). The Ling Six-Sound Test. *The Listener*, 52–53.

Macaulay, C. E., & Ford, R. M. (2013). Family influences on the cognitive development of profoundly deaf children: Exploring the effects of socioeconomic status and siblings. *Journal of Deaf Studies and Deaf Education, 18*(4), 544–563.

McConkey-Robbins, A. (2005). Clinical red flags for slow progress in children with cochlear implants. *Loud and Clear, 1*, 1–8.

Mischook, M., & Cole, E. (1986). Auditory learning and teaching of hearing-impaired infants. *Volta Review, 88*(5), 67–81.

Oller, D. K., Eiler, R. E., Neal, A. R., & Schwartz, H. K. (1999). Precursors to speech in infancy: the prediction of speech and language disorders. *Journal of Communication Disorders, 32*(4), 223–245.

Paffhouse, K. (2018). This handout provides tips for supporting a child's development of Theory of Mind. *Hearing First*. https://www.hearingfirst.org/m/resources/456

Peterson, C. C., Wellman, H. M., & Slaughter, V. (2012). The mind behind the message: Advancing theory-of-mind scales for typically developing children, and those with deafness, autism, or Asperger's syndrome. *Child Development, 83*(2), 469–485.

Rotfleisch, S., & Martindale, M. (2012). How do you know if a child is making appropriate progress in auditory-verbal therapy and education? In W. Estabrooks (Ed.), *101 frequently asked questions about auditory-verbal practice*, (pp. 348–352). Alexander Graham Bell Association for the Deaf.

Simser, J. I. (1993). Auditory-verbal intervention: Infants and toddlers. *Volta Review, 95*(3), 217–229.

Templin, M. (1957). *Certain language skills in children: Their development and interrelationships*. University of Minnesota Press.

Tomblin, J., Barker, B., Spencer, L., Zhang, X., & Gantz, B. (2005). The effect of age at cochlear implant stimulation on expressive language growth in infants and toddlers. *Journal of Speech, Language, and Hearing Research, 48*, 853–867.

Vaughan, P. (1976). *Learning to listen: A book by mothers for mothers of hearing-impaired children*. General Mills Publishing.

Walker, E. A., Ambrose, S. E., Oleson, J., & Moeller, M. P. (2017). False belief development in children who are hard of hearing compared with peers with normal hearing. *Journal of Speech, Language, and Hearing Research, 60*, 3487–3506.

Wiig, E., Secord, W., & Semel, E. (2020). *Clinical Evaluation of Language Fundamentals—Preschool* (3rd ed.). NCS Pearson.

Wilkes, E. (2001). *Cottage acquisition scales for listening, language, and speech*. Sunshine Cottage School for Deaf Children.

Zimmerman, I. L., Steiner, V. G., & Pond, R. E. (2011). *Preschool Language Scales* (4th ed.). Pearson.

Chapter 4

Assessment of English Language, Speech, and Listening

Maura Martindale

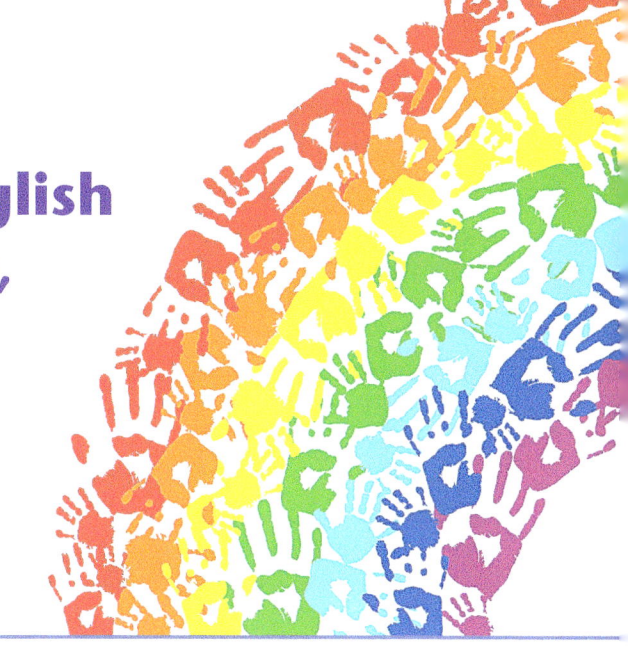

Key Points

- Assessment is essential for measuring and evaluating children's progress over time and for setting goals.
- Standardized instruments can provide data at a fixed point in time and can be used to compare the child with others in a sample population.
- Informal checklists and language sampling can augment and triangulate standardized tests, allowing for ongoing assessment and multiple sources of data.
- Assessments of morphological and pragmatic development allow for a broad picture of a child's progress in overall language development.
- Each stage of the proposed model contains tables and case studies with skills and evidence by a child at that stage and can be used as a checklist.
- Goal setting can occur when assessments are completed and the data is analyzed.
- A report of the data and an evaluation will be presented to the parents as well as other members of the child's team.

There are a number of terms frequently used in a discussion of assessments.

Terms and Definitions

- Assessment: Any procedure (formal or informal) used to obtain information about student performance.
- Measurement: A process of assigning numbers to individuals or their characteristics according to specified rules. This quantifies the value judgment.
- Tests or test instruments: A particular type of assessment. It generally fits this description:
  - Consists of a set of questions
  - Administered during a fixed time period (e.g., 1 hour)
  - Given under reasonably comparable conditions for all children
- Evaluation: The decision-making process that is ongoing and based on the information gained from assessments

of student learning (Linn & Gronlund, 2000).
- Mean Length of Utterance (MLU): The average number of morphemes calculated from 100 utterances in a language sample (Singleton & Shulman, 2014).

Regular assessments and evaluations are essential to identify children's strengths and weaknesses, and to document progress over time. The process is diagnostic as well as formative and summative. This chapter will focus exclusively on the assessment of spoken language, speech, and listening as it relates to the proposed model. Other domains such as overall child development are well explained and detailed in other texts.

General Tips for Assessment of Children

Here are some general tips to consider when thinking about conducting assessments:

- Reach out to other members of the child's team to decide which professional will administer which instruments and when. Avoid overtesting, or repeated administrations of the same assessments over a narrow time period, by different professionals. Results might lack reliability or validity. Reaching out provides a good opportunity for collaborative decision making.
- Choose your instruments/tests carefully. Read the manual to be certain that this instrument will yield the most essential information for parents and professionals in any given domain and at specific stages of growth.
- Be aware of the age range that the instrument is intended for, particularly for formal, standardized, and norm-referenced instruments.
- Allow parents to observe. Discuss what their role will be in the process ahead of time. Parents sometimes want to help their child by inadvertently saying, for example, which picture to point to. Strategic seating can help.
- Parents sometimes want to know the words or phrases or sounds on the assessment ahead of time to teach these to their child. Explain that the results need to be a legitimate reflection of their child's growth. Preteaching will skew these results.
- Gain informed parental consent in writing prior to assessing a child (typically required in many school programs and clinical settings).
- Find out at the time of assessment if the child is hungry, thirsty, tired, sick, hurt, upset, or needs to use a restroom. Any one of these may impact the validity and reliability of the results. Reschedule if necessary.
- Check hearing technology prior to assessments so that the child's responses are more likely to reflect their best efforts and auditory access to spoken language.
- Make sure that you have enough time, per the manual, to complete the instrument as recommended and/or required. The manual should indicate if breaks are permitted.
- Have forms and materials prepared ahead of time. Follow the protocol as described. If possible, practice administration of assessment on an adult or child not in therapy to develop an easy flow.
- Be careful of your own facial expressions and gestures, such as nodding or shaking your head after a response is given. For encouragement, simply use

phrases such as, "You are working hard on this. Thank you."

- In reviewing the results with parents, focus on strengths as well as areas that you will work on together. As you read in Chapter 2, on hearing the testing results, you may bring up stressful feelings and anxiety for the parents, particularly if the evaluation as a whole or in part shows less than age-appropriate outcomes. Practice ENUF (Empathizing, Nonjudgmental, Unconditional, Feeling focused)!

Assessment and evaluations should be ongoing, not a one-and-done experience. Professionals should consider administering a variety of assessment types throughout the year, including standardized instruments, informal checklists, lists of skills, and hierarchies, as well as informal data collection, such as language samples, checklists, and observations. This allows for triangulation of the data collected, or multiple sources of data, to provide the broadest picture of the child's level of functioning and language acquisition style. Informal assessments are often conducted best when initially working with the family. This allows time for you and the child to get to know one another, and for the child to become comfortable and trusting of you, before bringing out the standardized instruments. This is also the case with infants and toddlers for whom more informal assessments are best.

Formal, Standardized Tests for Assessment

More discussion about standardized tests is needed. Many advantages include relative ease of administration and scoring, and the ability to administer them quickly. There are hundreds of them available, in English, for purchase and it can be difficult to choose which ones to invest in for children with hearing loss. There are lists and lists of tests for language, speech, and listening that fill numerous catalogs. New ones often come on the market as well. In the end, there is no perfect test that meets all needs or stages of learning.

Many companies of commercially produced tests change editions throughout the years, adding new features, calculating new norms to include diverse populations, and extending age ranges. Many are very expensive. It is not always possible for schools, programs, and professionals to purchase them all. In addition, many professionals have limited access to or funding for upgrades to purchase new editions on a regular basis. If the protocols call for face-to-face individualized administration, professionals who are using remote learning for therapy may not be able to follow the instructions in the manual with fidelity, thus the scores are in question. For these reasons, it is wise to have a team approach to assessments, allowing for as much useful data as possible from a variety of sources.

For children with hearing loss, these tests can be useful in noting specific deficits at a given moment in time, and in relation to typically hearing peers. The normed populations of tools for typically hearing children do not usually have norms for children with hearing loss. The manuals usually limit how often any test can be administered over the course of a year or years. Photos or pictures used in older instrument editions may become so dated over the years that the illustration is completely unknown to today's children (e.g., rotary phones versus cell phones). The pictures may reflect items from middle-class homes, and the child's family may not have the item in question or be able to afford it, or it may not be part of their cultural heritage. This is something to keep in mind when choosing formal instruments.

A good resource to learn more about published, formal assessment instruments in English, covering a wide range of domains, can be found in the Mental Measurement Yearbook, published every 3 years by the Buros Center for Testing at the University of Nebraska—Lincoln (Carson et al., 2021).

Checklists, Observations, and Questionnaires

There are a number of checklists and auditory questionnaires that have been developed specifically for children with hearing loss and that can assist parents and professionals in assessing a child's auditory behaviors at home and school settings. They are readily available via the internet and inexpensive, thus eliminating costly purchases of curriculum materials. Checklists are typically arranged hierarchically, listing skills that are progressively more difficult, allowing parents and professionals to choose goals. Their disadvantage is that the professional and parents will need to craft goals and activities to focus on needed skills. A few of them are:

> https://teachertoolstakeout.com/0299-checklists (Stredler-Brown & DeConde, 2001, 2003).
>
> https://successforkidswithhearingloss.com/for-professionals/listening-inventory-for-education-revised-life-r/ (Anderson et al., 1998).
>
> PEACH+: Parent's Evaluation of Aural/Oral Performance of Children and Ease of Listening (Ching & Hill, 2005).

Brain Functions for Listening and Spoken Language

Assessing auditory brain functions for listening and spoken language will be comprised of ongoing diagnostics of three specific areas (Daniel et al., 1999). These are: auditory processes for using sound meaningfully, auditory processes for learning to talk, and auditory processes for learning language (see Chapters 6–11 for goals associated with each area). Within each area, the professional and parents need to note what the child can do by seeking answers to questions. Does the child demonstrate:

- Auditory attention: Is the child selecting focused attention to sound?
- Auditory memory: Is the child recalling the sequence of sounds, words, and phrases?
- Auditory discrimination: Is the child able to tell one sound from another, which will lead to auditory recognition?
- Auditory integration: Is the child able to integrate sound into all activities?
- Auditory feedback: Is the child able to listen to their own speech sounds while talking?
- Auditory recognition: Is the child able to associate a sound with a symbolic function of the sound? Do they recognize a series of sounds with meaning?
- Auditory sequencing: Is the child able to retain sounds in their correct order (e.g., words, phrases, sentences)?
- Auditory comprehension: Is the child able to understand the linguistic structures of a language?
- Auditory retrieval: Is the child able to use words stored in their memory?
- Can the child express thoughts and use spoken language for spontaneous, expressive communication?

- Auditory application: Is the child able to apply all these functions for use in learning literacy or other content areas?

The case studies at the end of Chapters 6 to 11 will provide you with real-life examples of how these questions are answered for the children under discussion.

Assessing Spoken Language

Spoken Vocabulary/Semantics

There are many assessments that were developed strictly to assess receptive and/or expressive vocabulary, both formally (e.g., *Peabody Picture Vocabulary Test*, 2018) and informally. Other instruments have a subsection for assessing vocabulary as part of a test battery (e.g., *Test for Auditory Comprehension of Language*, 2017). However, for children at the prelinguistic and single-word stages, who understand and express up to about 250 words and some phrases, professionals and parents typically keep lists of words that are understood, imitated, and spontaneously expressed by the child (see Chapters 6 and 7). Receptive understanding usually precedes expressive language.

Beginning vocabulary words can be divided into categories and subcategories, such as:

nouns (e.g., animals, body parts, foods, drinks, clothing, toys);

places (e.g., grocery store, doctor's office, dentist, department store, relatives' homes);

verbs (e.g., run, walk, eat, sleep, sit, open);

location words (e.g., in, up, down);

folks at home (e.g., mommy, daddy, names of siblings, names of pets, grandparents);

vehicles (e.g., car, truck, airplane, helicopter);

animals (e.g., dog, cat, bird, horse);

pronouns (e.g., my, mine);

household items (e.g., spoon, cup, chair, bed);

adjectives (e.g., hot, cold, big, little); and

questions (e.g., who, what, where).

By keeping track of vocabulary in an organized manner, it will become clear which beginning vocabulary categories are emerging and which ones are not (Ling & Ling, 1977).

Children at these beginning stages also learn to understand and express phrases, which they may understand and/or express as a single word, such as "bye-bye," "night-night," "all gone," "sit down," "wanna," and "no more." Keeping a running tally of these emerging vocabulary words and phrases is another way to assess a child's progress over time and to keep a record for your reporting and planning. This is a road map to the word combinations stage. Many of the words and phrases, particularly those specific to home such as the names of pets, are often not found on formal assessments. Be aware that it is common for early vocabulary learners to engage in *overextensions*, using one word for an entire category of words, such as all animals are doggies (Rescorla, 1980). By acknowledging a child's actual emerging vocabulary words and phrases, we gain a more complete picture of how listening to and using spoken language is progressing and in what contexts. In addition, children at these early stages still need to learn about multiple meanings of a single word, such as "bark" like dog bark or bark of a tree, or "fly" like an airplane or insect (see Table 5–1). For additional lists of beginning words and phrases, see tables in Chapter 6.

Language Sampling

Some of the most useful, ongoing assessments that work well for this model are language samples (Nippold, 2021). In addition to formal, standardized instruments, a sample of the child's rich, real-world listening and spoken language abilities can be inexpensively obtained for analysis. Thus, we can triangulate data gathered from multiple sources and gather a vibrant view of spoken language development. If a child is receiving therapy via remote learning, language sampling allows for data gathering at any point in time and space.

Language sampling allows professionals to observe not only what is learned, but also how the child is acquiring language in day-to-day life. The data gathered from a language sample aligns well with activities of daily living (ADL), which form the foundation of the proposed model. The child is learning listening and spoken language during daily conversations and interactions with family and peers. Sampling in many settings beyond the therapy setting is recommended.

Another advantage of language sampling is that the sample itself can be gathered from sources other than the professionals. The child's listening and spoken language can be assessed within a number of contexts, such as playing with peers or siblings, specific school settings, and events such as birthday parties. The richest conversations with peers, siblings, and family members often reveal nuances and complexities that do not emerge in a therapy setting. One of the disadvantages of listening to conversations gathered on audio in homes is the possible addition of background noises (e.g., dogs barking, babies crying, appliances running). It can make it difficult to make out small but salient aspects of the interactions such as morphemes.

Language samples that are gathered from parents of children for whom a home language differs from the spoken English of school and therapy can provide valuable insights into the child's transition to English, while maintaining their home language. Is there evidence of code switching in the sample? Is there evidence of code mixing or using two languages within one utterance (Poplack, 1980)? In other words, does the sample contain two expressive languages? This is not considered error, but rather typical of those who are becoming bilingual. It is not the intent to provide a deep discussion of bilingualism here, but to make sure the language samples are viewed within a cultural context and in line with the parents' goals (Poplack, 1980).

The therapy setting sample should not be discounted; however, there are constraints of time and space, particularly for those professionals who are teaching in school settings. Professionals will need to elicit various forms of language usage during therapy with carefully crafted conversations, such as storytelling or retelling a story, giving directions from the house to the store, playing board games, explaining how to make a sandwich, or beginning pretend play scenarios. High-quality audio recordings are recommended so that the conversation flow is not interrupted with note taking. Playback, when you have time to transcribe what was said and the context, is the next important step. A team of listeners can be helpful when the sample is lengthy.

The analysis of a language sample can seem daunting. Initially, as professionals, we may need to refresh ourselves on parts of English speech and syntactic structures prior to analysis, such as recalling the various types of clauses. There are computer software programs that can support your analysis, such as *SALT (Systematic Analysis of Language Transcripts)* (2003), with free downloads available. Nevertheless, a program such as this may not be available to individual professionals, schools, centers, or university preparation programs. *Language sampling with children and adolescents: Implications for intervention* (Nippold, 2021) is an excellent resource that provides the reader with examples and exercises to recall the complexity of the English language that you learned earlier in your education.

There are tools developed specifically to assist professionals who are gathering and analyzing language samples from children with hearing loss. The forms, videos, materials, and manuals that accompany these tools can assist professionals in identifying strengths and areas of need by noting syntactic structures' emergence and use. Three of them, which are relatively inexpensive, are:

- Moog and Kozak-Robinson. (1983). *CID teacher assessment of grammatical structures.* Central Institute for the Deaf.
- Moog and Biedenstein. (1998). *Teacher assessment of spoken language.* The Moog Center for Deaf Education.
- Wilkes, E. M. (2001). *Cottage acquisition scales for listening, language, and speech (CASLLS)* (2nd ed.). Sunshine Cottage School for Deaf Children.

After you have transcribed the sample, word for word, you can note on one of the forms which structures are present consistently, which are used inconsistently, and which structures are missing or used in error. Because the syntactic structures are hierarchical, such as the acquisition of verb tenses, the professional can use the list of structures to choose goals in spoken language based on the child's needs. It must be acknowledged that this is time consuming, particularly the very first analysis of a child who is new to you. This time needs to be weighed against the wasted years on goals that are cut/pasted from web-based or computer program goal banks. Those goals might fit nicely into educational plans, but might not move the child toward advanced spoken language acquisition commensurate with typically hearing peers.

Are you comfortable with the parts of speech delineated on the assessment forms noted earlier? It is acceptable to admit that you do not really remember present progressive versus past progressive. Take time prior to administering assessments and engaging families in therapy sessions to reacquaint yourself with these structures. Precision is important, and we want families and other professionals to focus on what will achieve the child's goals.

Mean Length of Utterance (MLU)

One of the useful calculations that come from the analysis of a language sample is the calculation of the child's MLU, which is the average use of words and/or morphemes in the sample. This measure can be calculated for children at any age, although for older children, we want to elicit their very highest degree of complexity with cognitively challenging contexts. There are both free and bound morphemes. A free morpheme has meaning on its own, such as *dog, car, run, jump, over,* and *big*. A bound morpheme does not have meaning independently and must be connected to a free morpheme, such as *pre, -un, -ing, -es, -est,* and *-ed* (Singleton & Shulman, 2014). The calculation is made by dividing the number of morphemes by the number of utterances, and the number of words by the number of utterances. Calculating both allows for the professional and parents to track progress over time and target structural errors (Miller & Chapman, 1981). As the child moves toward becoming a competent communicator, a higher and more complex MLU is anticipated.

Calculation of morphemes is important to measure and document the child's flexibility with newly acquired vocabulary, such as adding morphological structures at the ends of a regular verb to indicate tense (e.g., *walked, walking,* or *walks*). When morphemes are acoustically located primarily in the high frequencies, such as in *walk**ed*** and *walk**s***, the child with hearing loss with limited or no high-frequency access may experience delays in morphological development compared with typically hearing peers. This is where *acoustic highlighting* can be helpful for the child as well as assuring adequate access to high frequencies (see Chapter 5).

Pragmatic Functions

Whether communicating with peers and other children, family members, teachers, and other adults in their environment, it is also important to assess a child's conversation skills. Professionals need to assess these skills in both quality and quantity of language exchanges with peers and adults. Conversational norms differ from culture to culture—another reason to be aware of a family's culturally acceptable and unacceptable conversation norms. For example, in one culture, maintaining eye contact while conversing is considered typical and even polite, while in another culture, it may be considered rude. Children need to learn how to adjust their conversational behaviors, depending upon their relationship to the other speaker (Ochs & Schieffelin, 1983). How a child talks to a peer (e.g., "I really want more ice cream") differs from how a child speaks to a teacher (e.g., "May I please have more ice cream?"), so this concept may need to be explicitly taught by professionals and parents.

An excellent checklist of pragmatic or conversation skills was developed for children who have hearing loss at the John Tracy Clinic (McGinnis, 2018) and can be found on the companion website for this book. The "serve and return" strategy within Chapter 5 describes how to incorporate pragmatic skill development within therapy sessions. There are overall questions to guide your assessment of a child's pragmatic or social conversational skills, such as does the child:

- Make age-appropriate greetings? Are the greetings acceptable for the time, place, and social relationship with conversation partners?
- Use natural gestures?
- Initiate a conversation?
- Ask and answer age-appropriate questions?
- Establish and maintain topics? Change topics appropriately?
- Take turns in the conversation? If so, how many exchanges?
- Respond to requests for clarification?
- Modify spoken language in line with time and place?
- Offer information or actions that contribute to the conversation?

- Close conversations using age-appropriate language?

Goals for pragmatic skills should be included in therapy plans, for therapy sessions, home, and school. They are generally taught implicitly; i.e., within a conversation. Role playing and positive behavior supports can contribute to the development of these skills. The professional-parent-child dialogues at the end of Chapters 6 to 11 provide examples of how to implicitly interweave pragmatic skills into a conversation.

Speech Assessment (Phonetic and Phonologic)

For children who are following in progression with typical speech development that is aligned with their typically hearing peers, professionals may discover that extensive sessions of speech therapy are not necessary. Regularly scheduled phonetic level (i.e., phonemes in isolation or in syllables) and phonologic level assessments (i.e., phonemes in words and phrases) of suprasegmentals (e.g., duration, intensity and pitch, rhythm, stress, intonation) and segmentals (e.g., vowels, diphthongs, consonants and consonant blends) are essential to ensure the child is progressing in speech production (see tables in Chapters 6–11). The goal of speech assessment is to measure the child's speech intelligibility, something to remind parents about.

For children who are remedial in speech acquisition, there are a number of tools to gain this information (Ling, 1976, 2002). The speech assessments developed specifically by Ling were designed for children who have hearing loss. Unlike those developed for typically hearing children who may have a speech impairment, the Ling tools assess suprasegmentals, vowels, and diphthongs in addition to consonants and consonant blends, in isolation, at the syllable level, and in running speech. It will be important to look beyond speech sounds in single words, via elicitation or imitation. This cannot be achieved by showing the child a single picture and asking for a single-word response. How are speech sounds articulated within a conversation? One way to save time is to audio record the child talking, thus collecting a language sample, and at the same time, transcribe the sample into the International Phonetic Alphabet (IPA).

Ongoing speech errors that occur regularly in running speech need attention, thus increasing intelligibility. For children who are older, late starters, or who have been identified with another disability, the seven stages of the Ling system (2003) provide an order for direct teaching of phonetic and phonologic skills that builds on previously acquired speech sounds.

How to Align Assessment Data With the Proposed Therapy Model

As you will see in the tables in Chapters 6 through 11, there are numerous lists of observable skills for language, speech, and listening, which can be used as informal assessments both by the professionals and the parents via observations. Under "Putting It All Together" in the chapters for each stage of the model, you will find a detailed case study, along with a running dialogue between adults and the child in question. For each case history, results of formal assessments and those skills that were observed from the tests are provided. This provides you with an idea as to which assessments fit best at each stage and which specific skills to assess. You will also find references of specific instruments in these chapters and on the many tables throughout the chapters. This is not an all-inclusive list, but it will provide some guidance for you.

Prelinguistic Stage

Auditory Abilities Evidenced in the Prelinguistic Stage (Table 6–1); *Language and Speech Skills Evidenced in the Prelinguistic Stage* (Table 6–2); Ling Six-Sound Test (2003); *LittlEARS* (2004); *Receptive-Expressive Emergent Language Scale* (REEL) (2003); *Integrated scales of development* (2010); ASHA milestones (1997–2021; https://www.asha.org/public/speech/development/chart/); *Infant-Toddler Meaningful Auditory Integration Scale* (IT-MAIS) (2001).

Single-Word Stage

Auditory Abilities Evidenced in the Single-Word Stage (Table 7–1); *Language and Speech Skills Evidenced in the Single-Word Stage* (Table 7–2); Ling Six-Sound Test (2003); *LittlEARS* (2004); *Receptive-Expressive Emergent Language Scale* (REEL) (2003); *Integrated scales of development* (2010); ASHA milestones (1997–2021; https://www.asha.org/public/speech/development/chart/); *Infant-Toddler Meaningful Auditory Integration Scale* (IT-MAIS) (2001).

Emerging Word Combinations Stage

Auditory Abilities Evidenced in the Emerging Word Combinations Stage (Table 8–1); *Language and Speech Skills Evidenced in the Emerging Word Combinations Stage* (Table 8–2); Ling Six-Sound Test (2003); MLU and language sampling; *Receptive-Expressive Emergent Language Scale* (REEL) (2003); *LittlEARS* (2004); *Preschool Language Scales* (2011).

Communication With Childlike Errors Stage

Auditory Abilities Evidenced in the Communication With Childlike Errors Stage (Table 9–1); *Language and Speech Skills Evidenced in the Communication With Childlike Errors Stage* (Table 9–2); Ling Six-Sound Test (2003); *Receptive-Expressive Emergent Language Scale* (REEL) (2003); *Test for Auditory Comprehension of Language* (TACL) (2011); *Test of Auditory Processing Skills-3* (2005); *Preschool Language Scales* (2011); *Peabody Picture Vocabulary Test* (2007); *Structured Photographic Expressive Language Test—Preschool 2* (2003); MLU and language sampling.

Competent Communicator Stage

Auditory Abilities Evidenced by a Child who Is a Competent Communicator (Table 10–1); *Language and Speech Skills Evidenced in the Competent Communicator Stage* (Table 10–2); Ling Six-Sound Test (2003); *Preschool Language Scales* (2011); *Test for Auditory Comprehension of Language* (TACL) (2011); *Clinical Evaluation of Language Fundamentals—P* (2020); *Compass test of auditory discrimination* (2021); MLU and language sampling; *Clinical Evaluation of Language Fundamentals—Preschool* (CELF) (2020); *Test of Auditory Processing Skills-3* (2005); *The child language data exchange system* (1984).

Advanced Communicator Stage

Auditory Abilities Evidenced in the Advanced Communicator Stage (Table 11–1); *Language and Speech Skills Evidenced in the Advanced Communicator Stage* (Table 11–2); Ling Six-Sound Test (2003); *Test of Auditory Processing Skills-3* (2005); *Clinical Evaluation of Language Fundamentals (2020); Test for Auditory Comprehension of Language* (TACL) (2011); MLU and language sampling; *The Test of Language Development—Primary* (2008).

The reader will note that at each of the stage assessments, the Ling Six-Sound Test (2003) is included. A deep discussion of this assessment of a child's detection of, and access to, all speech frequencies using this test can be found in Chapter 1, *Speech Acoustics*.

Reporting Your Findings

The next step after gathering and analyzing data from multiple sources is to report the child's current level of performance to parents and other members of the educational team in a clear summary of the outcomes. In addition to sharing scores, areas of strength, and areas of need, summarize the stage of spoken language, listening, and speech acquisition in terms that are understandable to everyone by using examples. Remember that not everyone knows what an embedded clause is or what constitutes a prepositional phrase. Providing examples can assist parents in understanding vocabulary that is often used in education. The assessment forms developed for children with hearing loss mentioned earlier provide examples for you on the forms themselves.

In a written report, use professional language and avoid describing your impression of the child's personality by avoiding using words such as *funny*, *happy*, or *cheerful*. The audiologist and/or the parents can provide you with a history related to age of identification of the hearing loss, hearing technologies, degree and type of loss, and details from hearing tests. Keep the focus on the child, not on yourself. Divide your report into sections and subsections for easy reference.

Goal Setting Based on Data Gathered and Analyzed

Determining each child's current level of performance is a required part of lesson/session planning, as well as needed for establishing longer-term goals. This is a major part of your therapy plans going forward as you choose strategies and activities most likely to meet the child's targeted goals. Goal selection for auditory learning and spoken language, including vocabulary growth, need to be detailed for maximum carryover from therapy to school, to peers, and to family life. If goals are set too low, the child may achieve them within a few weeks or months of the document, thus necessitating an addendum to include long- and short-term goals. If they are too cursory or too narrow, other professionals may not know what to focus on, wasting valuable time and efforts. Assume that other professionals and paraprofessionals, as well as parents, will be reading and using your goals as a touchstone for their planning as well. Explanation of the child's goals for other professionals who are unfamiliar with the language you use in describing your goals, at required meetings, will most likely be needed.

Each of the therapy-focused chapters (6 to 11) contain lists of potential goals in all relevant domains related to listening and spoken language. Potential goals are presented in each therapy chapter based on stages and presented in tables, for example:

Auditory goals for auditory attention, detection, discrimination, memory

Auditory goals for development of the speech production system

Auditory recognition, sequencing, and comprehension

Auditory retrieval and expressive communication

Using the tables, it is logical to move from one stage to another. For example, if the child can auditorily understand two-element directions, the next goal would logically be three-element directions (e.g., "go to the bathroom, wash your hands, and brush your teeth"). Include specific goals for vocabulary, receptive and expressive language, and speech (phonetic and phonologic), using typical development as a guide. Make certain all goals and objectives are written using measurable and observable verbs such as *write*, *spontaneously expressed in full sentences*, and *point to the correct item*, avoiding words such as *think* or *appreciate* that cannot be sensed except by the child demonstrating in some way that they can be seen, heard, or felt.

Summary

This chapter describes how both formal and informal data gathering will guide professionals and parents in monitoring a child's progress and movement over time toward becoming an advanced communicator, commensurate with abilities and across all environments. Assessment data from multiple sources triangulate the information, allowing for a more complete picture of the child's strengths and areas of need. Samples of assessments for each stage of the model were presented, with full knowledge that there are many other excellent tools that could be used as well. The intension of the chapter was not to present every tool currently available, but to provide examples, knowing full well that new editions and new tools will be developed and are continually being developed in the years after the publication of this book chapter.

Discussion Questions

1. What are the advantages and disadvantages of standardized language assessments?
2. What are the advantages and disadvantages of language sampling?
3. Why would a professional want multiple sources of data from multiple assessments in a given domain?
4. What are the advantages and disadvantages of gathering a language sample from home or during therapy?
5. What are the advantages and disadvantages of using checklists and parent questionnaires to assess children's progress?

References

American Speech-Language-Hearing Association (1997–2021). *Developmental norms for speech and language.* https://www.asha.org/public/speech/development/chart/

American Speech-Language-Hearing Association Task Force on Central Auditory Processing Consensus Development (1996). Central auditory processing: Current status and implications for clinical practice. *Journal of Audiology, 5,* 41–52.

Anderson, K., Smaldino, J., & Spangler, C. (2011). *The Listening Inventories for Education—Revised.* http://successforkidswithhearingloss.com/wp-content/uploads/2011/09/LIFE-R-Instruction-Manual.pdf

Brown, V. L., Bzoch, D. R., & League, R. (2020). *Receptive-Expressive Emergent Language Test* (4th ed.). Western Psychological Services.

Carrow-Woolfolk, E. (1999). *Test for Auditory Comprehension of Language-3.* Western Psychological Services.

Carson, J. F., Geisinger, K. F., & Jonson, J. L. (2021). *Mental measurement yearbook.* University of Nebraska Press.

Ching, T. Y. C, & Hill, M. (2005). PEACH+: Parent's Evaluation of Aural/Oral Performance of Children and Ease of Listening. *Journal of the American Academy of Audiology, 18*(3), 220–235.

Cochlear Corporation. (2010). Integrated Scales of Development. In *Listen, learn, talk.* (pp. 16–31). Cochlear Limited.

Daniel, L., Daniloff, R., & Schuckers, G. (1999). A language rehabilitation program for children with cochlear implants. *Journal of Louisiana Applied Health Professionals, II,* 35–44.

Dawson, J., Stout, C., & Eyer, J. (2005). *SPELT-P 2, Structured Photographic Expressive Language Test—Preschool.* Janell Publishing.

Dunn, L., & Dunn, D. (2007). *Peabody Picture Vocabulary Test* (4th ed.). Pearson.

Hammill, D. D., & Newcomer, P. L. (2019). *Test of Language Development.* Western Psychological Services.

Ling, D. (1976, 2002). *Speech and the hearing-impaired child.* Alexander Graham Bell Association for the Deaf.

Ling, D. (2003). The Ling Six-Sound Test. *The Listener,* 52–53.

Ling, D., & Ling, A. (1977). *Basic vocabulary and language thesaurus for hearing-impaired children.* Alexander Graham Bell Association for the Deaf.

Linn, R. L., & Gronlund, N. E. (2000). *Measurement and assessment in teaching* (8th ed.). Prentice Hall.

Martin, N. A., & Brownell, R. (2005). *Test of Auditory Processing Skills* (3rd ed.). World Publishing.

McGinnis, M. (2018). *McGinnis Pragmatic Skills Checklist.* John Tracy Clinic.

McWinney, B., & Snow, C. (1984). *The child language data exchange system.* Carnegie Mellon.

Miller, J. F., & Chapman, R. S. (1981). The relation between age and mean length of utterance in morphemes. *Journal of Speech and Hearing Research, 24*(2), 154–161.

Miller, J. F., & Chapman, R. (2003). *SALT: Systemic Analysis of Language Transcripts.* [Computer software]. University of Wisconsin—Madison, Waisman Center, Language Analysis Lab.

Moog, J., & Kozak-Robinson, V. (1983). *CID Teacher Assessment of Grammatical Structures.* Central Institute for the Deaf.

Moog, J. S., & Biedenstein, J. (1998). *Teacher Assessment of Spoken Language.* The Moog Center for Deaf Education.

Nippold, M. A. (2021). *Language sampling with children and adolescents: Implications for intervention.* Plural Publishing.

Ochs, E., & Schieffelin, B. B. (1983). *Acquiring conversational competence.* Routledge & Kegan Paul.

Poplack, S. (1980). Sometimes I'll start a sentence in Spanish y termino en español: Toward a typology of code-switching. *Linguistics, 18,* 581–618.

Rescorla, L. A. (1980). Overextension in early language development. *Journal of Child Language, 7*(2), 321–335. 10.1017/S0305000900002658

Rossetti, L. M. (1990). *Rossetti Infant-Toddler Language Scale.* LinguiSystems.

Sindrey, D. (2021). *Compass Test of Auditory Discrimination.* Supporting Success for Children With Hearing Loss.

Singleton, N. C., & Shulman, B. B. (2014). *Language development: Foundations, processes and clinical applications* (2nd ed.). Jones & Bartlett Learning.

Stredler-Brown, A., & DeConde, C. (2001). *Functional auditory performance indicators.* Colorado Department of Education, Special Education Services Unit.

Tsiakpini, L., Weichbold, V., Kuehn-Inacker, H., Coninx, F., D'Haese, P., & Almadin, S. (2004). *LittlEARS Auditory Questionnaire*. Med-EL.

Wiig, E., Secord, W., & Semel, E. (2020). *Clinical Evaluation of Language Fundamentals—Preschool* (3rd ed.). Pearson Publishing.

Wilkes, E. M. (2001). *Cottage Acquisition Scales for Listening, Language, and Speech* (2nd ed.). Sunshine Cottage School for Deaf Children.

Zimmerman, I. L., Steiner, V. G., & Pond, R. E. (2011). *Preschool Language Scales* (4th ed.). Pearson Publishing.

Zimmerman, S., Osberger, M. J., & Robbins, A. M. (2001a). *Infant-Toddler Meaningful Auditory Integration Scale*. Advanced Bionics.

Zimmerman-Phillips, S., Osberger, M. J., & Robbins, A. M. (2001b). *Meaningful Auditory Integration Scale*. Advanced Bionics.

Chapter 5
Therapy Basics

Sylvia Rotfleisch and
Maura Martindale

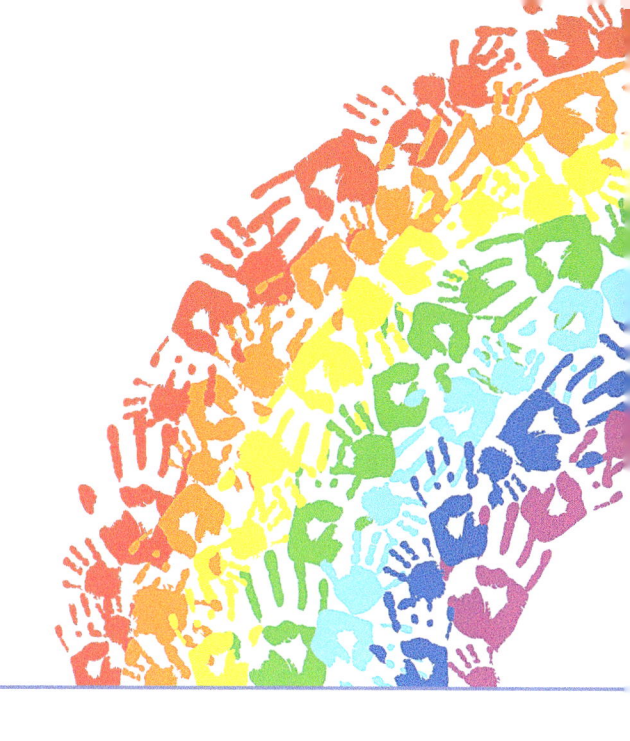

Key Points

- Spoken language is acquired naturally during all activities of daily living.
- Therapy domains will follow the same sequence of development as typically developing hearing children will.
- Therapy should be fun! This enhances engagement, retention of skills, and carryover into daily life.
- Spoken language emerges from listening and engaging in conversations.
- Hearing technologies, when set correctly, need to be worn during all waking hours.
- Auditory-based strategies are an integral part of all therapy activities.

What Should Therapy Look Like? Fun!

It can be tempting during sessions to think of language and speech development as isolated from how children learn. Children who enjoy going to therapy think of it as fun and engaging, using toys and activities that they enjoy! Therapy should be fun and should be set up so that the children are active learners, engaged, and interested in the interaction and the play activity. If you play and interact appropriately with a child, then you have built in enjoyment and therapy sessions won't be a drudgery for the child or parent. It will also help the parents understand that therapy is an all-day activity, making use of everything we do. A basic principle to remember is that everything we do has language, especially within the developmental world of children (Curtis & Carter, 2008).

The Chocolate Chip Cookie Theory

A way to conceptualize for parents how listening, speech, and spoken language are combined is the chocolate chip cookie analogy (Rotfleisch, 2001). The chocolate chip cookie theory uses the example of baking cookies to illustrate the important points and principles in the habilitation of the deaf and hard of hearing learning spoken language. In this analogy, one compares the ingredients in the recipe for baking cookies to the skills needed to become a competent communicator through a listening and spoken language approach. The process of mixing the cookie dough is used to show the need for all components to mix together to implement therapy goals. This cookie dough is what we aim for in our sessions with children. All the elements of listening and spoken language should be integrated into the "dough."

Consider the different ingredients in the recipe for a chocolate chip cookie and the possible variations in recipes that result from both a change in ingredients such as including nuts, using semisweet rather than milk chocolate chips, choosing butter rather than shortening, and even using different baking equipment. Though the resulting cookies are different, they are still essentially chocolate chip cookies. However, we can tell from the flavor if the cookie has the perfect quantity of butter, not enough sugar, or an inadequate amount of chocolate chips. Once baked, it is not possible to separate the sugar from the flour from the eggs. One might separate out a chocolate chip, but by the time it is pulled out with our fingernail, it would hardly resemble the initial chocolate chip.

When looking at the "recipes" of the required skills for a child who is deaf or hard of hearing, "bakers" may use different variations or components. Typically, the obvious "ingredients" include auditory processes, receptive and expressive language, pragmatics, speech, and those that reflect their unique "equipment" or experiences such as behavior management, preschool, or sibling interactions. Just like the variability in cookie recipes, the "ingredients" may vary, but we are still "baking" or working toward becoming a competent spoken language communicator.

Consider again that the "baked cookies" and "cookie dough," and the "ingredients" or skills for developing listening and spoken language, cannot really be separated from each other. They are combined, as in the cookie dough. We need all the elements in the right balance. It does not matter how clear the articulation is if the child does not have the language and pragmatic skills for communication. It does not matter if the language is age appropriate if the child does not listen to participate in a conversation, respond appropriately, and use language for real communication. It does not matter how age appropriate the language is if the articulation and speech are so poor that people are unable to understand the message.

When working with young children, we interact in a manner that necessitates overlapping of skills. When we announce to the child a simple command or stereotypic phrase within their comprehension, such as "Time for lunch," the child must attend to the auditory signal and discriminate the sounds as different at the level of their abilities to be able to comprehend the message. A baby or toddler will typically demonstrate auditory comprehension by responding appropriately to the adult's conversational contribution by moving toward the table or saying "mmm" to indicate it is time to eat. Just as with chocolate chip cookies, it is not clear where the butter ends and the sugar begins. We are not separating audition from speech from expressive or receptive language when we are interacting with the child. There is an interaction with all these components in a successful communicative act and all ingredients need to be integrated. This can be easily accomplished when involved with the child in natural and typical everyday situations.

This analogy can be summarized in a formula: E = mc² or "English equals milk and cookies too" (Rotfleisch, 2001). Where the ingredients for the chocolate chip cookies are flour, sugar, butter, eggs, baking soda, chocolate chips, salt, and nuts (as long as you do not have a nut allergy), the ingredients for spoken language are auditory processes, receptive language, expressive language, pragmatic functions, and speech production.

General Tips for the Sessions

Each family is unique, so your therapy plans need to be tailored to the individual child and parent. Before sharing the details of specific activities, here are some general tips for keeping in mind.

- Variety and balance of activities. Be prepared with a balance of activities for daily living (ADL) (e.g., eating, changing clothes, cleaning up, gardening, opening mail, playing dress-up, washing the dishes) and allow the child and parent to choose some games or toys. Almost anything can be used to achieve listening and spoken language goals.
- Maximize audition.
  - We should have the child with hearing loss focus on hearing by strategically positioning parents and professionals behind or next to the child.
  - Model working as close to hearing aids and/or cochlear implants as possible, reminding parents of the 6 dB rule (see Chapter 1).
  - Use audition first when presenting materials. Tell the child that you are going to introduce an object to play with, without letting him see it, such as a toy car. Then pause and bring out the car.
- The unexpected teachable moment. Be ready for the unexpected, such as a spilled cup of juice, a broken toy or missing game piece, the need to change a diaper, a truck passing by, or a sudden change in the weather. All of these events present ways to incorporate your goals into the session and for problem solving.
- Singing. Incorporate singing and fingerplays into sessions, often using them as transitions from one activity to another. Find out what songs the family enjoys and in what language. Music and singing are whole brain activities. Sing as much as possible by making up songs as well.
- Greetings. Use greetings and closings as language time too. These are great times to establish joint attention and begin the conversation.
- Children are busy. Toddlers are often busy learning how to walk, and all children prefer active learning, so be careful about forcing a child to sit for long periods of time. Use walking (and falling) as opportunities to listen to and learn verbs.
- Books. Incorporate reading and books in your sessions. Ask about commercial books and homemade books that the family has at home or plan a trip to the local library. Many times, children like to read the same book over and over, which is an important emergent literacy event. Rereading leads to predictability!
- Questions. Model asking a variety of questions! In addition to providing rich variations in pitch, it sets up the interaction for conversation and meaningful turn taking.
- Praise, praise, praise. All learners benefit from feedback, particularly authentic

praise for parents. They may be feeling a bit overwhelmed and not feeling secure about what to do. Point out specifically what they are doing right!
- Comprehensive records. Keep good records! You will be asked to share information about your sessions in a variety of settings and meetings, and in reports. You will want to provide specific goals, outcomes, degree of attainment, and results of your time with families, maintaining confidentiality at all times.
- Avoid exaggerated facial features. Speak naturally when speaking to children with hearing loss and guide families to do the same.
- What if the session goes wrong and a child's behavior needs attention? It is always best to prevent behavior issues with careful planning for maximum engagement and interest. Keeping the child's developmental level in mind, set boundaries and rules for your sessions, such as not grabbing materials away from parents or professionals.
- Have fun. Above all, *have fun*! It leads to higher levels of engagement, thus increasing the learning!

Tools, Strategies, Building Materials

Turn Taking or Serve and Return

Turn taking, also referred to as *serve and return*, communicates a message of conversation. We take turns. In the tennis analogy, you serve by using your voice and the ball is in the other person's court. They must return it. This is done with physical and vocal turns. We encourage vocal turns to promote listening and spoken language. With nonverbal children, speaking to them, or serving, and then waiting for their return, is a strategy that will be used for an extended period of time. Initial turns from children who aren't using their voices could begin with turns evidenced by action or movement. The success of the communication is the intrinsic reward and will lead to more turns, attempts, and willingness to initiate communications. We are letting the child know "I want to talk to you. I really care about what you are saying." At the same time, we are letting the child know that talking is happening all around us and is expected from the child as well. For these reasons, we are careful not to talk when children are talking. In the same way, they need to listen and wait for their turn in conversations during sessions and ADL. Joint attention and turn taking need to be pointed out to parents as basic language development behaviors.

Infant- and Child-Directed Speech (IDS, CDS)

Parents and adults will typically speak to prelinguistic babies and young children in a manner that is also referred to as *parentese*. This is also known as *child-directed speech* (CDS) or *infant-directed speech* (IDS) (Song et al., 2010; Wang et al., 2017). Parentese incorporates a voice that is slightly higher pitched with shorter phrases, more inflection, and many repetitions. In this style of interaction, the adult intentionally uses exaggerated suprasegmental aspects of speech to produce strong intonation patterns with up and down pitch control, and changes in duration of the sounds. For the child with hearing loss, this focuses on the lower frequency sounds that the brain is interested in listening to at early stages of establishing serve and return communicative turns. Professionals and parents will describe their child's actions in real time using this style of speaking.

Narrating

Narrating is essential in interacting with a new or even experienced listener. Think of it like a radio broadcast of a sporting event. If a child is getting dressed, the parent or caregiver will use phrases such as "You're putting on your shirt. Now put one foot into your pant leg and help me pull them up. Then we will put on your socks. Which color socks do you want today? Where are your shoes? Here they are! You are putting your foot into one shoe and I am going to tie the laces." Eventually, parents do this automatically wherever they are and whatever the child is doing. You can see the connection of ADL with narration. The dialogues in each of the succeeding chapters will provide a wealth of ideas on how narration can be integrated into sessions.

The Expectant Pause

The expectant pause is a critical element that comes into play in establishing serve and return and expanding multiple consistent turn taking. The expectant pause incorporates silence, eye contact, facial expressions, and body language such as leaning forward or tilting your head. Adults playing with the child with hearing loss determine the balance between speaking and pausing. This balance gives the message that it is time for the baby to take a turn. Too long a pause can risk loss of the volley. Speaking too soon could interrupt the child who was about to vocalize.

Waiting, Waiting, and Sometimes . . . More Waiting . . .

Once children have communicative intent and especially when they have some expressive vocabulary, we can intentionally set up a situation and tempt the child to use their words to achieve success. When we know the child has the word *ball* receptively, we can playfully hold it and bounce it or toss it in the air with a narration such as "I have a ball. Bounce, bounce, bounce. Do you want the ball?" Then wait to give children the understanding that you said something and now it is their turn. This is a strategy that pairs well and automatically with narrate, serve and return, expectant pause, and up the ante.

We never want to frustrate the child in this sort of situation, just tempt and facilitate with the understanding that what the child says is important. This can be seen as the initial implementation of "use your words" and might not be immediately successful. Adults must patiently wait for a verbal turn but understand that this is not a call for a battle of wills by withholding an object to cause frustration or for insisting on imitations. From an early stage of verbal communicative intent, this is the prompt that conveys the message that it is your turn to talk and that I want to know what you want to say. We are striving for communication, not imitation. When the child is not able to be successful, we can achieve positive closure by providing an appropriate comment that shows the meaning (Dickson, 2010).

Waiting continues to be essential even as the child grows into a more skilled communicator. As adults, we have an extensive knowledge of our native vocabulary and language, so we respond very quickly. If adults do not respond to us in approximately 3 seconds or so, we begin to think they were not listening, they misunderstood, or they are ignoring us. However, all children, but especially those with hearing loss, are constantly being introduced to new vocabulary and language, so they cannot process as quickly as adults. All too often adults will say something to a child, wait an adult processing time of 3 seconds, and then assume the child did not hear, did not understand, or was ignoring, so they will repeat. In many cases, the adult's repetition has interrupted the child's processing.

Suggesting that parents think about how long it would take them to answer a question in the foreign language they learned in high school or having them silently count to 10 on their fingers can help them recognize how long it may take for the child to answer. We, as professionals must model for and stress to parents the importance of waiting so that the child has ample time to process, formulate a response, and reply. We will never find out what children know if we do not give them the time to think and then respond.

Blah, Blah, Blah Ginger

When we are speaking to young listeners, they are hearing the key words and their repertoire of key words needs to grow and expand. There was a comic by Larson of *The Far Side* cartoon with two panels (2003). The first one is "What we say to dogs" and the bubble says, "Okay Ginger! I've had it! You stay out of the garbage! Understand Ginger? Stay out of the garbage or else!" The following panel is titled, "What they hear" and the bubble says, "Blah blah GINGER blah blah blah blah blah blah blah blah GINGER blah blah blah blah blah blah blah Ginger." This is the strategy where parents will learn to sprinkle *mommy* and the child's name within sentences and phrases to facilitate learning to learn words. As children learn their names and the word for their mother, they will then be able to learn to pull those words out when embedded in sentences and learn more words by the way words start or finish.

Teach children to listen and pay attention to words they understand within sentences and phrases, and that will teach them how to learn their first words. Speak to children with hearing loss with phrases and sentences as appropriate and they will use that input to understand word boundaries and learn how to determine sound combinations at the beginning or the ending of words. Key words that children learn will act as wedges within phrases, beginning with their name and a version of *mama*. This helps them to identify and learn new words. This teaches the child to learn new words, rather than teaching them a list of selected words—the same as "give a person a fish" or "teach them to fish."

Joint Attention

One of the first and most important behaviors to promote language development in all children is the development of joint attention. This involves the caregiver and child interacting together, paying attention to the object or toy that is being discussed. This facilitates the normal progression of communication development and provides auditory input with some reinforcement of what is being discussed by virtue of the presence of the object that is the subject of the communication. Auditory-based therapy does not forbid any visual input or speech reading, but dictates that natural interactions be facilitated. When auditory-only input is necessary, the situation can always be manipulated to meet that need (Tomasello & Farrar, 1986).

Auditory Closure

Auditory closure allows the parents to have the child fill in the blank. Parents often do this naturally as they start to say something, then in midsentence allow the child with hearing loss to complete the phrase or sentence. It can be used effectively in many activities. When singing, we can pause to have the child contribute the key word in the song. During reading, we can use a book that is familiar to the child and predictable. This is naturally incorporated when the book has a pattern that can be said or completed. In everyday activities, we can look for predictable language or words such as "Let's wash your hands with soap and . . . " or "Please sit down on your . . . " or as simple as "Mommy will pick you . . . "

Auditory Sandwich

For students who are older, who are transitioning to listening and spoken language, who are bilingual learners, or who need some visual prompts to connect the auditory signal with meaning, a strategy called the *auditory sandwich* has been employed by many professionals (Koch, 1999). It consists of presenting a message via audition alone, then presenting the message again accompanied by a visual prompt such as a gesture, picture, or object, and finally putting the message back into audition only. As soon as the child is able to respond to the auditory message alone, the visuals should be dropped. This strategy has the potential to bridge the gap for students who are struggling in their ability to process auditory information.

Listening Hoop

A listening hoop is recommended and used by some professionals to present information through audition only and prevent lipreading. Using a hand cue (Estabrooks, 2012) is a technique that has been long associated with auditory-verbal therapy to obstruct the view of the mouth or to prompt a response or turn from the child with hearing loss. However, this technique may block a portion of the auditory information and will make it more difficult for the child with hearing loss to access the auditory event. Professionals can use a listening hoop with an acoustically transparent fabric such as a speaker cloth. Neither hand cues nor listening hoops model or foster natural interactions. They would not be recommended for use by the parent or when fostering a parent-child interaction. This strategy might be effective or necessary with an older child during a structured listening activity or assessment if the child with hearing loss insists or tried to rely on speechreading.

Enhancing Perception

The basic premise is that a child with hearing loss will have speech production abilities that reflect their auditory access and perception. When promoting listening and spoken language, we look for emerging and accurate perceptions of speech features. When a child demonstrates errors in perception, as evidenced through their discrimination, identification, or production of a speech feature, we aim to enhance the perception. When we work auditorily, we directly work to correct the perception, not the production.

New listeners' ability to attend, discriminate, remember, and comprehend different words can depend on a variety of elements within the auditory signal.

A young child at a level with initial skills is typically able to discriminate words such as *hot* versus *hot dog* versus *happy* based on suprasegmental information of the different number of syllables and the stress pattern. Words such as *hat* versus *hot* can best be discriminated based on the different vowel content. Words with consonants that vary by manner of production such as *hat* versus *mat*, or words that have voicing differences such as *bat* versus *pat*, would more easily be discriminated than words with place cue differences such as *cake* versus *take* or *mat* versus *gnat*.

However, a child may or may not be able to discriminate words where the place cue difference is not within their production abilities but might be within their discrimination skills. The child with emerging abilities should have the appropriate skills reinforced. Providing many contrasts in meaningful contexts, at the level of success, will reinforce and expand current skills. New and more difficult contrasts should be introduced and facilitated in the areas of attention, discrimination, memory, productions, and comprehension by contrasting phonemes that are being misperceived and confused. Often isolating the phoneme out of the word, and appropriately acoustically highlighting it (see Acoustic Highlighting), enhances the correct perception, discrimination, and production. Correcting and enhancing the child's perception allows for better perception and production matching needed for auditory feedback and will lead to use of the feedback loop and correction of phoneme production.

Acoustic Highlighting

Acoustic highlighting (Pollack, 1964) is a technique that makes a particular sound or word more salient. Think of it as having one red rose in a bouquet of white roses, which makes the red one stand out and be more apparent. There are a variety of different ways to accomplish this. When we take a word out of natural interactions and language, we always put it back in the natural language. Acoustically highlighting a word can be accomplished by manipulating the suprasegmentals; for example, making the word louder or longer or a different pitch. By playing a natural game to incorporate intensity contrast, we could use whispering for going to sleep while playing with a baby doll and then using a loud sing-song voice to wake up the baby. An unvoiced consonant is more salient when it is whispered either on its own or within the word or phrase. Specific strategies for acoustic highlighting are addressed by speech features in Table 5–1.

A word of caution: When isolating the feature, do not distort it an unnatural way in interactions. You could isolate an /m/ by saying "mmmm" and then saying "milk." Another example would be with an unvoiced /p/ by whispering "puhpuh-puh," then putting it back in the word *push* and then into the sentence or phrase —"Let's push, push, push!" We are not teaching the child *p- p- p-* connected to the word *push*, but instead focusing the listening on *p- p- p-* and then modeling the word correctly as *push*. After highlighting the sounds, always put them back in a natural context for the child to have the opportunity to match the speech feature that was isolated. Do not pair the highlighted feature with the word in a way that distorts or changes the word (e.g., elongated *mmmmilk* or like a stutter in *p-p-p-push*).

We can use acoustic highlighting in a way that is natural when we stress a word

Table 5–1. Sample Acoustic Highlighting Strategies Illustrated by Speech Feature

Feature	Strategy	Example
Suprasegmentals: Duration, Intensity, Pitch (DIP)	Highlight by using contrasting DIP or a sing-song-y voice. It is easy to change the DIP in any word, phrase, or sentence.	Use phrases preferably with meaning and cognitively appropriate for the child. "How big is baby? Soooo big!" "Give me a high five." "Where's your nose?"
Duration	Contrasting pairs with added inflection incorporating meaning (e.g., short versus long versus interrupted)	*Up up up* versus *down* *Nooooo* versus *yes*! *Open* versus *push push push* *Mooooo* versus *hop hop hop* *Stop* versus *round and round and round*
Intensity	Contrasting pairs with added inflection incorporating meaning (e.g., loud versus quiet or whispered)	Playing with a toy *Shhh* versus *wake up*
Pitch	Contrasting pairs with added inflection incorporating meaning (e.g., low pitch versus high pitch)	Playing with toys or books using pitch for different characters such as father, mother, child Low-pitched *moo* for a cow and high-pitched *peep peep peep* for a bird *Tickle tickle tickle* (high pitch) versus *bang bang bang* (low pitch) Walking game with different pitches for tiny steps, medium and big steps, or other movements: *walk, run run run run, jump jump jump*
Vowels	Highlight by using DIP or a sing-song-y voice. It is easy to change the DIP to make a vowel louder, quieter, longer, high pitched, etc. Have the child listen to contrast between vowels (e.g., *hot* versus *hoot* versus *heat*)	*Moooooo* *Ch ch oooo ooooo*
Consonants by Manner (that are continuants)	Nasals, fricatives, and semivowels can be elongated or isolated	"Mmmmm that's good" "Listen: *ssss*, like a snake. *Ssss*." *Sunny*
Consonants	Can be repeated in same and/or different vowel contexts to allow the child repetition to highlight specific sounds for most errors, or two sounds can be used to contrast the difference	Explain that *cheetah* with a *chee chee chee* is a different sound than *tee tee tee*
Consonants Voicing	Whisper for unvoiced consonants so the vowel is less salient and the consonant is audible or eliminate the vowel	*P p p* (e.g., *pop pop pop*) when playing with bubbles

by making it longer. It is not unusual for us to use duration, intensity, and pitch (DIP) to stress a sound, for example when adults are using IDS and saying, "Nooooo, don't touch that!"

Life in Slow Motion

We have talked about language that is directed to the child. Narrating is a wonderful way to incorporate this style of talking. Teach parents to look at activities for the multiple elements involved rather than just the overall activity. This is a strategy best used when there is time to seize the moment and turn it into a teaching moment and not when everyone is late to get to school, work, and getting on with life. We can consider the child's cognitive level in addressing the elements of the activity (Lunenburg, 2011).

For example, when putting on a child's shirt, look at how the shirt has sleeves and a hole for the head, a top and bottom, an inside and outside, and that it can be inside out and upside down. We find the hole, put it over the child's head, and then have a game of peek-a-boo before we pull, pull, pull, the shirt down over the child's head, unless of course it gets stuck. Then we magically find face parts emerging. Some clothes are more interactive than others, but they are what you make of the slow-motion activity. Shirts have different colors, sizes, pictures, designs, or decorations. They have seams, tags, sleeves, stains, holes, buttons, collars, and so much more. This of course is just example of how one simple activity can be an entire therapy session if you go in slow motion and break it down into the variety of elements that can make getting dressed or any other daily activity a learning and very language-engaging situation.

The Three-Act Play

A very successful playwright was being interviewed and was asked to what he attributed his tremendous success. He went on to explain that it was very simple. In the first act, he told the audience what was going to happen. In the second act, it happened. In the third act, he told them it happened. Through everyday life, we make it a goal to tell the child what is going to happen, explain the activity while it is occurring, and finally discuss the events that have been completed. This gives us an easy way to maximize exposure to language and listening opportunities inherent in the event. Parents are encouraged to use this strategy. Act One: "We are going to wash your hands." Act Two: "We are washing your hands." Act Three: "We washed your hands." When parents incorporate the three-act play instead of just doing the activity, they build in an introduction to the activity and the conclusion and completion of the activity. This strategy allows for consistent exposure to verb tenses (e.g., future, present, and past) while incorporating and reinforcing the use of narration. This is a particularly good strategy when facilitating the present progressive verb form, which is an early emerging morphemic structure.

Expansion

Expansion is an effective strategy to facilitate many skills and goals. When the child with hearing loss says a word or word approximation, the caregiver responds by using that word and a few others as appropriate to expand on the communicative contribution. The words can be combined with others to produce a phrase or short sentence. There are many correct ways to expand children's utterances depending on their language level. If the child says "milk," we can respond, "Do you want milk?" or "Drink your milk" or "The milk is all gone." At a more advanced stage, the child might say, "more milk cup," and the parent could respond, "I am pouring more milk in the cup" or "You want more milk in the cup" or "You have more milk in your cup." This strategy reinforces the children's communication by responding using their word or words. Again, remember we are facilitating communication, not imitation. This makes it clear that their language was understood and, at the same time, expands the utterance and works toward increasing the child's attention, discrimination, auditory memory, vocabulary, and language (Weybright, 1985).

Upping the Ante

It is important to realize the improvements and steps that the child is making and be positive about them with the child and ourselves. However, it is important to be aware of the long-term goals and to know how to get the child there. That is part of upping the ante every step of the way in every aspect. We must celebrate the progress, but also help the parents recognize the next goal.

Correcting Is OK

People interacting with a child who has a hearing loss are often unaware of the child's potential and are just amazed when the child is talking at all regardless of what is being said or how it is expressed. It is important to know that correcting a child's grammatical errors or pronunciation is OK when done appropriately. This issue of correcting must be dealt with in a sensitive manner. Often expanding and repeating the child's communicative intent with a complete sentence or using the correct grammatical structure will facilitate a correction over time.

Dangling Carrot

Explain to parents how it is our job to encourage the child's current language, very slowly, to the next level. This strategy promotes spoken language, so that when talking to the child, we must be close enough to the child's current level to ensure successful communication but, at the same time, we must promote a slightly more advanced level with the goal of moving the child to the next language stage. This is another way to use expansion by exposure and modeling more complex language.

Vocabulary Expansion

Too often, students with hearing loss stagnate in vocabulary development, particularly past the preschool years. For parents, knowing that their child has a vocabulary of more than 100 words can be very exciting. At that level, communication has become effective, and we all end up in a comfort zone that must be left behind to move the child forward in the development. We need to help the parents and child to move out of the comfort zone of their first 100 or few hundred vocabulary words. Celebrate that accomplishment, but realize we do not want to be stuck there. Use a variety of words in sessions and don't simplify language constantly, or else we risk vocabulary stagnation. Table 5–2 provides some easy strategies to use in intervention and to teach parents as ways of promoting ongoing expansion of vocabulary and preventing vocabulary stagnation.

Table 5–2. Preventing Vocabulary Stagnation

Strategy	Implementation Examples
Convergent Thinking	
Parts of the whole	Begin with a known or familiar object and look for related vocabulary that converges in on the item (e.g., car: steering wheel, tires, wheels, flat tire, hubcaps, jack, bolts, trunk, front seat, driver's seat, passenger seat, "shotgun"; dog: paw, tail, fangs, fur, whiskers, collar; bird: wings, beak, tail, feathers, claws)
Divergent Thinking	
Categories and associated concepts	Begin with a known or familiar object and look for related vocabulary that diverges from the item (e.g., car: vehicles; transportation; land, water, and air vehicles; commercial transportation; cargo; freight; private vehicles)
Synonyms	
Be the thesaurus—introduce and use Tier 2 level words	You can decide to banish a word (e.g., big: large, huge, gigantic, massive, enormous; said: asked, questioned, stated, whispered, mumbled, grumbled, commanded, demanded, yelled)
	Expand using Tier 3 vocabulary (e.g., truck: pickup truck, semitruck, cement mixer, tow truck, back hoe)
Antonyms	
Use opposites and negative concepts	If it is not big, then it could be medium, tiny, petite, miniscule, microscopic. Learn basic and advanced opposites: big/small, old/new, tall/short, full/empty, wide/narrow, broad/slim, sharp/dull, bright/dim.
Homonyms	
Multiple meanings: homographs (spelled the same)	Homographs, multiple meanings for a word (e.g., trunk: of a tree, of an elephant, of a car, trunk for storage; down: feathers from a duck, down from the ladder; fly [noun]: fly of your pants, the insect that is a fly; fly [verb]: an airplane can fly)
homophones (sound the same)	Homophones (e.g., wait and weight; stair and stare; their, there, and they're)
Eliminate Nonspecific Words	
Do not use words that aren't clear in their meaning related to an object or placement.	Eliminate: here, there, this, that, thing, stuff
	Use specific words or descriptions when there aren't words to describe items by color, pattern, material, texture (e.g., The plastic tip of the shoelace helps thread the shoelace through the eyelets; The plastic container belongs next to the small cardboard box)

Table 5–2. *continued*

Strategy	Implementation Examples
Speak the Unspoken Portion	
Don't assume the missing word is known	Include the "unspoken" part (e.g., Wash your hands <u>in the sink</u>, wash your hands <u>with soap and water</u>. Dry your <u>wet</u> hands <u>with a towel</u>)
Emotions	
Go beyond the basic happy and sad	Anxious, frustrated, annoyed, frazzled, determined, jealous, scared, disgusted
Concepts	
Spatial and directional	Refuse to use here, there; instead use specific prepositions and descriptive words (e.g., behind, between, besides, middle, corner, clockwise, counterclockwise; Put the book on the top shelf beside the ball; The bird flew out of the nest and down to the ground)
Temporal/time concepts	Before, after, later, while, during, today, tomorrow, yesterday, week, day, month
Shapes, dimensions, measurements, and comparatives	Circle, square, triangle, oval, straight, curved, long, short, thick, thin, tall, taller, tallest, heavy, light, narrow
Quantity and ordinal concepts	Numbers, first, second, third, last, next, one by one, each, a few, several, once, twice, double, triple
Activity or Object-Specific Vocabulary	
Vocabulary that belongs to specific situations	Card games: shuffle, deal, dealer, cut the deck, draw pile, discard pile Swimming: strokes, laps, dive, float, shallow, deep, plunge, wade
Captivate Sensory Experience	
Vocabulary related to the senses	Descriptive words that create vivid pictures to captivate our senses (e.g., <u>sight</u>: bright, blurry, dingy, shiny; <u>smell</u>: fragrant, aroma, acrid, foul; <u>touch</u>: rough, smooth, coarse, hot, cold; <u>taste</u>: sweet, spicy, bland, bitter, delicious; <u>hearing</u>: soft, loud, crackling, buzz, clang, blare)
Words With Hidden Information	
Inferential words	Look for words and expressions that imply additional information, particularly emotions (e.g., pacing the floor implies nervousness, reluctant to try implies concern, trembling implies fear)

Summary

Keeping the sessions fun and positive will make a more lasting impression on children and their parents. There are multiple other strategies than those listed here that you may develop or have developed over the course of your practice. You may also find that the terms we used here are different than terms that you currently use for the same strategies. Finally, in your planning with the parents, keep your eye on the next stage of listening and spoken language with the idea of moving forward.

Discussion Questions

1. Of the tips presented, which one(s) would you find most challenging?
2. Using the vocabulary expansion table (Table 5–2), think of two activities that would promote expansion for each section.
3. Reading over the strategies and tools, what activities of daily living align with each one?

References

Curtis, D., & Carter, M. (2008). *Learning together with young children: A curriculum framework for reflective teachers*. Redleaf Publishing.

Dickson, C. L. (2010). *Sound foundations for babies*. Cochlear Corporation.

Estabrooks, W. (Ed.). (2012). *101 frequently asked questions about auditory-verbal practice: Promoting listening and spoken language for children who are deaf and hard of hearing and their families*. Alexander Graham Bell Association for the Deaf.

Koch, M. (1999). *Bringing sound to life*. York Press.

Larson, G. (2003). *Blah, blah, blah, blah Ginger. The complete Far Side* (1st ed.). Andrews McMeel.

Lunenburg, F.C. (2011). Early childhood education: Implications for school readiness. *Schooling, 2*(1), 1–8.

Pollack, D. (1964). Acoupedics: A unisensory approach to auditory training. *Volta Review, 66*, 400–409.

Rotfleisch, S. (2001). E = mc^2 (English equals milk and cookies too!). *The Listener*, (Fall), 39–42.

Song, J. Y., Demuth, K., & Morgan, J. (2010). Effects of the acoustic properties of infant-directed speech on infant word recognition. *Journal of the Acoustic Society of America, 128*(1), 389–400. https://www.ncbi.nlm.nih.gov/pmc/articles/PMC2921436/

Tomasello, M., & Farrar, T. (1986). Joint attention and early language. *Child Development, 57*(6), 1454–1463.

Wang, Y., Bergeson, T. R., & Houston, D. M. (2017). Infant-directed speech enhances attention to speech in deaf infants with cochlear implants. *Journal of Speech, Language, and Hearing Research, 60*(11), 3321–3333.

Weybright, G. (1985). *Oh, say what they see: An introduction to indirect language stimulation techniques*. Educational Productions.

Chapter 6

The Prelinguistic Stage

Sylvia Rotfleisch

Key Points

- We begin at the critical foundation stage.
- The child in the prelinguistic stage will learn foundational skills in the development of listening, speaking, and principles of conversations before they say their first word.
- At the prelinguistic stage, the child develops early listening skills, awareness that sound has meaning, use of vocalizations, and initial receptive language.
- Goals should be incorporated into activities of daily living by the family, which will incorporate the culture of the family.
- Goals should be incorporated into play and adapted to the child's age, cognitive and developmental stages, and interests.

Basic Characteristics of the Prelinguistic Child

Listening

This child is a new listener or is listening with new technology and is still at very basic detection and auditory attention foundation skills levels. Early responses to sounds by the new listener could be widening eyes or stopping an ongoing action such as moving, sucking, or vocalizing at the onset or cessation of a sound event. A perceived sound might elicit different reactions in a toddler or older child. An older child is more mature and may search for the sound source; vocalize in response to it; or touch, point to, or remove their technology. Responses initially will be to sounds that are loud enough and adequately above thresholds levels so that the child becomes aware of them (Madell et al., 2018). A child with hearing loss with new auditory access will demonstrate variability in reactions and in the consistency or lack of consistency of their responses to sounds. The order of emergence of the various speech features will depend on the degree of hearing loss and auditory access provided by technology (see Speech Acoustics, Chapter 1). Early auditory abilities typically evident and/or emerging in the prelinguistic stage are indicated in Table 6–1. Skills listed are not sequential.

Language

Children at the prelinguistic stage have no word approximations but will move into the next level with the emergence

Table 6–1. Auditory Abilities Evidenced in the Prelinguistic Stage

- Quiets when listening.
- Responds to loud sounds (babies: e.g., eyes widening, cessation of activity such as moving or sucking; older children: e.g., looks for sound, points to ear, looks interested).
- Responds and attends to voices with increasing consistency.
- Enjoys toys or items that make noises (babies: e.g., rattles, squeakers; older children: e.g., phone, electronic items).
- Responds to musical sounds (e.g., humming, singing, music, musical or electronic toys).
- Creates sounds to listen to (e.g., bangs on tables or other objects, drops items, plays with a toy to make sound).
- Responds to environmental sounds (e.g., phone, airplane, doorbell, vehicles, dog barking).
- Vocalizes in response to speech.
- Attempts to localize sound.
- Recognizes different voices.
- Tracks speech between people.
- Recognizes mood of speaker based on vocal quality of speaker.
- Moves in rhythm with music.
- Discriminates some phrases based on rhythmic structures.
- Understands some words and responds by performing appropriate gestures (e.g., up, bye-bye).
- Recognizes stereotypic phrases announcing routines and anticipates what will happen.
- Responds to and recognizes own name.
- Listens when spoken to.
- May be calmed or quieted by calm, soothing voice.
- Frightened or disturbed when hears an angry voice.
- Vocalizes along with singing, though not using real words.
- Identifies animals or vehicles based on characteristics and associated sounds that will be specific to culture or home language (e.g., choo choo for train, meow for cat).
- Recognizes the intonation of a question.
- Understands a few names and words.
- Responds to voice by using voice to take turns even though not using real words.

Sources: REEL (2020); LittlEARS (2004); ASHA Milestones.

of their first word approximation. They initially may or may not have some limited comprehension of words that will reflect previous auditory access. They will progress through skills (see Table 6–2) and toward the next stage as they are provided with consistent auditory access and the listening skills emerge. Children at the prelinguistic stage will recognize their names and "mama" after a period of exposure to the auditory message. They understand simple phrases that are part of their daily routine and common first words, such as "daddy" or "bye-bye." Receptive and expressive language abilities evidenced or expected to emerge in this stage are included in Table 6–2, Language and Speech Skills Evidenced in the Prelinguistic Stage. Skills listed are not sequential.

Speech

Speech at this stage is an integral component of expressive skills and behaviors as included in Table 6–2. The child at this stage might be producing speech sounds in the form of cooing, babbling, or jargoning. You might witness the child using some gestures or gestures combined with vocalizations for communicative intent and emerging pragmatic functions. However, children with hearing loss who have not had auditory access and/or have not been focusing on listening and spo-

Table 6–2. Language and Speech Skills Evidenced in the Prelinguistic Stage

Audition and Auditory Comprehension of Language	Expressive Language/Vocalization and Communication
• Quiets or smiles when spoken to. • Seems to recognize voices and quiets if crying. • Looks at speaker and smiles. • Responds to changes in tone of voice. • Responds appropriately to friendly and angry tones. • Responds to own name. • Vocalizes with intonation. • Emergence of naming insight. • Understands simple instructions/ requests with use of vocal or physical cues (e.g., "Come here," "Want more?"). • Responds to "no." • Recognizes names. • Is aware of the social value of speech. • Recognizes words for common items (e.g., *cup*, *shoe*, *juice*).	• Begins to imitate sounds. • Laughs. • Makes pleasure sounds (e.g., cooing, gooing). • Cries differently for different needs. • Vocalizes excitement and displeasure. • Babbles sound more speechlike with different sounds, including /p/, /b/, and /m/. • Enjoys games like peek-a-boo and pat-a-cake. • Uses gestures: reaching, waves bye bye, rejects objects, lifts arms to be picked up. • Babbles with inflection. • Babbles with both long and short groups of sounds (e.g., *ma*, *tata*, *upup*, *bibibibi*). • Uses speech or noncrying sounds to get and keep attention. • Gestures to accompany rhymes or songs. • Uses suprasegmentals (i.e., duration, intensity, pitch) to develop control in vocal play.

Sources: REEL (2020); LittlEARS (2004); ASHA Milestones; Lanza and Flahive (2008).

ken language might be nonvocal at this stage. Additional information regarding expected initial speech production abilities is addressed in the speech development section of Chapter 3.

Goals for the Prelinguistic Stage

Developing an Appropriate Therapy Plan by Addressing Strengths and Areas of Need

The normal sequence of development will be followed to develop listening skills and appropriate speech and language abilities. Goals for the prelinguistic stage focus on:

- facilitating and monitoring early listening skills,
- developing an awareness that sound has meaning,
- facilitating appropriate use of vocalizations,
- facilitating foundations of receptive language, and
- facilitating initial word approximations.

Select appropriate goals based on your assessment results, which identify the child's strengths and needs (see Chapter 4). With the understanding of speech features and the acoustics parameters related to an audiogram, you can monitor for emerging skills. Based on the hearing loss, you predict and prepare for areas of potential difficulty (see Chapter 1).

Goals must be individualized within the stage to meet the needs of the child. Consider this when determining goals related to speech development. You must look at the child's current level of vocalizations. If the child is producing reduplicative babbling, you can select goals to expand the current stage and to facilitate progression to the next. However, with a child who is not vocalizing, you will begin with turn taking and facilitating the use of voice as a turn before progressing through the stages of babbling.

The reactions and responses to sounds can be subtle and will be discussed further. This child will have listening and vocalizing skills that mirror each other. Vocalizations will emerge as a reflection of the auditory access and attention to sounds. You will pick goals in the developmental sequence aligned with assessment results. You might select an auditory goal to discriminate vowels and the suprasegmentals (duration, intensity, and pitch [DIP]) or one that addresses consonants of different manners; likely a plosive and/or a nasal will emerge.

The auditory needs will be reflected by the child's use of those features. The attention, discrimination and identification of the features, allows for the production of those features. Goals will address the child's understanding that vocal tones reflect the speaker's mood (Table 6–3, Goal 4a; Table 6–5, Goal 16). As that auditory ability emerges, the speech and language goals (Table 6–4, Goals 9, 10; Table 6–6, Goal 22) will facilitate productions with vocal tones that reflect the child's mood and carry a pragmatic message. The need to integrate these skills with each other is apparent as we see how the skills promoted in these goals are connected to each other.

Typical Goals for the Prelinguistic Stage

Typical recommended goals for children with hearing loss at the prelinguistic level are included in Tables 6–3 to 6–6. Goals

Table 6–3. Auditory Goals for Understanding Sound as Meaningful in the Prelinguistic Stage

Auditory Attention, Detection, Memory, and Discrimination

1. Monitor and facilitate attention to:
   a. speech sounds
   b. voices of caregivers
   c. variety of sounds including loud, sudden noises
   d. voices of different quality and tones
   e. environmental sounds
   f. music/singing
2. Localize voices and environmental sounds.
3. Develop and reinforce a one- to two-item auditory memory.
4. Monitor and facilitate auditory discrimination of a variety of aspects of speech:
   a. suprasegmental aspect of speech: duration, intensity, and pitch (DIP)
   b. variety of vowels and diphthongs to include a variety of mid- and low-frequency vowels
   c. Ling six sounds /m/, /u/, /ɑ/, /i/, /ʃ/, /s/
   d. frontal and bilabial consonants /b/, /p/, /w/, /m/ with vowel variety
   e. consonants by manner of production and voicing cues
5. Integrate listening naturally while engaged in various activities.

Table 6–4. Auditory Feedback and Speech Production Goals in the Prelinguistic Stage

Auditory Goals for Development of the Speech Production System

6. Facilitate stages of babbling in appropriate sequence and quality of productions (e.g., cooing, reduplicative, canonical).
7. Facilitate and monitor increase in variety of vocalizations and phrase babbling.
8. Facilitate use of vocalizations as turns.
9. Facilitate use of vocalizations with communicative intent.
10. Facilitate and monitor control of suprasegmental aspects of speech (duration, intensity, pitch).
11. Expand vowel productions to include a variety of mid- and low-frequency vowels.
12. Facilitate babbling of various consonants including frontal and bilabial consonants /b/, /p/, /w/, /m/ with vowel variety.

are organized based upon defined skills related to the brain functions necessary for learning to use audition for language development (see Chapter 3). The goals included in these tables should not be considered the definitive set of goals for all children at this stage; neither should they be considered an exhaustive list of possible audition goals for the prelinguistic child with hearing loss. Goals must

Table 6–5. Auditory Goals for Language Comprehension in the Prelinguistic Stage

Auditory Recognition, Sequencing, and Comprehension
13. Facilitate recognition of sounds and their differing sequences and patterns.
14. Identify objects for animals and vehicles by associated sounds that vary in suprasegmental qualities and vowel content.
15. Discriminate stereotypic phrases on the basis of DIP patterns and known words.
16. Discriminate vocal tones as a reflection of speaker's mood.
17. Facilitate responses (vocal or physical) that indicate comprehension of the adult's communicative intent.
18. Stimulate receptive language beginning with their name, *mommy* (or noun used to refer to parent), and names of family members.
19. Stimulate receptive language in the areas of repeatedly encountered functional activities of daily living (ADL) words (e.g., *up, down, drink, wash, all gone, more*), stereotypic phrases (e.g., "time to eat," "let's read a book," "wave bye bye"), nouns, verbs, and adjectives.
20. Monitor and record receptive vocabulary.

Table 6–6. Auditory Goals for Developing Expressive Language in the Prelinguistic Stage

Auditory Retrieval and Expressive Communication
21. Facilitate and reinforce vocalizations as communicative intent and communicative turns.
22. Facilitate and reinforce appropriate control of vocal speech features (e.g., DIP, vowels, some consonants) in appropriate situations as communicative turns and intent within each successive babbling stage.
23. Encourage use of voice and babbling phrases, productions, and speech approximations for a variety of pragmatic functions (e.g., requesting, protesting, responding, turn taking, attention getting).

address the specific errors and needs determined during comprehensive assessment as well as from observation and informal diagnostic work.

How Do We Work on These Goals?

Professionals must have a knowledge base and multiple appropriate strategies (see Tables 6–7 and 6–8) applicable to the prelinguistic child with hearing loss. The knowledge and strategies included are the basis for you to guide and coach the parent as the primary person to develop their child's listening and spoken language abilities. Knowledge areas and strategies applicable to the prelinguistic child with hearing loss are identified in Tables 6–7 and 6–8.

Key strategies for the professionals to model and facilitate are the use of infant-

Table 6–7. Knowledge Areas in the Prelinguistic Stage

- Hearing technologies being used
- Effective trouble shooting of technology
- Speech acoustics: initially related to prelinguistic stage (e.g., low frequency including DIP, vowels)
- Initial stages of development of audition
- Initial stages of development of speech and babble
- Initial stages of development of receptive language
- Initial stages of development of expressive language
- Ling six sounds
- Reading and the beginning of literacy

Table 6–8. Optimal Strategies to Implement in the Prelinguistic Stage

- Infant- and child-directed speech/caregiver ease (IDS, CDS)
- Acceptance of vocalizations
- Serve and return
- Expectant pause
- Singing
- Reading
- Stereotypic phrases
- Narrate
- 24/7 and activities of daily living (ADL)
- "Blah, blah, blah Ginger"
- Auditory maximizing strategies: joint attention, positioning to support audition
- Sound-object associations
- Chocolate chip cookie theory

therapy sessions the parents will be learning strategies and implementing them in the sessions. These strategies should rapidly carry over into natural daily interactions. Parents will rapidly start to sound like the professional, that is, like you. You will help them to understand how to develop listening and spoken language with their child with hearing loss.

Early in the prelinguistic stage, auditory development is integrally tied to the stages of vocalizations and the development of auditory comprehension of language (i.e., receptive language.) We know that infants require listening experience to develop adequate language and literacy development (Yeung & Werker, 2009). The developing and emerging skills are interconnected and, like the chocolate chip cookie theory (see Chapter 3), are blended together. During intervention, remember the cookie dough. You should always be integrating the child's listening and spoken language skills and transitioning them into natural interactions.

Parents and professionals will be using infant- and child-directed speech (IDS, CDS) when playing and interacting with the child with hearing loss as the basis for facilitating the auditory goals targeted (Bergeson, 2012; Tables 6–3 to 6–6). Parents and professionals will watch the child with hearing loss for various behaviors (Table 6–1). As these behaviors emerge and become consistent, they are an indication that the child is aware and attending to sounds (Friederici & Wessels, 1993). Full-time use of technology and auditory access is essential to begin to build the foundational auditory skills (Marschark et al., 2019).

Parents and professionals will facilitate the appropriate use of voice through interactions with the child. Children beginning to listen will not show interest to

directed speech (IDS) with optimal use of DIP, simplified language, and serve and return for facilitating turn taking. During conversation not intended for them, but when the voice changes to IDS, they are likely to respond and attend to the voice (Song et al., 2010; Wang et al., 2017). The child will begin to vocalize and you and the parent will encourage this by verbally responding, smiling, and making eye contact. Those interacting with the child with hearing loss should understand that cheering the child for using their voice might encourage the child to use their voice again, particularly for the older child who is a new listener. However, that is not the natural or logical consequence of a communicative contribution, and over time this does not develop the foundational building blocks of communication. You must explain and model serve and return with the child's initial vocalizations. Explain to the parent that, though the child might show some improvement with that sort of reward, this behavior does not evolve into a strategy for working on next stages of conversational abilities.

Guide the parents to use some words repeatedly during the prelinguistic stage and to speak in complete but short sentences. This will naturally occur if it is incorporated into daily activities that are repeated (see Activities of Daily Living [ADL] formula; see Chapter 2). This allows the child to develop some comprehension of first vocabulary words. The child will listen to the repeated words and sounds, think about the sound, and keep that idea in their brain. This is their short-term auditory memory. Everyday interactions allow the child to hear words that are becoming familiar, understand them, and keep the word in their auditory memory. This ability will be apparent as the child begins to understand some words or sound-object associations. The child might then look or reach for the specific item or person. The child can keep the concept in their mind and lift up their hands as the mother says "up, up, up."

Additional suggested activities for you to use and to guide and coach the parents are included in Table 6–9. Some additional tips for the parents of a child just learning to listen to encourage initial use of technology are listed in Table 6–10. When monitoring responses to sounds, there are many factors that can be considered to determine if the child's behavior indicated a valid response to sound. Some of these factors are addressed in Table 6–11.

Targeting and Incorporating Goals

Auditory Attention, Detection, Memory, and Discrimination (Table 6–3)

Once the child is showing consistent awareness to sounds, watch for indications that they are paying attention to a variety of types of sounds (Mandel et al., 1995). This goal includes low-, mid-, and high-frequency speech sounds that are specific on the audiogram, such as the Ling six sounds (see Chapter 1). Sounds at this stage must include various features of speech, including both the suprasegmentals of DIP and the segmental aspects including vowels, diphthongs, and the various features of consonants. Discrimination and emerging comprehension can be witnessed by a child's simple actions. The child could show understanding as: they hold their finger to their mouth for "shhh" and put the baby doll to sleep; they look at or reach for the toy train when you say "ch ch oooo"; or they hold

Table 6–9. Guide and Coach Parents To:

Implement optimal strategies for prelinguistic stage (Table 6–8)

Listen!

- Monitor child's responses to sounds.
- Talk about the sounds you hear.

Talk, talk, talk!

- Speak in the language that is natural in the home.
- Use infant- and child-directed speech (IDS, CDS).
- Respond consistently to the child's noises and attempts at interactions.
- Talk to the child and imitate sounds they make.
- Allow the child a chance to take a turn and contribute to the conversation.
- Teach actions (e.g., clapping, shaking, peek-a-boo, blowing kisses, waving bye bye).
- Narrate what is happening throughout the day (e.g., "Mommy is putting on your shoes," "Jacob is drinking water," "Mmm, the apple is so good").
- Talk about the who, what, where, when throughout the day and during ADL (e.g., "We are at the park. Billy can go in the swing. Mommy is pushing Billy. Billy is going back and forth," "We are at the store. I need to get some milk. Let's find the milk. Here, mommy found the milk. Mommy is holding the cold milk. Jenny, touch the cold milk. Mommy put the milk in our cart").
- Teach sound-object associations using lots of intonation and inflection.

Play, play, play!

- Laugh and make faces back at the child.
- Play age- and cognitively appropriate activities.

Sing

- Sing songs or do simple games with culturally appropriate actions (e.g., peek-a-boo; Twinkle, Twinkle Little Star; Wheels on the Bus; How big is baby?; I'm going to get you!).

Read

- Read 10 books to your child every day.

Source: Adapted from ASHA (https://www.asha.org/public/speech/development/01/).

up their arms when the mother says "up up up." The child might be attending to the durational aspects and differences as well as the segmental aspects that are salient as they learn to attend and discriminate the sounds of speech.

Table 6–10. Tips for Encouraging Initial Use of Technology

- Use a matter-of-fact approach with technology.
- Don't make pulling out technology a game for the child to get attention.
- Smile when child is touching or pointing at technology.
- Provide toys for both hands for youngsters to distract them from pulling out their technology.
- Use your voice when the technology comes off so they understand they can't hear without it (or sing a song or play the sound from a toy they know).
- Use your voice when replacing the technology so they can hear when the sound comes back on and, if applicable, the difference between hearing through one versus two devices.
- Try to catch the child about to take off their technology and gently guide it back on while smiling and saying, "push push" or "yes, those are your hearing aids."
- Encourage the child to try to put their own technology on by replacing a headpiece or pushing in the earmold.
- When one device falls off, you can vocalize "bah bah bah" and they can learn to hear the difference with one device off and how it sounds when you replace the second device.
- Look disappointed when technology is off and express the concept "but you can't hear me without your hearing aids" by pointing to ears, speaking, or using an object that makes noise.

Table 6–11. Factors to Consider When Assessing Initial Responses to Sounds

Do observers agree that it was a response?

Was the response close enough in time to the auditory event?

Was it just coincidence?

How reliable did the response seem based on the robustness or subtlety of the reaction?

Has the child responded previously to that particular sound or intensity level?

Were there previously evidenced responses that were similar or different to the current evidenced response?

Did the sound event have elements that would predict an awareness by the child due to intensity of the sound or the frequency of the sound?

Based on hearing experience and the technology, does it seem plausible that it was a response?

Auditory Feedback and Development of the Speech Production System; Auditory Retrieval and Expressive Communication
(Tables 6–4 and 6–6)

Early in the prelinguistic stage, auditory development is integrally tied to the stages of vocalizations and the development of auditory comprehension of language, which is also referred to as receptive language.

Time for a Conversation . . .

The child with hearing loss says, "beh" and the mother makes eye contact, leans forward, shrugs her shoulders, and responds, "I don't know, Jake." He is very quiet. She waits and he says, "behdah" in response. Mother says, "Mommy will get Jake a snack." Mother does not really know what the child is saying but she is providing positive reinforcement to the child's vocalization by taking a turn, guessing or predicting what the child might want, or telling the child what is going to happen and creating a conversation. In this simple interaction the mother has incorporated multiple strategies and used "cookie dough" to target all of the initial goals. In this interaction, the mother is also able to incorporate auditory Goals 3 and 4 as listed in Table 6–3. The parent has facilitated vocalizations and encouraged an increased variety of sounds by accepting any vocalization by the child with hearing loss and facilitating more vocalizations.

Serve and return strategies and the expectant pause will promote initial vocal turns. These vocal turns will evolve into the child producing consistent, spontaneous vocalizations with communicative intent. Essentially, for the child who has no language, we are looking at encouraging various levels of babbling (see Table 6–4), up to and including jargoning or babbling phrases (see Chapter 3, Tables 1–23 and 3–10). An initial turn might just be a simple neutral vowel production that is reinforced enthusiastically to encourage repetition and an increase in vocalizations. The more the child vocalizes, the more we understand what is getting to the child's brain. The more the child vocalizes, the more opportunities they have to expand and increase their variety of productions.

Strive to have the child use utterances that sound like phrases or sentences even though they are not using real words at this stage. While playing a game or taking turns with a specific vocal prompt such as when playing peek-a-boo, the parents and professionals can pause and wait as an encouragement for the child to vocalize and then pull off the blanket hiding the person. While playing with stacking blocks in a tower or stacking toy rings, the parents and professionals can say "up, up, up" or "more" with each additional piece being moved. Then you pause, waiting for the child to vocalize or approximate the acoustic event. This simple pause can provide the child with an opportunity to vocalize as a turn and to develop the realization that their voice has power. As the child learns to take turns in these vocal games, the approximations can be monitored for development of different speech features.

These activities promote all of the previous listed speech and expressive language goals, as well as comprehension of language as targeted in Goals 13 through 20. Once again, use the chocolate chip cookie theory to integrate multiple skills in the development of listening and spoken language.

Language Comprehension Development of Auditory Recognition, Sequencing, and Comprehension (Table 6–5)

Allow the child's brain appropriate time to go through the needed steps to begin to respond to their name and understand other highly repeated words. All children will have many words receptively before their first expressive word. Goals in this area are to facilitate and monitor this expected comprehension to determine if the child is making progress and when it might be appropriate or unrealistic to expect the child to progress to their first word and the next stage of spoken language development. The cookie dough principle is strongly illustrated as comprehension is developed upon the foundations of audition, and Goals 3, 4, and 5 in Table 6–3 are not isolated from the following goals. Listening will promote language comprehension.

Activities of Daily Living (ADL)

Daily routines and the auditory ritual as discussed in the strategies sections (see Chapter 5) and the ADL formula will promote recognition and comprehension for the prelinguistic child with hearing loss. When parents are consistent in their use of specific auditory rituals, they provide opportunities for the young prelinguistic child to begin to pay attention to the different segmental and suprasegmental features of the acoustic event. This promotes understanding of the different auditory rituals related to their daily routines. Support the parents in simple activities that are elements of routines you see in your intervention sessions, from greeting when they arrive and leave; opening doors; being picked up or put down; sitting down or standing up; holding adults' hands; and taking, giving, or sharing items.

Routines vary according to families and their situations, but a good place to begin is with the basic human needs of eating, sleeping, love, and nurturing and assist the parent in expanding to personal care such as washing, brushing teeth, and getting dressed. With the parent, examine the stereotypic phrases, key words, or songs that they would naturally use (Table 6–12). Parents who are struggling with these elements of interaction could be helped by having parents collect their stereotypic phrases at home and discuss them with the professional in a subsequent session.

Professionals can assist in increasing the family repertoire if needed by modeling some typical childhood songs, such as a "clean up" song, "this is the way we wash our hands," or a lullaby. Support and help parents to make up their own family songs using familiar tunes that will signal the upcoming event. This allows the child with hearing loss to anticipate what will happen, know their world is predictable, and be more secure and confident in their world.

Start by combining the child's name and mommy in the "Blah, blah, Ginger" example since we know those are the first words a child understands. This strategy will facilitate starting to listen to and learn those names and other key words. If we apply the ADL formula, the names and key words can be repeated many times within that activity. Narrating the actions of what the adult and child are doing allows for this while acoustically highlighting the important two to three words. Simple narration for dressing the child could be: "Mommy has Brian's shirt." "Mommy put the shirt on Brian." "There

Table 6–12. Stereotypic Phrases

Sample Stereotypic Phrases to Use at the Prelinguistic Stage	
All done	Wave bye bye to Daddy
Blow a kiss	Shhhh night night
Pee-yoo, what a stinky diaper	Daddy's/mommy's home
So hungry; let's eat	Clean up clean up
Brush brush your teeth	Let's wash those dirty hands
I'm coming to get you	SO dirty!
Last one down is a rotten egg	Uh oh, it fell down
Oh no, what a mess	Let's get in the car
Who is first?	My turn

is Brian." "Mommy has your socks." While washing the child: "Mommy is going to wash Rachel." "Let's wash Rachel's face." "Rachel has a dirty nose." "Mommy made your nose clean." "Rachel has a dirty chin." "Mommy is washing your chin, Rachel." (Tomasello et al., 2010).

Talk! Talk! Talk!

But what to say? Parents should be talking, but remember to facilitate their use of IDS and CDS, and provide some guidance as to what to say. Listen to the interaction and reinforce the elements that are helpful in facilitating the targeted goals. Encourage the parent to work on serve and return, but balance that with also providing the play-by-play narrative of what is happening at the time (see Chapter 5). In this case, the parents should provide some typical preliminary words that work with daily activities and simple play activities (Table 6–13). The parent learns that they need to provide input that is slightly above the level of the child with hearing loss to promote the next stages of development. Parents can babble back and forth with the prelinguistic child with hearing loss, but they must also provide some words for the child to learn word boundaries and phoneme patterns and to promote the comprehension of key words. Again, while using these strategies and language, we are also targeting all the auditory skills as included in Goals 1 through 5. Note that many of the short words are repeated to allow the child with hearing loss opportunities to hear the sound as it is repeated and used in a pattern or contrast such as "up, up, up" and "*dooooown!*"

Therapy should be fun and engaging, and should use toys and activities that the child enjoys (Chapter 5). Follow the child's interests and select activities that appeal to their cognitive, developmental, and play stages. You could select a variety of toys such as cars, puzzles, dolls, building toys, Play-Doh, drawing materials, dollhouses, and toy kitchen items. Modify the language to be appropriate to the prelinguistic language stage and applicable to the activity. Remember ADL activities will be applicable for all the children and their families.

Table 6–13. Preliminary Words: Examples to Use at the Prelinguistic Stage

Verb Phrases			
sshh, go to sleep		sit down	
up, up, up		down	
wash, wash, wash		blow	
walk, walk, walk		round and round	
pop		bounce, bounce the ball	
shake, shake		uh-oh, it fell down	
have a drink		knock, knock	
close		open	
push, push		pull	
Adjectives			
hot	more	dirty	soft cold
broken	dirty	wet	mmm, that's good
People and Objects			
Mommy		Daddy	baby shoes
watch—tick tock		eye	nose mouth
doggie		bottle	blanket

Source: Bortfeld et al. (2005).

Keep in mind that the suggested words and phrases are not unique to specific toys and that all the phrases and words can be integrated naturally throughout the day. Stacking cups could go "up, up, up, and down," but that language is also for when the child is being picked up or the spoon falls on the floor, or the airplane is up, up in the sky. Spinning a toy, drawing circles with a marker, swinging a child around, or mixing cupcake batter can all be used to reinforce round and round (Wang et al., 2017). Remember that when mixing up the cookie dough we can work on speech production Goals 6 through 12 and expressive language Goals 21 through 23 by simply pausing between the repetitions of a vocal prompt such as "up." Help the parents use the suggested language naturally and applied to the ADL formula.

Sound-Object Associations

Reinforcing and assessing the earliest auditory skills for the child with hearing loss who is new to listening we use a quick shortcut to help us monitor what is getting to the child's brain and is discriminable. You want the child to understand that a specific sound is associated with a specific animal or vehicle (Vaughan, 1976). This will simultaneously promote the auditory goals of discrimination of the suprasegmentals, vowels, and some consonants as noted in Goals 3, 4, and 5. See Table 6–14 for a list of sound-object associations. Keep language, home environments, and cultural diversity in mind. What the rooster says in English might be different in Spanish. Children in some environments might not have exposure to

Table 6–14. Sound-Object Associations

Animals		Vehicles
Cat: meow	Dog: woof woof	Boat: papapapa
Cow: moo	Horse: neigh	Car/truck/bus: beep, beep
Pig: oink oink	Lamb: ba-a-a-a	Airplane: aaaah
Duck: quack, quack	Fish: (no sound)	Train: ch, ch ooo oo
Rabbit: hop, hop, hop	Bird: peep peep	
Rooster: cock-a-doodle-doo	Chicken: cluck	
Frog: hop, hop, hop		

Source: Stockall and Dennis (2012); Vaughan (1976).

some of these items in real experiences, only with toys, books, or pictures. However, another child might go and collect fresh eggs from the chickens before breakfast.

Putting It All Together: Case History

Rachel was identified at 4 months with a profound bilateral sensorineural hearing loss and was aided binaurally. She was implanted at 1 year of age after a trial with hearing aids. Her hearing aids provided limited access to low-frequency sounds, which was evidenced in her use of the suprasegmentals and low-frequency neutral vowels. Initial stimulation of the cochlear implant (CI) was at the age of 1 year, 1 month. Rachel tolerated the implants from the initial fitting and wore them all of her waking hours. Rachel has now been listening with her CIs for 1 month. She plays appropriately with toys, interacts with adults, and has met age-appropriate developmental milestones in the areas of gross motor, fine motor, and cognition skills (Rotfleisch, 2009).

Auditory Processes for Using Sound Meaningfully

Auditory Detection and Attention

Rachel shows good responses to a variety of sounds using her cochlear implants. She will listen to music and voices. She has been observed to point to or touch her ear when she hears a sound. She is not yet responding to all of the Ling sounds. She shows inconsistent awareness of the fricative /ʃ/ and the higher-frequency consonants, such as the plosive /k/ and nasal /ŋ/ manners. No consistent response has been noted to the fricative /s/.

Auditory Discrimination

Rachel has begun to discriminate some of the suprasegmental aspects of speech, including duration, intensity, and pitch, as noted in her spontaneous productions and imitations. In therapy sessions, it was noted that when she vocalized with a vowel and was provided with an auditory-only response of a nasal /m/, she changed from the vowel production using an oral resonance to a nasal sound using a nasal resonance.

Auditory Processes for Learning to Talk

Auditory Feedback

Rachel has increased her spontaneous vocalizations and has used her voice to take conversational turns with adults in the sessions on many occasions. She has begun to modulate the suprasegmental aspects of speech, including duration, intensity, and pitch, in her spontaneous productions. Her vocalizations tend to be of an appropriate intensity, and she does vary her pitch. She is producing a few vowels, including but not limited to: /ʌ/ ("u" as in *but*), /ɛ/ ("e" as in *bed*), and /u/ ("oo" as in *boot*).

At this time, she is not producing any consonants consistently. She has produced the consonants /m/, /p/, and /b/ and will occasionally combine them with a vowel.

Auditory Processes for Learning Language

Auditory Comprehension and Auditory Retrieval

Standardized language testing indicated an age-equivalent score for Rachel of 9 months in receptive language and 7 months in expressive language. She will vocalize and playfully chatter and, though she doesn't use words, she sometimes seems to be using phrases and sentences with intonation patterns of statements or questions.

Rachel demonstrates excellent eye contact and has used her voice to take turns with her mother and the professional on many occasions. She has begun to show awareness that using her voice is an effective means of getting attention and eliciting a response to her needs. She will vocalize to get her mother's attention. She understands a few words (*mommy*, *Rachel*, *up*, *bye bye*). She has just begun to imitate some durational cues and vowel content for words or phrases produced by her mother but is not using any one consistently.

The Intervention Session

(Rachel is sitting on the blanket pulling rings from a stacking toy)

(Mother walks toward Rachel)

Mother (in an excited sing-song-y voice): Hi Rachel

(Mother pauses and waits for a response)

(Mother walks closer to Rachel)

Mother (talking slightly louder, repeats exactly the vocal pattern): Hi Rachel

(Baby stops what she's doing and looks at mother, who is now sitting in front of her. Mother leans down toward baby)

(Baby looks up at her mother's face, mouth, and then eyes)

Rachel (vocalizes a very short sound): Ah

Mother (with lots of intonation and excitement in her voice): Hiiii Rachel. You heard mommy. I heard Rachel.

Rachel: Ah

(Mother smiles again, still maintaining eye contact, and responds immediately)

Mother: I know, Rachel. Let's play.

(Smiling back at her mother, continuing to make eye contact)

Rachel coos: Aaaah

(Mother turns around to get a toy from behind her)

Mother: OK, Rachel. Let's play!

Professional: Perfect; this is just what we want. You are using your voice in a very fun way for her to listen to—all that "motherese" we have been talking about. You spoke to her and paused for her to take a turn and she did—I think three times. Then as soon as she responded with her voice, you answered her. We are setting up her foundations for basic communication: turn taking, pausing, and listening. We want to encourage this as much as possible. I talk, you listen, then you talk and I listen. Let's see if you can get several more turns. Be sure to remember to pause long enough to give Rachel the opportunity to vocalize.

Analysis of Session

In discussion of the therapy session, we will analyze which goals are being addressed in the described interval of therapy. For purposes of this discussion, goal numbers are indicated in parentheses and refer back to numbering used in Tables 6–3 through 6–6. Through these few turns, the mother had the baby attend to her voice (Goals 1a, b) and used lots of inflections to get her attention and to have her listen to the suprasegmental aspects of speech (Goals 1a, b, d; 4a, b). She is establishing some turn taking by immediately responding to the child's vocalizations. Mother is encouraging her use of voice to babble or coo and to have Rachel use her voice to communicate her excitement and responses whenever she vocalizes. This will provide reinforcement and encourage her to vocalize more (Goals 7, 8, 9, 21, 22, 23). The professional reinforced the mother's behaviors, which we want to encourage, and explained how to proceed to the next stage. The professional is being very positive and telling the mother all the good things she is doing, to encourage the mother to repeat those behaviors.

(Mother holding the toy behind her but turning to look at the baby)

Mother (using with a question intonation contour): Yeah Rachel! What should mommy and Rachel play?

Rachel: Ah

(Mother still holding a toy train behind her back but making eye contact with the baby)

Mother: Rachel, do you want to play with the choo choo?

Rachel: Aah

Mother: Yes?

(Mother pauses, holding up the toy train in front of the baby and between them as they had been in mutual gaze)

Mother: Ok! Here's the choo choo.

(Baby reaches toward the toy)

Rachel: Aah

Professional: OK, let's see if we can get her to change the duration. Remember the suprasegmental aspects: duration, intensity, pitch. Let's try to get her vocalization to sound more like yours. Maybe—but maybe not—she will use the duration information. Duration is usually the first suprasegmental feature that the child will play with. Since we know she will sometimes do a longer vowel sound, she may do that or she may try to imitate the pitch change, or she may change the vowel if she listens and realizes what you are saying isn't the same as the "ah." We know she has been doing some different vowels. So try acoustically highlighting the "oooo" so that THE most interesting thing you are saying is "ch ch ooooo" and see if she will pay attention to the difference in the sounds. But she may not change anything. Go ahead and try.

(Mother holding the toy between them)

Mother (making her voice sound like the whistle on a train with an up and down intonation contour): The train goes Ch ch ooooo.

(Baby reaching for the toy)

Rachel: Ah

(Mother moving the train to hold the baby's interest)

Mother: Ch ch oooooooooo.

Rachel: Aaaaah

Professional: OK! Did you catch that?

Mother: What?

Professional: I think that might have been a longer duration attempt and that's great! All the other times when she talked to you, she made a short sound, but this last one was really longer. Also, that was great using her hearing first. You told her what we are going to play before you showed her the toy. You had her listen and then reinforced the auditory message, what you told her by showing the toy. This is a great strategy to use regularly. Now you are both going to look at the train and talk about it and she knows you are talking about the train. You are both paying attention and looking at the train. We call that joint attention. She doesn't have to look at you when you are talking. Let's see if she will do it again…but she may not. Remember to pause to let her know it is her turn.

Analysis of Session

In these turns, the baby is listening to the durational information which the mother is making to characterize the train. She uses her voice with a different quality, almost like singing (Goal 1b). Rachel is being repeatedly provided with the auditory signal, which has very specific suprasegmental patterns and vowel content, and is learning to pay attention to the sound, hear it as different, and approximate the sound (Goals 1a, b; 4a, b; 9; 10; 11). Rachel will learn to associate the sounds with the given object, and other objects will be associated with different suprasegmental patterns and speech patterns (Goals 13, 14).

The professional is reinforcing the concept of the suprasegmentals and reminding the mother about the order of acquisition, what the baby has done before, so we can expect or try to elicit it again. She explains the concept of joint attention and the auditory strategy of talking to establish auditory integration. The baby doesn't need to be looking at the mother when she speaks. The professional reinforces the need to pause but mostly has a positive attitude and tells the mother all the great things that she has done.

> Mother: Ch ch oooooo.
>
> Rachel: Oo ooooo
>
> Professional (with enthusiasm looking at the baby): Yeah Rachel, ch ch oooooo says the train!
>
> (Rachel looks toward the professional)
>
> Professional: FABULOUS job, mom! She did a short sound and a longer sound! She changed and used the right vowel. We want Rachel to know how excited we are about that. She is trying to imitate the duration information she is hearing by using her voice. Do it some more so she can keep listening to the different vowel. Then we will try to change it to a different duration and different vowel for the rabbit.
>
> Mother (making the sound louder, longer and with the same sing-song-y pitch as previously): Ch ch oooooo.
>
> Rachel: Ah aaaaaah
>
> Mother (with the same intonation pattern used previously): Ch ch oooooo.
>
> (Rachel looks at the toy but does not respond)
>
> Mother (same intonation pattern): Ch ch oooo that's the choo choo.
>
> Rachel: Ooo
>
> Mother: Oooooo
>
> Rachel (reaching for the toy): Oooo
>
> (Mother smiles and as she holds the train in front of the baby within her reach, giving the toy train to the baby as she reaches the train. Mom keeps her hands on the train as well)
>
> Mother (enthusiastically): Ch ch ooooo. That's the train. Does Rachel want to hold the train?
>
> Professional: Ch ch oooooo says the train. FABULOUS job, mom! So did you catch what happened?
>
> Mother: Yes! She actually listened to the sound and changed it.
>
> Professional: You are right, mom! You are teaching her to listen and hear the different vowels and different durations of speech sounds and then to say what she is hearing. That is fantastic. She is learning to listen and change the sound because she is engaged with you and you are working on her conversation so she wants to talk to you and grab the train. This is the beginning of her auditory feedback loop.
>
> (Mother and professional both laugh)
>
> Mother: Ch ch oooooo, that's the train. It says choo, choo.
>
> (Baby is busily playing and looking at the toy)
>
> Mother (points to her ear, pushes on the train to make the whistle toot as the baby looks at her)
>
> Mother: Rachel! Listen.
>
> (Rachel's eyes widen and she looks toward the toy)
>
> Mother: Rachel! Good listening.
>
> (Mother points at her ear and then Rachel's ear while nodding her head up and down and smiling)
>
> Mother: I know you heard that, didn't you? Mommy hears that!

(Tooting the train whistle as the baby is playing with the toy train. Again, mother points at her ears and then Rachel's ear, shaking her head up and down and smiling.)

Mother: Listen again. Mommy hears that!

Professional: OK, now let's take out the rabbit and you say "hop, hop, hop." Remember to say it and get her listening before you show it to her—the same as you did with the train.

(Mother is holding the toy rabbit behind her but turning to look at the baby and making eye contact)

Mother (calling the baby and using with a question intonation contour): Rachel! What should Rachel and mommy play?

Rachel (looking up from the toy train): Uh

Mother: Hop, hop, hop. Should mommy and Rachel play with the bunny rabbit?

Mother: That's the bunny. The bunny goes hop hop, hop.

Rachel: Ah

(Mother holds up the toy rabbit in front of the baby and between them as they had been in mutual gaze)

Professional: That was nice, you called her and she turned to you and vocalized. You told her about the rabbit before you took it out. Try to do just the hop, hop and make it important so maybe she will try to imitate that.

Mother: Hop hop hop.

Rachel: Aah aah aah

Mother: Hop hop hop.

Professional: That is great, she changed the duration to a short, repeated sound. Let's go for the vowel. I remember that you told me she has done this vowel in her babbling. I'm going to make the vowel the most important thing for her to listen to by acoustically highlighting it. We can do this with a vowel by making it a bit longer, or a bit louder. Let's see if we can get her to change it. hOp hOp hOp hOp

Rachel: Aah aah aah

(Baby reaches for toy as mom moves the rabbit as if it is hopping through the air)

Mother (moves the bunny in a hopping motion in front of the baby as she moves forward grabbing the toy): hOp hOp hOp hOp.

Rachel: Aah aah aah

Mother (still waving the bunny in the air): hOp hOp hOp hOp.

Rachel: Aaw

Mother: hOp hOp hOp hOp

Professional: That's it! She changed the vowel and is trying to say the right one, but we lost the duration. OK! Don't give her the toy yet. Let her listen and play with the sound and her voice and match what she hears (her perception) with what she says (her production). But if she seems frustrated, give her the toy.

Mother (holding the bunny in the air in front of the baby but high up out of her reach as they both look at the toy): hOp hOp hOp hOp.

Rachel: Aaw

Mother (moving the bunny down and looking at the baby): hOp hOp hOp hOp.

(Rachel continues to look at the toy)

Rachel (reaching again for the toy and moving toward it and grabbing it): Aaw aaw

Mother (with excitement, looking at the baby): Hop hop hop! That's the rabbit. Hop hop hop!!!

Mother (turns to the professional): She really hears that, doesn't she?

Professional: She sure does, and even more than that, you are teaching her to hear sounds as different—long, short, repeated, different vowels. And you are teaching her to use her hearing for auditory feedback to start with a good foundation for her speech intelligibility! Rachel! Hop hop hop!

Rachel: Aw aw

Mother: Hop hop hop hop, yeah, I heard that!

Rachel: Aw aw

Analysis of Session

The mother is continuing to incorporate the goals as mentioned earlier with turn taking, attending to voice, listening to a variety of suprasegmental patterns, encouraging communicative intent, and reinforcing the sound-object association. She uses a variety of strategies such as joint attention, parent speech, expansion, acoustic highlighting, and pausing. At this time, we are focusing on her approximation by duration and the change in vowel. The next step would be to get both features correct. As the baby is not able to produce the "ch" sound, a reasonable production would be the correct duration and the vowel: "oo oo ooooo." As we play with the train, Rachel listens to the train whistle (Goals 1a, d; 13; 14) and we facilitate localization responses (Goal 2). She continues to listen to the three parts of the sound, which is associated with the train and the noun, working on her auditory memory (Goals 1d; 4a, b; 13; 14). Through acoustic highlighting and repetition, the baby showed auditory discrimination ability for the vowel she was producing and the vowel she was hearing from her mother and the professional (Goals 3; 4a, b).

The auditory input allowed Rachel to discriminate the duration information and the vowel and we encouraged the use of her vocalization as the pragmatic functions of turn taking and requesting with communicative intent (Goals 3, 4a, 9, 10, 11, 21, 22, 23). This type of activity will lead to the baby developing auditory recognition of the sounds and comprehending what objects are being indicated by their associated sounds and then by the word (Goals 3; 4a, b, d; 13; 14). In addition, the baby is learning to listen while actively engaged with holding, manipulating, and looking at an object (Goals 1a, b, d; 3; 5).

The professional is positively reinforcing the child and the mother in this scenario. The child vocalizes in response to the model, the behavior of the mother, and the mother's interaction. The mother is then told to continue to see if she can elicit several more of her productions to reinforce the auditory feedback loop—where the child hears the signal and produces the same sound using her emerging ability to match her perception and her production. The professional encourages auditory integration while she and Rachel are engaged in playing to allow the child to integrate listening with other activities. The child is learning to listen while doing other things as well. The professional then directs the mother to use a toy that will have a different durational pattern and a different vowel.

This baby is demonstrating some consistent and basic responses to a variety of sounds, learning to listen to the durational information in speech and to some vowel variety. All these skills need to be expanded and then developed into the next level of skills. Rachel is showing the progression from attending to these sounds, to discriminating them, and to producing them. She must now learn to attend to and discriminate intensity, pitch, and additional vowels and learn to produce and control these aspects of speech. Through everyday interactions and sound-object associations, Rachel will soon move to the next stage of spoken language development. She will attribute meaning and therefore facilitate naming insight and comprehension, and some auditory retrieval and protowords will emerge, moving her out of the prelinguistic stage.

Summary

The professional's knowledge base and work guiding and coaching the parent to understand relevant elements of auditory, speech, and language skills and strategies to promote development in these areas at the prelinguistic stage will help the child to achieve the outlined goals from this stage of language development. The achievement of these goals provides a strong basis for the child with hearing loss to progress to the next level of listening and spoken language abilities. Behaviors that are indicative of the child emerging into the next stage of development are indicated in Table 6–15.

Table 6–15. By the End of the Prelinguistic Stage, the Child Should:

> Demonstrate access to and respond to variety of sounds and speech features.
>
> Show comprehension of a few different words.
>
> Use voice in babbling with communicative intent.
>
> Use a word approximation or protoword.

Discussion Questions

1. How do you determine if a child is at this stage?
2. How would you illustrate the chocolate chip cookie analogy to the parents of a child with hearing loss at this stage?
3. Select a goal from one of the Tables 6–3 through 6–6. How would you explain to a parent to use a specific ADL to target the goal? Consider and identify other goals would be naturally included in that selected ADL.
4. What activities could you do with an older child to work on the goals at this level?
5. Consider a child with additional disabilities or needs and discuss an activity that you could work on to target a selected goal at this level.

References

American Speech-Language-Hearing Association Task Force on Central Auditory Processing Consensus Development (1996). Central auditory processing: Current status and implications for clinical practice. *Journal of Audiology, 5,* 41–52.

American Speech-Language-Hearing Association (n.d.). Developmental norms for speech and language. https://www.asha.org/public/speech/development/chart/

Bergeson, T. R. (2012). Spoken language development in infants who are deaf or hard of hearing: The role of maternal infant-directed speech. *Volta Review, Research Symposium, 111*(2), 171–180.

Bortfeld, H., Morgan, J. L., Golinkoff, R. M., & Rathbun, K. (2005). Mommy and me: Familiar names help launch babies into speech-stream segmentation. *Psychology Science, 16*(4), 298–304.

Brown, V. L., Bzoch, D. R., & League, R. (2020). *Receptive-Expressive Emergent Language Test* (4th ed.). Western Psychological Services.

Friederici, A. D., & Wessels, J. M. (1993). Phonotactic knowledge and its use in infant speech perception. *Perception and Psychophysics, 54*, 287–295.

Lanza, J. R., & Flahive, L. (2008). *Guide to communication milestones: Concepts, feeding, morphology, literacy, mean length of utterance, phonological awareness, pragmatics, pronouns, questions, speech sound acquistion, vocabulary*. LinguiSystems.

Ling, D. (2003). The Ling-Six-Sound Test. *The Listener*, 52–53.

Madell, J. R., Hewitt, J. G., & Rotfleisch, S. (2018). Chapter 25: Red flags: Identifying and managing barriers to the child's optimal auditory development. In J. R. Madell, C. Flexer, Wolfe, & E. C. Schafer (Eds.). *Pediatric audiology: Diagnosis, technology and management* (3rd ed., pp. 267–276). Thieme.

Mandel, D. R., Jusczyk, P. W., & Pisoni, D. B. (1995). Infants' recognition of the sound patterns of their own names. *Psychological Science, 6*, 314–317.

Marschark, M., Duchesne, L., & Pisoni, D. (2019). Effects of age at cochlear implantation on learning and cognition: A critical assessment. *American Journal of Speech-Language Pathology, 28*, 1318–1334.

Rotfleisch, S. (2001). E = mc^2 (English equals milk and cookies too!). *The Listener*, (Fall), 39–42.

Rotfleisch, S. (2009). Auditory verbal therapy and babies. In L. Eisenberg (Ed.), *Clinical management of children with cochlear implants* (pp. 435–493). Plural Publishing.

Rotfleisch, S., & Martindale, M. (2012). How do you know if a child is making appropriate progress in auditory-verbal therapy and education? In W. Estabrooks (Ed.), *101 frequently asked questions about auditory-verbal practice* (pp. 348–352). Alexander Graham Bell Association for the Deaf.

Rossetti, L. M. (1990). *Rossetti Infant-Toddler Language Scale*. LinguiSystems.

Song, J. Y., Demuth, K., & Morgan, J. (2010). Effects of the acoustic properties of infant-directed speech on infant word recognition. *Journal of the Acoustic Society of America, 128*(1), 389–400. https://www.ncbi.nlm.nih.gov/pmc/articles/PMC2921436/10.1121/1.3419786

Stockall, N., & Dennis, L. R. (2012). The dirty dozen: Strategies for enhancing social communication of infants with language delays. *Young Children, National Association for the Education of Young Children, 67*(4), 36–41.

Tomasello, N. M., Manning, A. R., & Dulmus, C. M. (2010). Family-centered early intervention for infants and toddlers with disabilities. *Journal of Family Social Work, 13*(2), 163–172.

Tsiakpini, L., Weichbold, V., Kuehn-Inacker, H., Coninx, F., D'Haese, P., & Almadin, S. (2004). *LittlEARS Auditory Questionnaire*. MED-EL.

Vaughan, P. (1976). *Learning to listen: A book by mothers for mothers of hearing-impaired children*. General Mills Publishing.

Wang, Y., Bergeson, T. R., & Houston, D. M. (2017). Infant-directed speech enhances attention to speech in deaf infants with cochlear implants. *Journal of Speech, Language, and Hearing Research, 60*(11), 3321–3333.

Yeung, H. H., & Werker, J. F. (2009). Learning words' sounds before learning how words sound: 9-Month-olds use distinct objects as cues to categorize speech information. *Cognition, 113*, 234–243.

Chapter 7

Single-Word Communication Stage

Sylvia Rotfleisch

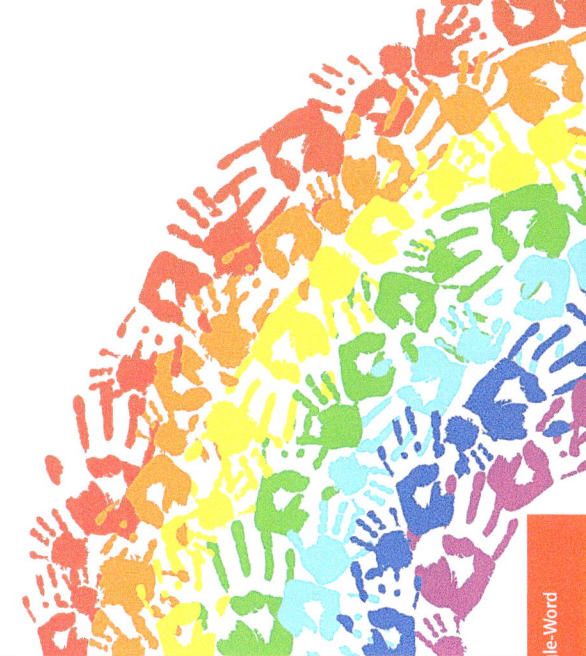

Key Points

- Initial word approximations emerge and indicate foundation skills of listening and spoken language are developing.
- At the single-word stage, the child will learn to attend to, remember, and discriminate sounds and words and learn to comprehend more language.
- The child will use an increased variety of vocalizations with different speech features, which will be used in emerging word approximations.
- Goals should be incorporated into activities of daily living by the family, which will incorporate the culture of the family.
- Goals should be incorporated into play and adapted to the child's age, cognitive and developmental stages, and interests.

Basic Characteristics of the Child at the Single-Word Stage of Communication

Listening

This child has had adequate exposure to the auditory signal to master basic detection skills, understand that sounds have meaning, and provide some predictability to their life. With this understanding comes an increase in attention to various sounds as the child is figuring out which sounds are of significance to them—or not. A child at this stage will show interest in infant-directed speech (IDS) and known auditory rituals. The child has typically learned that the technology provides important information and is showing stronger signs of bonding with it. From this point, the child will continue to learn the significance of new sounds, new language, new auditory patterns, and rituals that are important, but will typically begin to learn to ignore sounds that are of no particular significance (Hogan et al., 2008). This can sometimes be confused with lack of detection of sounds and must be monitored.

The child with hearing loss who has begun to use word approximations is learning that sounds are differentiated by a variety of features and attends to differences in suprasegmental features, vowels and some consonant manners (Obenchain et al., 1998). The order of emergence of the various consonant features will depend on the hearing loss and on the auditory access provided by the child's technology (see Speech Acoustics in Chapter 1). These beginning auditory abilities typically evident and/or emerging in the single-word stage are indicated in Table 7–1. Skills listed are not sequential.

Language

Children at the single-word communication stage are showing emerging understanding when spoken to and are starting to speak or vocalize to express needs. It is typical for children to use babbling as communicative attempts and contributions. The child at this stage has begun to use their first word approximation, which is also referred to as a *protoword*. First words, for typically developing children as well as for children with hearing loss, are not clearly articulated, but are a rela-

Table 7–1. Auditory Abilities Evidenced in the Single-Word Stage

- Listens to songs and stories for a short time.
- Turns when you call their name.
- Listens to simple stories, songs, and rhymes.
- Follows one-part simple direction (e.g., "Put that down," "Come here," "Stop that," "Wave bye-bye").
- Demonstrates a one-item auditory memory.
- Localizes sounds from varying directions and distance.
- Monitors own voice.
- Imitates words and sounds.
- Discriminates suprasegmentals (DIP).
- Discriminates vowels.
- Understands/recognizes different vocal tones of speakers as a reflection of mood.
- Recognizes sounds by sequences and patterns.
- Recognizes familiar songs (will independently do appropriate actions/gestures).
- Discriminates and identifies stereotypic phrases and auditory routines.
- Discriminates a variety of speech features including several vowels and consonants of different manners of production (e.g., nasal, plosive, semivowel, fricative).
- Able to listen while engaged in an activity.
- Knows certain sounds go with specific animals or objects specific to culture and home language.
- Can listen to a voice with competing sounds.

Sources: REEL (2020); LittlEARS (2004); ASHA Milestones (2021); Integrated Scales of Development (Cochlear) (2012).

tively consistent approximation so that a parent can recognize them. Parents will identify the word approximations, saying, "*Baba* is how he says *bottle*." They can be used consistently for an object, person, or action but they are not true words as recognized by linguists.

At this stage, the child has learned to understand and extract some key words that they hear consistently in their environment. They are learning how to learn words by figuring out word boundaries and sounds that begin words or end words in their home language (Bortfeld et al., 2005). The child with hearing loss will continue to develop receptive skills and vocabulary at a more rapid rate than expressive skills at this stage of development (Zaidman-Zait & Dromi, 2007). Typically, children will understand about 50 words when they are able to produce about 10-word approximations (Gleason & Ratner, 2009). Receptive and expressive language abilities evidenced or expected to emerge in this stage are included in Table 7–2 (Language and Speech Skills Evidenced in the Single-Word Stage). Skills listed are not sequential.

Table 7–2. Language and Speech Skills Evidenced in the Single-Word Stage

Audition and Auditory Comprehension of Language	Expressive Language/Vocalization and Communication
• Understands words for common items and people (e.g., *daddy*, *ball*, *cup*, *shoe*, *juice*). • Points to a few body parts when asked. • Responds to simple questions such as "Who's that?" or "Where's the car?" • Understands and follows simple requests. • Points to pictures in a book when named. • Uses gestures (e.g., waves "bye" or "hi," reaches for "pick you up," shakes head "no"). • Brings an item when requested. • Knows family members' names. • Selects a known item correctly from a group. • Shows more comprehension than expression. • Receptive vocabulary increases by a word per month and then a word or more per week. • Understands simple expressions and comments (e.g., *stop*, *no*, *all done*). • Understands yes/no questions.	• Uses one- or two-word approximations (e.g., *hi*, *more*, *dada*, *mama*). • Imitates words and sounds. • Points to objects to show them to others. • Indicates wants by combining voice with gestures. • Uses culturally appropriate sound-object associations for animals, vehicles. • Talks to toys and objects. • Attempts to vocalize with a familiar song. • Uses words to indicate doesn't want something (e.g., *no*). • Uses some words when requested (e.g., "say 'hi'" or "say 'bye bye'"). • Says new words—slow emergence initially and then more regularly. • Uses jargon utterances that might have real words embedded. • Starts to name pictures in books. • Begins to use expressions (e.g., *uh oh!*). • Learns some two-word expressions (e.g., *all done*, *clean up*). • Demonstrates a variety of pragmatic functions using words. • Imitates words and sounds.

Sources: REEL (2020); LittlEARS (2004); ASHA Milestones (2021).

Speech

Speech at this stage is an integral component of expressive skills (see Table 7–2) and behaviors. It is typical for a child at this stage of speech development to imitate some sounds heard. Production abilities are primarily evidenced by the progression through the stages of babbling (Chapter 3, Babble Skills; Table 3–10). Speech babble skills can continue and some initial speech production abilities can be expected to emerge as the first words develop. Canonical babble, including reduplicative and jargoning, initially will include bilabial consonants such as /p/, /b/, /m/, and /w/ and then expand to other consonants. The use of one or more of these initial consonants can be expected in some of the first words. The first words any child says are not expected to be clear. These first words are more appropriately described as approximations.

The child with hearing loss is learning to listen and discriminate the suprasegmentals and to produce vocalizations that reflect what is heard. Control of speech productions is practiced in babbling and is initially evident with the emerging use of vowels and the use of vowels to modify and control the suprasegmental speech features of duration, intensity, and pitch (DIP). At this early stage of speech production, DIP creates intonation that allows the child to express pragmatic functions and moods. We can tell from the way the child uses their voice if they are content, sad, excited, or angry. Intonation can be used to ask a question, even if just a babble string or a single-word approximation. The child with hearing loss who had been nonvocal has begun to use their voice for word approximations and might be moving through some vocal play and/or the babble stages.

Goals for the Single-Word Stage

Developing an Appropriate Therapy Plan by Addressing Strengths and Areas of Need

The normal sequence of development will be followed to develop listening skills and appropriate speech and language abilities. All previous goals will be used as the basis for expanding to the next skills. Some goals from the prelinguistic stage might not be mastered and might be carried over initially in this stage. Goals for the single-word stage focus on:

- facilitating listening abilities through technology for attending, memory, and discriminating speech features,
- facilitating vocalizations with increased variety of speech features,
- facilitating comprehension of language, and
- facilitating expanded use of word approximations.

Select appropriate goals based on your assessment results that identify the child's strengths and needs (see Chapter 4). With the understanding of speech features and the acoustics parameters related to an audiogram, you can monitor for emerging skills. Based on the hearing loss, you can predict and prepare for areas of potential difficulty (see Chapter 1). Goals must be individualized within the stage to meet the child's needs. Consider, for example, when determining goals related to language comprehension. One child may show limited comprehension of stereotypic phrases, and the goal would focus on increasing that ability with and without context (Goals 16, 19).

However, with a child who understands many stereotypic phrases, you will expand that understanding but can use those phrases as the basis for increasing the auditory memory (Goals 5, 6, 20). You can help the child attend to and understand longer linguistic messages by combining a stereotypic phrase with another known word or phrase. For the child who understands "wave bye-bye," you can facilitate comprehension for two elements, combining the known phrase with a known name. The message "wave bye-bye to daddy," is more specific and requires that the child attend to and comprehend both the phrase "wave bye-bye" and the name.

Select goals that address the strengths and needs of the child to expand the listening and spoken language skills. The use of various speech sounds is an indication of the emergence of auditory discrimination of those speech features. Target additional discrimination abilities that will support production of additional phonemes to expand the child's current skills. The child has learned the significance of listening to words and has learned how to learn words. Choose goals for the use of vocalizations, to express pragmatic functions, to understand relevant words and phrases, and to use word approximations. Goals to increase auditory memory (i.e., attending to words) and to learn more words (i.e., expanding expressive use of word approximations) will provide the foundation skills for the stage of word combinations.

Typical Goals for the Single-Word Communication Stage

Typical, recommended goals for children with hearing loss at the single-word communication level are included in Tables 7–3 to 7–6. Goals are organized based upon defined skills related to the brain functions necessary for learning to use audition for language development (see Chapter 3). The goals included in these tables should not be considered the definitive set of goals for all children at this stage, neither should they be considered an exhaustive list of possible audition goals for children with hearing loss at the single-word communication stage. Goals must address the specific errors and needs determined during comprehensive assessment as well as from observation and informal diagnostic work.

How Do We Work on These Goals?

Professionals must have a knowledge base and multiple appropriate strategies (see Tables 7–7 and 7–8) applicable to the child in the single-word stage to accomplish the recommended goals. The knowledge and strategies included in these tables are the basis for you to guide and coach the parent as the primary person to develop their child's listening and spoken language abilities.

The parents will be learning strategies and implementing them during therapy sessions. Basic principles as used with the prelinguistic child continue to be the foundation for interactions. At the stage of single-word communication, you will use IDS with optimal use of DIP, use simplified language, promote serve and return, engage in natural interactions, and play as age and cognitively appropriate for the child.

You will support parents to use these strategies (see Table 7–8). The parent who began with these strategies in the

Table 7–3. Auditory Goals for Understanding Sound as Meaningful in the Single-Word Stage

Auditory Attention, Detection, Discrimination, and Memory

1. Attend to of a variety of speech features (evidenced by responses, discrimination and productions or imitations):
   a. suprasegmentals: Duration, intensity, pitch (DIP)
   b. vowels and diphthongs
   c. oral versus nasal resonances
   d. manners of consonant production
   e. places of consonant production
   f. voicing of consonant production
2. Discriminate speech features with decreased intensity or from increased distance:
   a. suprasegmentals
   b. vowels
   c. manners of consonant production
   d. places of consonant production
   e. voicing of consonant production
3. Indicate when technology is off or not working.
4. Reinforce and facilitate localization and consistent responses to name and other relevant auditory signals, including from increasing distances using technology.
5. Facilitate ability to attend for auditory-only recognition and comprehension tasks, including sentences and phrases of two to four words.
6. Expand and reinforce an auditory memory for two to four items.
7. Expand awareness and localization of environmental sounds that are part of auditory rituals.
8. Facilitate auditory discrimination of stereotypic phrases on the basis of rhythmic structure and known words.
9. Discriminate words consisting of varying syllabification (one, two, or three syllables) in a limited set using familiar words.
10. Facilitate and reinforce use of audition only for closed set discrimination.
11. Facilitate singing songs with accompanying actions and hand gestures.
12. Facilitate and reinforce use of audition to attend to voices when motorically or visually occupied in play and actively engaged in activities.

prelinguistic stage should be using them consistently. As their child reaches the single-word stage, you will introduce the parents to some new strategies. It is always important that strategies rapidly carry over into natural daily interactions. When the parent is new to listening and language intervention, they might not be familiar with strategies introduced at the earlier stage of prelinguistic language. They could be using some appropriate strategies but also some that do not

Table 7–4. Auditory Feedback and Speech Production Goals in the Single-Word Stage

Auditory Goals for Development of the Speech Production System
13. Develop and expand control in babbling (phonetic level) and word approximations (phonologic level) for: 　a. suprasegmentals: duration, intensity, pitch (DIP) 　b. vowels and diphthongs to include a variety of low-, mid-, and high-frequency vowels and diphthongs 　c. oral versus nasal resonances 　d. manners of consonant production 　e. fricative and affricate manners of production initially including, but not limited to, /h/, /ʃ/, /s/, and /tʃ/ with vowel variety 　f. places of consonant production within different manners of production 　g. voicing of consonant production within different manners of production
14. Facilitate and expand speech productions through auditory feedback loop using imitations, attempting to sing along, turn taking, and spontaneous vocalizations in prompted situations and spontaneously, and with modeling of language stimulus varying by suprasegmental aspects, vowels, and consonant content at phonologic level.

Table 7–5. Auditory Goals for Language Comprehension in the Single-Word Stage

Auditory Recognition, Sequencing, and Comprehension
15. Identify objects by associated sounds that vary in suprasegmental qualities and vowel content.
16. Develop and reinforce auditory recognition of stereotypic phrases on the basis of rhythmic structure, known words, and contextual cues.
17. Facilitate and expand comprehension of one- to four-syllable functional words and phrases.
18. Stimulate and expand auditory comprehension of language in the areas of functional words, phrases (e.g., *up, down, bye-bye, all gone, more*), nouns, verbs, and adjectives.
19. Develop and reinforce auditory comprehension of words and stereotypic phrases without contextual cues.
20. Develop and reinforce auditory comprehension of phrases based on one to two known words (directives and statements) (e.g., "give it to mommy," "show me your nose," "I see the doggie").
21. Monitor and record auditory comprehension of vocabulary every 2 months.

support listening and spoken language competence. Guide and coach them to understand more optimal strategies. Help parents so that strategies that are new to them quickly carry over into natural daily interactions with their child. Parents will soon start to sound like the professional. Help parents to understand knowledge

Table 7–6. Auditory Goals for Developing Expressive Language in the Single-Word Stage

Auditory Retrieval and Expressive Communication
22. Stimulate expressive language in the areas of functional words, phrases, nouns, verbs, and adjectives.
23. Facilitate vocal productions as a turn using word and phrase approximations in context, correct suprasegmental aspects, phoneme content, and syllabification.
24. Facilitate and expand consistent use of babbling and word approximations to communicate a variety of pragmatic functions (e.g., requesting, protesting, responding, turn taking, attention getting).
25. Facilitate and expand productions of functional words and phrases of one to four syllables.
26. Monitor and record expressive vocabulary every 2 months.

related to the next skills in listening and spoken language development with their child with hearing loss.

The parent and professional will use IDS or child-directed speech (CDS) to play and interact with the child with hearing loss, as they did in the prelinguistic stage. You should continue to be aware of the cookie dough theory (Chapter 5). Listening skills become linked to receptive abilities from this stage. The child must listen, attend, and remember the sounds they are accessing through audition. As we target speech production (see Table 7–4), it becomes part of the emergence of expressive language. The child listens to, understands, and expresses themselves by producing sounds. The consistent access to the auditory input of people talking to the child results in the emergence and expansion of comprehension of words and language.

The child has learned how to learn words. They continue to learn more words in this stage, as the parents continue to provide input appropriately. As their vocabulary develops, the child can keep more than one idea in their brain. This is their short-term auditory memory, which will expand to two items in this stage. They will understand these ideas and learn to keep more than one word in their auditory memory. You and the parents facilitate this ability through everyday interactions that allow the child to hear familiar words combined. For example, as the child develops more receptive vocabulary, they will understand "all done" and "bottle." The child will demonstrate the ability to keep these two concepts in their mind. We see when the child holds out the bottle to the parent in response to, "Are you all done with the bottle?" that they are holding the ideas of "all done" and "bottle" at the same time in their auditory memory.

Knowledge areas and strategies applicable to the child at the single-word stage are identified in Tables 7–7 and 7–8. Additional suggested activities for you to use and to guide and coach the parents are included in Table 7–9.

Table 7–7. Knowledge Areas in the Single-Word Stage

- Hearing technologies being used
- Effective troubleshooting of technology
- Speech acoustics—initially related to single-word stage (e.g., low frequency including DIP, vowels)
- Initial stages of development of audition
- Advanced stages of babble development
- Initial stages of development of expressive language
- Initial stages of development of receptive language
- Ling six sounds
- Reading and the beginning of literacy
- Developmental of initial morphemes

Table 7–8. Optimal Strategies to Implement in the Single-Word Stage

- Infant- and child-directed speech/caregiver ease (IDS, CDS)
- Acceptance of vocalizations
- Serve and return
- Expectant pause
- Singing
- Songs and rhymes with associated actions and gestures
- Reading
- Stereotypic phrases
- Narrate
- Three-act play
- 24/7 and ADL
- "Blah, blah, Ginger"
- Auditory maximizing strategies: joint attention, positioning to support audition
- Sound-object associations
- Dangling carrot
- Chocolate chip cookie theory
- Acoustic highlighting for initial morphemes

Targeting and Incorporating Goals

Auditory Attention, Detection, Memory, Discrimination, Auditory Recognition, Sequencing, and Comprehension
(Tables 7–3 and 7–5))

In this section, we explore a few suggested activities and their elements that will lend themselves to facilitating the listening goals and the comprehension goals.

Activities of Daily Living (ADL)

The parent and child with hearing loss interact throughout the day in natural routines. The child's waking hours are filled with family routines and activities related to the child's care and play. All of these events allow for an abundance of opportunities for the repetitive use of closed set language related to all that is part of daily life (see ADL in Chapter 2). Keep in mind that any activity can be divided into the preparation, the actual activity, and the completion. Also, remember to use the Three-Act Play (Chapter 5) for good use of a variety of verb tenses.

There is a never-ending source of vocabulary inherent in life. Be aware that specific activities have specific vocabulary and concepts. Dressing naturally involves body parts, items of clothing, plurals, and prepositions. We put clothing items on, we put body parts in! A very natural way to introduce or reinforce sequencing is with underwear before pants and socks before shoes. Further, exploit the natural and very specific language of a meal. You can include items in the kitchen, all the

Table 7–9. Guide and Coach Parents To:

Implement optimal strategies for single-word stage (Table 7–8)

Listen!
- Monitor the child's responses to sounds.
- Create auditory rituals and stereotypic phrases for activities of daily living (ADL).
- Play with sounds.
- Talk about sounds around the house (e.g., "Listen to the . . . ").

Talk, talk, talk!
- Speak in the language that is natural in the home.
- Talk to child while doing things and going places.
- Expand the word or word approximations the child says.
- Use a variety of words and short sentences with correct grammar as a model for the child to learn.
- Allow the child a chance to take a turn and contribute to the conversation.
- Talk about the who, what, where, when throughout the day and during ADL (e.g., "We are at the park. Billy can go in the swing. Mommy is pushing Billy. Billy is going back and forth," "We are at the store. I need to get some milk. Let's find the milk. Here, mommy found the milk. Mommy is holding the cold milk. Jenny, touch the cold milk. Mommy put the milk in the cart."
- Use a variety of verbs with -ing structure to describe actions and events (e.g., "You are drinking your bottle").

Play, play, play!
- Use plurals to demonstrate the difference between one and many (e.g., "You have a car. Here are lots of cars").
- Use sound object associations along with name of the object (e.g., "moo says the cow," "ch ch oo goes the train").
- Use prepositions and prepositional phrases (e.g., "put block in the box," "your spoon is on the table," "sit down on the chair," "the ball is under the blanket").

Sing
- Sing songs and do fingerplays with hand gestures.
- Make up songs to accompany actions that they are doing.

Read
- Read to the child every day.
- Find books with large pictures and a few words on each page. Talk about the pictures on each page.
- Encourage the child to point to pictures.
- Have their child point to pictures that you name.
- Ask their child to name pictures.

Theory of Mind
- Use thinking language (e.g., "I wonder where . . . ," "I think the boy is hungry"). Think aloud (e.g., "I . . . wonder, think, know, imagine, forgot, remember") during play and routines.
- Use thinking language during playtime.
- Incorporate imaginative scenarios into routine play (e.g., put toys in unusual place and ask, "What was your bunny thinking when he climbed in your shoe?").
- Follow child's lead and use feelings and tuning-in language (e.g., "You want the ball," "You were upset because you thought I was leaving," "I was upset because you grabbed my glasses").
- Describe wants and feelings of others. Look for opportunities and teachable moments to explain what people think and want (e.g., if you have ever seen another child having a tantrum).
- Discuss different likes and dislikes. Think about food for different people and animals (e.g., "Should we feed a banana to the horse or the monkey? Who might like the carrot? Do you like those? I don't like carrots!").

Sources: Compiled from ASHA: https://www.asha.org/public/speech/development/01/
http://www.hanen.org/helpful-info/articles/tuning-in-to-others-how-young-children-develop.aspx
Hearing First Theory of Mind handout

different foods, implements, utensils, and appliances.

Be sure to discuss if we are hungry, decisions about whether it is time to eat, where to eat, what to eat, preparing the food, and then cleaning up. Consider the variety of verbs related eating and food preparation. We barely scratch the surface of verb variety by using: *eating*, *chewing*, *swallowing*, *pouring*, *cutting*, *cooking*, *baking*, *drinking*, *mixing*, and *frying*. Use all the language to narrate and be sure to pause to encourage serve and return (e.g., "I'm thirsty. I think you could be thirsty. Let's go to the kitchen. We need a cup. Here's my glass. Your cup is on the table. You need a drink. Let's pour some water in my glass. I'm pouring in your cup. Here is your cup of water").

Talk! Talk! Talk!

Immerse the child in the sea of meaningful and interactive language. Talk about the here and now. Use short phrases to talk about what you are doing. Talk about objects. Let the child know where you are in the house and what things you or the child are playing with or using. Talk about where things are using prepositions (e.g., "Let's sit on the floor," "We can change your diaper in your room," "The socks are on your toes," "Let's read the book that is on the table"). As the child listens, encourage them to take a turn, babble, or say a word with communicative intent. The adult must remember to pause and wait to provide an opportunity for the child to take a turn.

Play! Play! Play!

Play is the child's work. This is the time to follow the child's lead. Modify the language to be appropriate to the single-word stage and applicable to the activity. Now you can reinforce turn taking with communicative intent and appropriately incorporating narrating. Talk about the toy. Name it. Talk about it. There will be excellent opportunities for prepositions and positional words as the toys go up, down, in, on, out—whether stacking blocks into a tower, putting puzzle pieces in their spaces, playing with a ball, or playing with toy cars or a stuffed animal. The three-act play (Chapter 5) fits here. Use verbs that are specific to the play activity and can be used with the *-ing* ending to facilitate the present progressive verb form. The child is pushing, pulling, lifting, racing, stopping, moving, dropping, throwing, bouncing, catching, rolling, and of course playing! You can make cleaning up part of playing.

What's Next?

Announce life. Narrate here too. Help the child anticipate and then predict what will happen. Understanding what is going to happen provides a sense of security, particularly for the child who is newer to listening. Stereotypic phrases are easily associated with daily routines. Once the child understands some of the language for the activity, we can add easily expand auditory memory by adding activities, items, and routines. This is the time to create and expand the closed-set language for the variety of different routines. For example, a bedtime routine can be used beginning with the stereotypic phrase (e.g., "Night-night time" and "Bedtime story time" soon combines with other closed-set familiar language for the bedtime routine: "Let's get your blankie, it's night-night time," "Let's get a book to read for your bedtime story while you can snuggle with your blankie").

Action-Packed Singing

Simple childhood songs with gestures, rhythm, rhymes, and repetition meet so many goals for children at this stage. We recommend using the ones that peers will be singing and learning, rather than some that might be made up or geared to children with hearing loss. Look for the ones that are natural to the child's culture, environment, peers, and siblings. Different cultures have their own songs and those are great. So many of these exist and they are very easy to find in books, videos, and online sources. You might begin with common ones such as *Wheels on the Bus* or *Twinkle, Twinkle Little Star*. Keep expanding to more songs, particularly as the child shows the ability to tell the difference between songs through audition only without seeing the actions first!

Success Breeds Success!

We all know those first word approximations are fabulous! Accept the words and the babble as a communication intent. This acceptance means success for the child with hearing loss. Success will foster more attempts and, therefore, more success. Be sure to foster interaction rather than imitations or cheering that the child said a word. Be the dangling carrot by using the accurate word targeted by the approximation. Add to it, clarify the meaning, and expand the auditory memory. For example, when the child says "buh" you can respond, "Yes, that is a book." Take the word and turn it to a short phrase: "We can read the book. Let's get the book." Any expansion is going to convey that you understood the message of their approximations. You celebrate their achievement and serve and return contributions and expand.

Books! Books! Books!

At this stage, the first steps toward literacy should be emerging, and consistently reading is essential. Depending on the age and cognitive level of the child with hearing loss, find books that appeal to the child, books with rhythm, books with rhyme, and books with repetition (see *The Reading Teacher's Book of Lists*). Read with enthusiasm. Read with energy. Read with intonation and different voices. Reading can be a full sensory experience. Let the child see, hear, touch, and even chew the book. Make reading part of the daily routine, and read many books every day.

Don't Forget the Obvious!

Adding to known language and the stereotypic phrases, we must expose children with hearing loss to the language that other children would overhear. To help with that we must add the understood but sometimes unspoken part of the message. For example, instead of saying, "We get the milk. We pour the milk. We wash the cup," expand to "Get the milk from the fridge. We pour the milk into the cup. We wash the cup in the sink." This expands to all the language we are providing to the child. They will go to sleep in their bed. Tuck them in, under the blanket. Put toothpaste on the toothbrush. Brush their teeth with the toothbrush.

Auditory Feedback and Speech Production Development of the Speech Production System, Auditory Retrieval, and Expressive Communication
(Tables 7–4 and 7–6)

Activities described earlier, for listening and comprehension goals, will be used to facilitate the goals in the areas of speech production and expressive communication. We do not use an activity for only one area of development or one goal. All the activities we have discussed are meant to be interactive and a starting point for natural interaction integrating listening, speech, and spoken language (see the chocolate chip cookie theory in Chapter 5).

Each of the suggested activities should be used to facilitate expressive language use and speech production for the word approximations. When reading books, we can use auditory closure to encourage the child to complete a word in a book with a pattern. We can point to a picture and ask, "Who's that? What do you see?" Use open-ended questions to encourage any response as a correct response. Singing allows the child to learn repeated patterns with intonation and to try to vocalize along; e.g., "all through the town, round and round." When announcing that it is snack time, if we add "What do you want to eat?" we set up serve and return and provide the opportunity for the child to respond. When the child gets the requested food, or a discussion that it is not time for a cookie, the return was successful, continuing with the use of preliminary words, stereotypic phrases, and sound-object associations (see Chapter 6; Tables 6–12, 6–13, and 6–14).

Serve and Return

The expansion of turn taking facilitates learning about conversational norms such as taking a turn and pausing to allow for a turn. We provide opportunities to use speech productions and word approximations to talk in a dialogue. The premise is, "You talk, I listen. I talk, you listen." The child does not need to say specific words at this time. Encourage and accept babbling as a turn rather than providing a word for them to imitate. Serve and return will foster communication, not imitation (see Chapter 5).

Speak Using the Auditory Feedback Loop!

Babbling back and forth can be interactive. Serve and return can be fun. When a child takes a turn makes a sound, then you change the sounds. This way you can encourage listening, and the child might change their productions. You can produce some strings of syllables, and at this stage the child will often imitates those different speech sounds. This allows for facilitation of the auditory feedback loop. You can monitor the sounds the child is beginning to discriminate, identify, and then produce through their auditory feedback loop. When baby says "babababa," we can use serve and return and respond by changing the suprasegmentals, the vowel, or consonant (e.g., *babadada* or *beebeebee*).

Accept the child's word approximation, say the word clearly to accept their communication, and let them be successful. Use the principle of enhancing perception (see Chapter 5) by repeating the word clearly and matching the clear production with the approximation, then let them hear the word embedded in a phrase or sentence. This allows for the child to develop an auditory feedback loop and transitions phoneme perception to production and from the phonetic level to the phonologic level. For example, when the little one says "mo" for more, you can respond with "Oh! More. You want more. You have no more. I will put more in your cup" or "read more books."

Play Dumb!

As the child's receptive and expressive language develops provide the opportunity and encouragement for them to use their emerging language. Use some enthusiastic encouragement and strategies to facilitate serve and return with communicative intent for different pragmatic functions. Step back from anticipating their every need and encourage them to use their approximations or voice along with gestures to express their needs. For example, when the child waves their hands in the air, you could anticipate that the child wants to be picked up. Then you would walk over and pick up the child. That didn't facilitate a verbal interaction. However, do not pick a word for the situation and insist on an imitation. This could drive the child to tears or set up a battle of wills (communication versus imitation; see Chapter 5).

Use the pause and quizzical look of expectation to encourage vocalizations. A pause can facilitate a vocal production with communicative intent. You could respond, "I see you. What do you want?" As the hands continue to wave, you can play dumb. Say, "Are your hands dirty?" and pause for a response. The child might vocalize to accompany the waving hands. If the child does not respond but continues to hold up their hands, you can ask "Up? Do you want to come up?" providing an option of a known word to consider as a turn. Then you can use the three-act play and as you pick up the child, provide the language that goes with the situation.

Putting It All Together: Case History

Billy, age 1 year 11 months, was identified at 10 months with a severe to profound sensorineural hearing loss in his right ear and a profound sensorineural hearing loss in his left ear. The diagnosis is possible enlarged vestibular aqueduct and he may have had typical hearing until 8 months of age. At that age, he sustained a bump to his head by falling outdoors as he was cruising along a gate. His parents noted several months later that he had stopped babbling and he was no longer frightened by loud noises that he had reacted to when he was younger. He was aided at 11 months and wore his hearing aids for most of his waking hours. He has been enrolled in weekly auditory-verbal therapy (AVT) sessions since he was aided. No consistent responses were noted with his hearing aids. At the age of 1 year 5 months, he underwent surgery for a cochlear implant in his right ear and was initially stimulated at 1 year 6 months. He uses his implant consistently and appears to be benefiting from the auditory information that it provides. He requests his implant as soon as he wakes up in the morning and often will not let his parents take off the device when he goes to sleep. His parents are pursuing a second implant for him at this time. Billy is cooperative, interacts well with adults during the sessions, and plays appropriately with toys presented to him. He has been receiving consistent programming by his CI audiologist for 6 months. All developmental milestones have been age-appropriate to date. He continues to attend weekly AVT sessions (Rotfleisch, 2009).

Auditory Processes for Using Sound Meaningfully

Auditory Attention

Billy is able to attend to a variety of auditory signals, including speech and environmental sounds. He is able to attend to a key word used at the beginning or end of a sentence or embedded within a short phrase or sentence when acoustically highlighted. He attends to a variety of stereotypic phrases, many of which are specific to his family and experiences.

Auditory Memory

Billy shows a consistent one-item auditory memory for one key word in a sentence. He is able to remember and repeat a series of three to five consonant and vowel combinations in words (e.g., *bang-bang*, *teddy bear*). He will repeat familiar key words placed at the beginning or end of a sentence or embedded within phrases when they are acoustically highlighted.

Auditory Discrimination

Billy is consistently responding to and discriminating all of the Ling six sounds (i.e., /m/, /u/, /ɑ/, /i/, /ʃ/, /s/), as evidenced by his pointing to the correct object or picture card when the sound is presented or by imitating some of the sounds. This is an indication that he is able to detect across the speech frequencies with his cochlear implant and is a good initial indicator for the development of the different speech sounds and for the continued development of receptive language. He demonstrates awareness to environmental sounds and responds to his name when called from a distance. He is also attending to different intensities of sounds (e.g., a whispered voice), voices, and music. He is able to attend to suprasegmental and segmental information through audition only. He attends to and discriminates familiar, context-related language when occupied in a play activity (e.g., "Turn it around," "Roll the ball"). He is able to attend through audition only to sentences with one to two familiar words (e.g., "Where is your hat?" "Shhh, the baby is sleeping"). He understands multiple stereotypic phrases that are used at home, and comprehends phrases based on one to two key words. His babbling and word approximations tend to be accurate by syllable and vowel content, as do many imitations or productions in response to a modeled word.

Auditory Integration

Billy is able to attend to suprasegmental and segmental information through audition only. He attends to and discriminates familiar, context-related language when visually or motorically occupied in an activity.

Auditory Processes for Learning to Talk

Auditory Feedback

At the present time, Billy uses a variety of vowel sounds consistently in his spontaneous babbling and word approximations. These include, but are not limited to:

/a/ ("o" as in *bomb*)

/i/ ("ee" as in *beep*)

/u/ ("oo" as in *boot*)

/au/ ("ow" as in *bowwow*)

/ai/ ("ye" as in *bye, bye*)

/o/ ("o" as in *boat*)

/ʊ/ ("oo" as in *book*)

/ɪ/ ("i" as in *big*)

/æ/ ("a" as in *bad*)

/ʌ/ ("u" as in *but*)

He has an increased variety and spontaneous use of consonants in a variety of manners of production. His phonemes are emerging in an appropriate sequence and are an excellent indication of good access to the auditory information through his cochlear implant. He most typically produces the following phonemes:

Plosives:
/b/ as in *bee*
/p/ as in *pea*
/t/ as in *tea*
/d/ as in *do*

Nasals:
/m/ as in *my*
/n/ as in *no*

Fricatives:
/h/ as in *hop*
/ʃ/ as in *she*

Semivowels
/w/ as in *we*
/j/ as in *you*

Auditory Processes for Learning Language

Auditory Recognition

Billy has acquired many new word approximations in the past months, which are indicative of his developing recognition of auditory patterns.

Auditory Comprehension and Auditory Retrieval

Billy's language abilities were assessed with a standardized evaluation, which indicated he has an age equivalent of 20 months in receptive language and 18 months in expressive language.

Billy has a growing expressive vocabulary of basic words that he uses spontaneously but that are not yet clearly articulated. He produces sounds for many vehicles and animals. Billy has about 30 words or word approximations, which he uses expressively at this time. These words include, but are not limited to:

more	*mommy*	*roll roll*
shoes	*uh oh*	*up*
hot	*ouch*	*pull*
shake	*Billy*	*moo*
help	*ball*	*bounce*
teddy bear	*shake*	*milk*
daddy	*ch ch ooo*	*airplane*
go	*train*	*no*
night, night	*thank you*	*open*
push	*bang, bang*	*bye, bye*
no	*aaah (airplane)*	*car*
airplane		

There are many more words in Billy's receptive vocabulary at this time. He does still use some jargoning in his communications, but the pragmatic intent and message he is attempting to communicate are generally apparent.

The Intervention Session

In this session, the professional guides and coaches the mother to structure the play activities in a way that will be of most benefit to her and Billy. Strength-based coaching allows the mother to determine goals and strategies that can be easily incorporated in the session. Throughout the session, the professional is able to reinforce their successes. Previous sessions with Billy have focused on consistent use of word approximations and vocal strings of jargon for communication and turn taking. Auditory attention and discrimination have been reinforced in sessions and used to improve his speech in word approximations, eliciting more accurate productions by number of syllables, vowel content, and the consonants he is able to produce. The mother reviews some of the strategies that have been used in the past weeks that she will incorporate in this session. In past sessions, she has consistently used expanding, pausing, accepting vocalizations, and using short phrases with intonation to narrate and take turns. In addition, she has also been focusing on using strategies for carryover at home in the daily routines of their home environment and to improve Billy's approximations.

> Mother (looking at several toys on the shelf beside the table and then at Billy): What should we play with next?
>
> Billy (looks at mom, then looks at the toys and returns to scribbling on a paper with markers): Puh.
>
> Professional: Billy, here are more markers. You can draw more. I'm going to talk to mommy. Round and round.
>
> Professional (turning around to initiate discussion with mom while Billy continues drawing): Alright, he is happy with the markers for right now. So, let's talk about what goals and strategies you want to be able to incorporate with the toys.
>
> Mother: We can certainly get him to use lots of his words with any of these toys. I know he wants the Play-Doh.
>
> Professional: OK, perfect. Let's try to hold back the Play-Doh and let him come out with the language first before you give it to him. Remember that, if your goal is to have him respond with words he knows, then you can use short sentences that include one to two of the familiar words he might say. What are some of the words he knows that you think relate to this activity?
>
> Mother: He knows *open*, *help*, *bang bang*, *roll*, and he is trying to say *Play-Doh*.
>
> Professional: So, he knows *open* and *help* and those are words you are about to use. You can say something like, "I'll help you open the Play-Doh." Try to acoustically highlight the words you think he can pull out from the phrase. Remember, if he is using these words spontaneously, he should recognize them and should be able to attend to them within those short sentences. And we have another goal incorporated while you are doing that. Those short sentences with words he knows will reinforce his two-item auditory memory at the same time. What else can did you want to work on?
>
> Mother: Listening to me while he is busy playing with the Play-Doh.
>
> Professional: Absolutely. We refer to that as auditory integration. Listening while engaged in another activity. That's a very important ability that should be reinforced. He was busy drawing and looked up at you when you asked what he wanted to play. It was great that he was paying attention. When you go back to picking the next toy, you can watch for that to reinforce that he was listening. Anything else can you think of? Or is that enough?
>
> Mother: I really want to practice making his speech clearer. I want to

do that more at home and teach that to my husband.

Professional: Sure, we can look at practicing that. We have talked about making his listening better and then that makes his speech better. We do that by enhancing his perception. Better attention and matching—perception and production—of what he hears from you with what he says and then reinforced by hearing himself say it. So, right off the bat, we can get him to listen and do better approximations for *Play-Doh* or *puzzle* or whatever he wants to play with. If it was Play-Doh, is that the best approximation you think he can do?

Mother: No, he can do a /d/.

Professional: His vowel seemed right and he did use only one syllable. If he was trying to say *Play-Doh*, then he didn't do the second vowel. That might be a good place to start. You can get him to listen and do better approximations. In listening to the two syllables, he may also perceive the /d/ and include that…or not. But two syllables would be an improved approximation.

Mother: OK, what should I do?

Professional: Ask him again, and he will probably tell you "puh" again. So, it's possible he means *puzzle*, even though we both know he likes Play-Doh much more than puzzles. So, play dumb! Let him know that you aren't sure what he means or that you think he means the puzzle because of what he said. Give him the two words again so he can listen to the contrast. Puzzle or Play-Doh? I bet he will protest if you try to give him the puzzle or say "no" if you let him know you think he wants the puzzle.

Mother: Isn't that mean to not give him what he wants if we know?

Professional: Well, do you REALLY know what he wants by what he communicated? He was drawing so he didn't point to anything, and it wasn't close enough for him to grab what he wanted.

Mother: Weeeellll, maybe not. So how do I tell him that I don't know what he means? He will not understand those words.

Professional: He will understand by the way you phrase it, your body language, and your intonation. You are letting him know that you know he wants a toy, but you aren't sure exactly which one. Then you can help him listen to the words again, so he can do a better approximation. Your wanting to understand should motivate him to communicate more clearly. You really want to understand, so let him know that with the interaction. You aren't not giving it to him to be mean, you are working on improving the communication, getting him to attend to the words, discriminate how they are different, and match his perception and production for his suprasegmentals, vowels, and consonants. THEN, you can give him what he REALLY wants, because you will know! That is a great way to work on a bunch of our goals!

Mother: So, I get a /d/ in *Doh*?

Professional: Sure, try to, but also, what about the number of syllables and the vowels he used? I know he can do that duration and so I think he should be able to get both vowels and the /d/. The /p/ isn't really a /p/ since it is in a /pl/ blend. So, he may reduce that to a /p/ the way he did before or he may just leave it out. But based on what we know he can perceive and produce, we could potentially get him to produce two syllables with the right vowels and a /d/ for the second syllable. Right?

Mother: For sure. So, if he doesn't do the /p/ I shouldn't worry about it for now?

Professional: Right—it might be too much unless he tries to put it in just as a /p/ like before. Get him to do the other sounds and syllables that you know he can do. Also, remember that once he has all the toys, he has the control. You have the most control while you have the object or while he needs your help. So, give him the toys slowly and not all the parts at the same time. That way he needs to ask for them and interact with you. OK!

Mother: Billy, what should we play with next? (Pointing at several toys on the shelf beside the table and then looking at Billy)

Billy (looks at mom, who then looks at the toys as he puts down his marker): Puh

Mother (making eye contact with Billy and pointing out each choice): I don't know what you mean. What should we play with? Cars? The puzzle? PLAY-DOH?

Billy: Puh

Mother (pointing at the puzzle and reaching with her hand like she is going to pick it up): Puzzle? You want to play with the puzzle?

Billy (shaking his head "no" and pointing at the Play-Doh): No!

Mother (shaking her head and then reaching toward the Play-Doh and grabbing several canisters with different colors of Play-Doh): No, not the puzzle. You want the Play-Doh! You want to play with Play-Doh?

Billy: Puh

Mother: It sounded like *puzzle*, but you want Play-Doh! You want to play with PLAY-DOH. Listen. PLAY-DOH.

Billy: Ah oh

Mother: Good try! Listen again. Play-Doh.

Billy: Ay-Doh

Mother (has several containers of Play-Doh and is holding them close to her body): Alright, I understand! We'll play with Play-Doh. What color do you want? We have so many! Which one?

Billy (jargoning with an excited voice): Ah be de wa de mah to wa

Mother (with lots of excitement and vocal play): I know, we have so many! Which one do you want?

Billy (babbles excitedly with similar intonation contour to the one mother just used, rapidly looking at his mom and then the Play-Doh and back at his mother): Ah be de wa de mah to wa

Mother (shows each different one as she names them): We have different colors: purple, blue, green, yellow.

Billy: Wah ba bauh

Mother: Yeah I know you WANT Play-Doh. Which one?

(Billy grabs at the purple canister)

Mother (holding up the purple, but not too close, in front of him and making eye contact): Oh, I think you want purple. It's not OK to grab. Use your voice. Just tell me that you want purple. This one is purple.

Billy: Puh, puh

Mother (hands him the Play-Doh container, sealed shut and puts the other Play-Doh away): Purple! You want purple! I thought so. Here is the purple Play-Doh.

Billy: Puh, puh

Mother: Yes, purple Play-Doh. I gave you the purple! You have purple Play-Doh.

Professional: FABULOUS! Nice getting him to listen while he was busy and then to improve his production. You really let him know you wanted to understand what he was saying. Your expansions were great. When he said one word, you used the same word in a sentence to let him know you understood what he communicated. That works on so many of his goals in that play interaction: his auditory memory, his attention, and recognizing words within phrases. You also were improving his communication by having him consistently use his word approximations and voice.

Mother (pauses for a long time, raises her eyebrows, leans forward, shrugs her shoulders in a quizzical, questioning manner): What should we do?

Billy: Open

Mother: Open the Play-Doh!

Billy: Open

Mother: Pull it open! OK, you pull it open.

Billy (holding it out, question intonation contour): Open

Mother: You need help. I can help open. Open the Play-Doh.

Billy: Hep

Mother: I'll help. Let's open the Play-Doh.

Billy: Open

Mother: Wow! It's stuck. We need to pull it open. I need to PULL...Pull, pull, pull!

Billy: Puh, puh, puh

Mother: Opening the Play-Doh. The Play-Doh is open!

Billy: Open

Mother: I pulled the Play-Doh open! What do you say?

Billy: An you!

Mother: Yeah! You're welcome!

Billy (showing Play-Doh and can't get it out of the container and, sounding frustrated, he babbles): Agah dehbe nata weena

Mother: Uh oh! The Play-Doh is stuck!

Billy: Uh oh!

Mother: What should we do?

Billy (holding out the Play-Doh for his mother to take it): Hep

Mother (puts her hand on the Play-Doh and turns it over): I'll help you. Let's shake, shake, shake!

Billy: Shay shay shay

Mother: Hmmmm, that's not working. What else can I do?

Billy: Shay shay

Mother: I did shake, but it didn't work. I can bang it on the table. Bang, bang, bang.

Billy: Ba ba ba

Mother: Bang, bang, bang on the Play-Doh. Listen, it's going to be loud.

Billy: Ba ba ba

Mother (smashes the container on the table repeatedly): I heard that! Bang, bang, bang.

Billy: Ba ba ba

Mother (gives the Play-Doh to Billy and he plays with it): I think we got it! Yeah.

Professional: FABULOUS! Great expansions and working on getting him to listen to two key items. He was listening to *bang* and *shake* and discriminating them with your model.

Billy (moving and gesturing with his hands as if he is rolling the Play-Doh): Oh oh oh

Professional (rummages in the basket of Play-Doh-related toys): Roll, roll, roll the Play-Doh. We need a rolling pin.

Billy (watching his mother as she looks for the rolling pin): Oh, Oh, Oh

Mother (finds the rolling pin and holds it out for Billy to take): There you go. Roll, roll, roll the Play-Doh.

Billy (as he attempts to roll the Play-Doh): Oh, oh, oh

Mother: Great! You are rolling the Play-Doh. My turn.

Billy (continuing to roll and seeming to not be listening): Oh, oh oh

Mother (reaching out for the rolling pin): Mommy's turn please.

Billy (babbles and keeps rolling, shakes his head and seems to be saying that he is not going to share): Na wahna agah dehbe mama

Mother: I know you want to roll the Play-Doh. It's Mommy's turn and then you can roll more.

Billy (shaking his head as he rolls out the Play-Doh): More

Mother (reaches for and gently takes the rolling pin as Billy releases it to her, not too certain that he wants to give it up): Roll more. You want to roll more. Mommy's turn now.

Billy (babbles as if he is reluctantly giving it to her but reminding her she has to give it back): Agah dehbe nata weena

Mother: Thank you! I will give it back. Roll, roll, roll. I'm rolling the Play-Doh.

Professional: Lovely turn taking, mom! He is mostly very engaged in what he is doing but still really listening to you whether or not he is looking at you. And you keep talking to him and pausing until he takes his turn. That is great. It is interesting that sometimes he takes a longer time, which means he may be thinking about what he wants to say, and then if it has a key word that you used, he is pulling it out of the phrase, remembering in his auditory memory, and using it spontaneously rather than more of an imitation. I also like the way he tells you like it is with his jargon. It's adorable!

Billy: More?

Mother: Ok, you want to roll more?

Billy (smiling and reaching for the rolling pin): More!

Mother (holding it out, raising her eyebrows, leaning toward him, and waiting for his response as she gets ready to let go of the rolling pin): Here you go.

Billy: An you

Mother: You're welcome!

Analysis of Session

In discussion of the therapy session, we will analyze which goals are being addressed in the described interval of therapy. For purposes of this discussion, goal numbers are indicated in parentheses and refer back to numbering used in Tables 7–3 through 7–6. This scenario helps to demonstrate the integration and overlap of multiple goals in the natural interactions. It is important to be certain that you are explaining things to the parent in a manner and at a level that they are able to understand (see Adult Learning Theory in Chapter 2). We feel it is critical that professionals explain to parents what they are doing and why they are doing it. New professionals and parents might want to initially limit their analysis to one to three goals. More experienced professionals will identify that some activities can address many goals simultaneously. Billy listens throughout this play activity and is tuned into his mother's voice (Goals 3, 12). The mother appropriately has him listen to the noise that is relevant to their activity, when they bang the Play-Doh container on the table (Goal 7). He attends to and discriminates a variety of suprasegmental features, vowels, and consonants, as we can monitor through his auditory feedback with his many spontaneous productions (Goal 1).

There is clearly an established conversational interaction in which he participates and uses his voice and phonemes in very controlled speech productions (Goals 1, 4, 13a–d, 23, 24). In addition, at this point of his auditory development, he shows an expanded use of one- to two-syllable functional words (Goals 15, 17, 18). Mother and Billy have very good turn taking and communication skills established at this time (Goals 1, 23, 24). He is aware of the suprasegmental aspects of her vocalizations and understands when she asks a question and the various ways for him to respond and vocalize (Goals 1, 13a–d, 14, 23, 24). As they continue to play, we have the opportunity to see Billy's auditory comprehension and retrieval abilities. He knows a variety of objects by associated sounds, which introduced meaning when he was younger and had emerging words (Goals 1a–f, 15). He understands words and phrases and questions with and without context based on one to two known words (directives and statements). This is evidenced when his mother asks a question or uses familiar words and he demonstrates he understands by reaching or looking for a toy or using word approximations for a variety of pragmatic functions (Goals 1a–b, 5, 6, 8, 17, 18, 19, 22, 23, 24, 25).

Professional: When you give him choices with the cookie cutters, you can do different sounds for the objects, the words, or both. Whatever you think he will be able to do. Also, remember we were trying to get him to listen to words that have different numbers of syllables and vowels. You can find different molds where we are contrasting the number of syllables (*dog*, *airplane*, *teddy bear*)—those give you one, two, and three syllables or the sounds he knows for the objects, like *aaah* for the airplane and *ch ch ooo* for the train. There are lots of different shapes in there. Let me model one for you, and you take over when you are ready.

Professional: Let's see—we could make an airplane that goes "aaaah" or the train that says "ch ch ooooo."

Billy: Aaaah

Professional (holds the airplane as she talks about it and hides the train in her hand, waiting for him to respond to her prompt and complete the phrase): Yes, the airplane goes "aaah." Or we could make a train that goes . . .

Billy: Sh sh ooooo

Mother: CH CH ooooo says the train. Billy, do you want the train?

Billy: Ayn

Mother (pauses and looks with expectation): The train goes . . .

Billy (reaching for the train and taking it from his mother and putting it on the Play-Doh): Sh sh ooooo

Mother: The train—CH Ch ooooooo. Push down and make the train.

Billy: Ayn

Mother: PUSH on the TRAIN.

Billy: Push

Mother: Push down on the Play-Doh.

Billy: Push

Mother: Push down. Push down on the train.

Billy: Dow

Mother: Let's push it out of the mold. Wow. Here's the choo choo train.

Billy: Ayn

Mother (turning to the professional to quickly make eye contact): I think he was trying to say "down." I don't think that is a word that he usually says.

Professional: Great, let's pay attention to see him try to approximate *down* again. Also, that was lovely turn taking. You also used some auditory closure very effectively by pausing and letting him finish the sentence. Let's see if we can get him to listen to the different words with different syllables. Maybe include the /n/ if he tries *down*.

Mother: I don't know how to do that. And I don't think that is a word that he usually says. It might be the first time he tried to say it.

Professional: Ok. So, getting the /n/ might be overshooting, but we won't know if we don't try and push for a bit more. Let me show you what I mean about the syllables, the number of sounds. I'm going to use different words—one syllable, two syllables, and three syllables.

Professional (turning to Billy, the professional takes three molds in her hand and shows them to Billy but doesn't give them to him yet): That's the car.

Billy: Aw

Professional: Yes, that's the car. I have the car. This is the airplane.

Billy: Upane

Professional: That is the airplane. This is the teddy bear.

Billy: Teddy beh

Professional (shows each one again as she says names them): Good listening, Billy. I heard you say *car*, *airplane*, and *teddy bear*. I have a car, an airplane, and a teddy bear.

Professional: So, I had him listening to the number of syllables and he actually did lovely approximations for them by syllable, vowel, and some consonants. Are there any sounds you think he can produce better?

Mother: I don't think so, I thought they sounded great and was surprised he didn't need you to repeat them for him to try to say them.

Professional: That's probably because we are giving him tasks in which we are setting him up for success. He knows those words. He CAN do syllables; he has great vowel variety and some nice emerging consonants, which he is mastering in word imitations and approximations. He has a great auditory feedback loop going for him. He is really listening! We are going to work on developing his two-item auditory memory. Ok, now have him pick two of the three items. Tell him which ones. If he gets only one of them, say both items again when you repeat it. If you just say the one he missed, then we are only making him listen to one item. We want him to pay attention to both because we are working on two-item auditory memory. I'll help you as you do it. This is a bit harder for him but he knows these items and loves Play-Doh, so this is a great place to practice.

Mother (Billy is reaching for the car, but mom, who now has the molds, is keeping her hands cupped so he can't get them yet): Billy, which do you want?

Mother (opens her hand to show him the toys but doesn't let him take them): You want the car. You can make the car. I want to make the teddy bear. Get the car and the teddy bear.

Billy (with a clear question intonation pattern): Teddy beh?

Professional: So that is very typical. He remembered and repeated the last one he heard, even though he really wants the car. So now he can keep *teddy bear* in his short-term auditory memory and concentrate on the other one. Repeat the directions again, "We need the car and teddy bear," but be sure to acoustically highlight the car since he didn't get that one.

Mother (acoustically highlighting *car*): Yes, but we need the car and the teddy bear.

Billy: Teddy beh

Mother (pauses and waits for him to process and acoustically highlights the word *car*): Yes, the car and the teddy bear.

Billy: Teddy beh

Mother (acoustically highlighting *car*): Yes, but we want the car and the teddy bear.

Billy: Teddy beh

Mother (acoustically highlighting *car*): Car and the teddy bear.

Billy: Ah

Mother (Billy reaches for the molds, she lets him take them): YES! The car and the teddy bear.

Mother: The teddy bear is for me. Thank you for the teddy bear, and you have the car. Let's put them in the Play-Doh. (She takes the teddy bear as he is playing with the car.)

Professional: So, what just happened there?

Mother: He picked two toys but I needed to repeat and repeat and repeat.

Professional: Good for both of you. You stuck to the two items, didn't forget what we were working on, and he did it. It did take some repetitions. You didn't have to repeat it that many times, and this is probably one of the first times we have really made him do that. So that would be a bit of a structured activity for a two-item auditory memory. But you were doing it all along with your two key words in short phrases that you were expanding for him.

Analysis of Session

Mother continues with many goals as discussed earlier with regard to attending, discriminating, and feedback. She makes certain that Billy is listening to her all the time by being very involved in the activity and expecting his consistent participation in the communication regardless of how exciting the activity is for him (Goals 4, 12). She contrasts words and short phrases with different syllables and suprasegmental patterns (Goal 1). She expects him to listen to her and take his role in the conversations (Goals 1, 5, 6, 13, 14). Mother makes good use of acoustic highlighting, auditory closure, joint attention, and expansions in this segment.

In this section, we see the emergence of new skills for both Billy and his mother. The mother is learning to have greater expectations for consistency in Billy's productions. She is learning to balance enhancing his listening, facilitating his production, and maintaining the balance of conversation such that the most important element remains the interaction and communication (Goals 1, 13, 14, 23, 24, 25). This requires her to monitor his discrimination of suprasegmentals, vowels, and consonants (Goals 1a–d, 6, 8, 9).

The natural evolution of these features is to develop auditory discrimination and comprehension ability for words and phrases based on those feature including ones of varying numbers of syllables, known words, and phrases (Goals 1a–d, 6, 8, 9, 13, 14, 15, 18, 19, 20). The mother is learning to facilitate Billy's two-item auditory memory in three different ways by having him listen to two familiar key words in phrases, expanding his language, and having him select two known items from a small set (Goals 5, 6, 9). These auditory processes of discrimination recognition and comprehension skills will facilitate the retrieval component. We are thereby stimulating spontaneous expressive language in the areas of one- to two-syllable functional words, and of functional words, phrases, nouns, verbs, and adjectives (Goals 22, 23, 24, 25) with consistent use of the speech phonemes within his repertoire (Goals 12, 13, 14).

Summary

In this model, we look at skills in a normal development and the progression to the next level of abilities. In the single-word stage, we are building on foundation skills introduced at the prelinguistic level. Billy demonstrates emergence of many of the skills designated in the goals at the single-word level (see Tables 7–3 to 7–6). Though development of receptive and expressive vocabulary is necessary for children to be able to combine words, we are not focused on only teaching words at this stage. We focus on audition at the levels of detection, attention, discrimination, feedback, identification, and comprehension. The child must refine their auditory abilities to attend to sounds that are less accessible (see Speech Acoustics in Chapter 1). Sounds can be imitated to allow us to determine not only detection but also discrimination and auditory feedback. Skills develop to include additional low-frequency elements of speech beyond those evidenced in the prelinguistic stage, including additional manners of production and cognate pairs to reinforce unvoiced and voiced phonemes. As speech perception develops, phoneme productions will expand to include a variety of manner, place, and voicing features. We do not isolate auditory goals; we combine and expand them. Auditory abilities and speech production will then transition to listening and spoken language.

Behaviors that are indicative of the child emerging into the next stage of development, Emerging Word Combinations, are indicated in Table 7–10.

Table 7–10. By the End of the Single-Word Stage, the Child Should:

> Demonstrate a two- to three-item auditory memory.
>
> Follow two-part related commands (e.g., "Get your shoes and give them to me").
>
> Have a consistently emerging receptive and expressive vocabulary on a weekly basis.
>
> Combine two words together to create an original phrase on at least one occasion (e.g., "more juice").
>
> Use a variety of consonants in words and word approximations.

Discussion Questions

1. How do you determine if a child is at this stage?
2. How would you illustrate the chocolate chip cookie dough analogy to the parents of a child with hearing loss at this stage?
3. Select a goal from one of the Tables 7–3 through 7–6. How would you explain to a parent how to use a specific activity of daily living to target the goal? Consider and identify other goals that would naturally be included in that selected ADL.
4. What activities could you do with an older child to work on the goals at this level?
5. Consider a child with additional disabilities or needs and discuss an activity that you could work on to target a selected goal at this level.

References

American Speech-Language-Hearing Association (1997–2021). *Developmental norms for speech and language*. https://www.asha.org/public/speech/development/chart/

Bortfeld, H., Morgan, J. L., Golinkoff, R. M., & Rathbun, K. (2005). Mommy and me: Familiar names help launch babies into speech-stream segmentation. *Psychology Science, 16*(4), 298–304.

Brown, V. L., Bzoch, D. R., & League, R. (2020). *Receptive-Expressive Emergent Language Test* (4th ed.). Western Psychological Services.

Cochlear Corporation. (2010). Integrated scales of development. In *Listen, learn, talk* (pp. 16–31). Cochlear Limited.

Gleason, J. B., & Ratner, N. B. (2009). *The development of language* (7th ed.). Pearson.

Hill, V. (Writer). (1939). *Wheels on the Bus* [Song]. https://www.lyrics.com/lyric/3100409/Raffi

Hogan, S., Stokes, J., White, C., Tyszkiewicz, E., & Woolgar, A. (2008). An evaluation of auditory verbal therapy using the rate of early language development as an outcome measure. *Deafness and Education International, 10*(3), 143–167.

Jones, G., Tamburelli, M., Watson, S. F., Gobet, F., & Pine, J. M. (2010). Lexicality and frequency in specific language impairment: Accuracy and error data from two nonword repetition tests. *Journal of Speech, Language, and Hearing Research, 53*, 1642–1655.

Ling, D. (2003). The Ling Six-Sound Test. *The Listener*, 52–53.

Lowry, L. (2015). "Tuning in" to others: How young children develop theory of mind. *Hanen Early Language Program*. http://www.hanen.org/SiteAssets/Helpful-Info/Articles/tuning-into-others.aspx

Macevoy, F. (1880). *Twinkle, Twinkle Little Star* [Notated music]. White, Smith & Co. https://www.loc.gov/item/sm1880.02994

Madell, J. R., Hewitt, J. G., & Rotfleisch, S. (2018). Chapter 25: Red flags: Identifying and managing barriers to the child's optimal auditory development. In J. R. Madell, C. Flexer, Wolfe, & E. C. Schafer (Eds.). *Pediatric audiology: Diagnosis, technology and management* (3rd ed., pp. 267–276). Thieme.

Obenchain, P., Menn, L., & Yoshinaga-Itano, C. (1998). Can speech development at 36 months in children with hearing loss be predicted from information available in the second year of life? *Volta Review, 100*(5), 149–180.

Rotfleisch, S. (2009). Auditory verbal therapy and babies. In L. Eisenberg (Ed.), *Clinical management of children with cochlear implants* (pp. 435–493). Plural Publishing.

Singleton, N. C., & Shulman, B. B. (2014). *Language development: Foundations, processes and clinical applications* (2nd ed.). Jones & Bartlett Learning.

Tsiakpini, L., Weichbold, V., Kuehn-Inacker, H., Coninx, F., D'Haese, P., & Almadin, S. (2004). *LittlEARS Auditory Questionnaire*. MED-EL.

Vickers, N., & Vickers, J. (1956). *Play-Doh*. Rainbow Crafts.

Weitzman, E., & Pepper, J. (2004). *It takes two to talk: A practical guide for parents of children with language delays*. Hanen Center.

Zaidman-Zait, A., & Dromi, E. (2007). Analogous and distinctive patterns of prelinguistic communication in toddlers with and without hearing loss. *Journal of Speech, Language, and Hearing Research, 50*(5), 1166–1180.

Chapter 8

Emerging Word Combinations Stage

Sylvia Rotfleisch

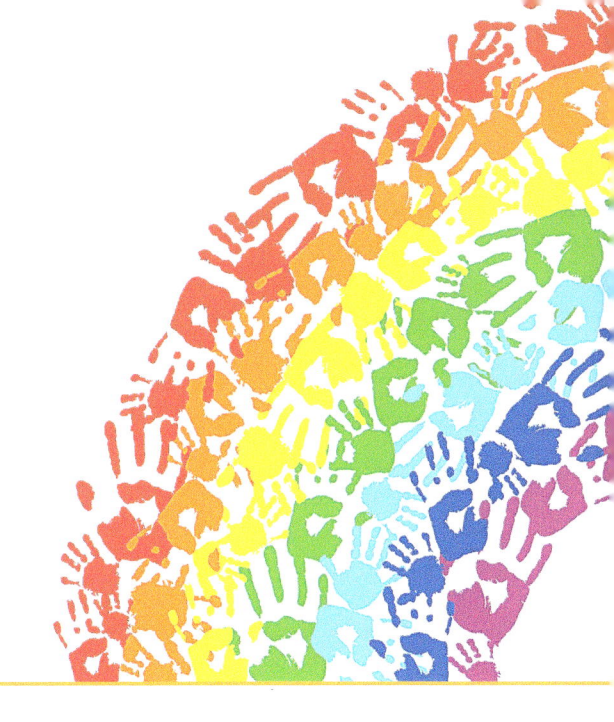

Key Points

- Sounds, language, and words have become an integral part of how the child communicates in the emerging word combinations stage.
- At the emerging word combinations stage, the child will attend to various features within longer auditory messages and show comprehension.
- The child will use an increased variety of speech features, words, and initial morphemes in their communications.
- Goals should be incorporated into activities of daily living by the family, which will incorporate the culture of the family.
- Goals should be incorporated into play and adapted to the child's age, cognitive and developmental stages, and interests.

Basic Characteristics of the Child With Emerging Word Combinations

Listening

Sound has become an integral part of this child's experiences and the auditory brain is developing the ability to discriminate, identify, and comprehend an expanding variety of speech features. The developing abilities include the expansion and reinforcement of the previously emerged abilities related to the suprasegmentals, vowels, and manners of consonants. The child's brain is learning the significance of speech features in the auditory signal to relay specific meaning. Productions of sounds and words approximations reflect what is heard. The child's abilities related to speech features expand to include additional consonants by manner, voicing, and place cues. These auditory skills allow the child to attend to and understand the importance of different sounds. They learn that quiet sounds, such word-final consonants, can change the meaning (e.g., *dog* versus *duck* versus *dot*).

The child attends to morphemes, which are phonemes with linguistic meaning. Comprehension emerges for prepositions *in*, *on*, and plural or possessive /s/. The order of emergence of the various consonant features can be dependent on hearing loss and the auditory access provided by the child's technology (see Speech Acoustics, Chapter 1). The child is able to hold multiple words in their short-term auditory memory, which demonstrates a two- to three-item auditory memory. These intermediate auditory abilities typically are evident and/or emerging in the emerging word combinations stage and are indicated in Table 8–1. Skills listed are not sequential.

Language

Children at this stage of listening and spoken language development demonstrate consistent expansion of their auditory comprehension of language and their expressive words and word approximations. The child's ability to construct two-word utterances using their expressive vocabulary begins with simple combinations. The child sees the book on the table and says, "book table." These utterances reflect a two-word auditory memory and the cognitive understanding that the meaning of their communication changes when combining two words together. Another type of combination will emerge,

Table 8–1. Auditory Abilities Evidenced in the Emerging Word Combinations Stage

- Remembers two critical items of information (two-item auditory memory) and/or sequences two events (e.g., "Show me the big dog," "Get a book and give it to me").
- Auditory memory and attention expand to two- and three-part complex commands, both related and unrelated (e.g., "Go to your room, get a book and give it to me" and "Take off your jacket and get your cup").
- Recognizes many different songs.
- Listens from a distance and with other degraded signals (e.g., recorded songs, some noise).
- Listens/attends to longer sentences.
- Attends to smaller words and morphemes such as prepositions (e.g., *in*, *on*,) pronouns (e.g., *he*, *she*), verb markers (e.g., *-ing*), negation (e.g., *not*, *no*).
- Attends to variety of different word-final sounds and morphemes within words and phrases.
- Begins to have incidental hearing (e.g., overhears familiar words in conversations not directed at them).
- Shows increasing attention and discrimination to the suprasegmentals and vowels.
- Recognizes the intonation of a question.
- Discriminates and identifies a variety of consonants that have different speech features (e.g., manner, voicing, and place).

Sources: REEL (2020); LittlEARS (2004); ASHA Milestones (2021); Integrated Scales of Development (2012); Madell et al. (2018).

referred to as a *pivot schema*. In this combination, there is a key word and a subsequent spot that can be filled by a variety of words. The key word controls the meaning and function of the utterance.

Typical early combinations could use words such as *more*, *hi*, and *no* as the pivot word. Once a pivot combination has emerged, it will be practiced by modifying the combination. The child will manipulate these types of combinations (e.g., "hi dog," "hi mama," "hi ball," "hi grandma," "more cracker," "more milk," "more up," "more book," "no book," "no more," "no down," "no dada"). Expressive vocabulary will typically expand to about 300 words or more as the child learns to use utterances from the initial two-word combinations and then advances to three- and four-word combinations. First morphemes are expected to emerge such as -*s* plural forms and the use of the prepositions *in* and/or *on* (Chapter 3, Table 3–7). The child's mean length of utterance (MLU) will go from 1 to 3 and possibly higher in this stage. Receptive and expressive language abilities that are evidenced or expected to emerge in this stage are included in Table 8–2, *Language and Speech Skills Evidenced in the Emerging Word Combinations Stage*. Skills listed are not sequential.

Table 8–2. Language and Speech Skills Evidenced in the Emerging Word Combinations Stage

Audition and Auditory Comprehension of Language	Expressive Language/Vocalization and Communication
• Understands opposites (e.g., go/stop, big/little, up/down).	• Combines two words together (e.g., "more apple," "no bed," and "mommy book").
• Follows two- to three-part related directions (e.g., "Go to your room, get your jacket, and put it on").	• Asks questions (e.g., "What's that?" "Who's that?" and "Where's kitty?").
• Follows two-part unrelated requests (e.g., "Take off your jacket and get some water").	• Has a word for almost everything from daily life and routines.
• Seems to understand everything.	• Talks about things that are not in the room.
• Understands new words quickly.	• Uses increasing number of phonemes in spontaneous productions of words, such as /k/, /g/, /f/, /t/, /d/, /n/.
• Understands meanings of words when looking at books or pictures.	• Uses prepositions such as in, on, and under.
• Understands several verbs and can point to them in pictures or do the action.	• Uses two or three words to talk about and ask for things.
• Understands several prepositions.	• People who know child can understand what they say.
• Understands increasing number of body parts (e.g., chin, eyebrow, elbow).	• Asks "Why?"
• Understand yes/no questions.	• Puts three words together to talk about things.
• Understands size differences and some descriptive words (e.g., big, dirty, wet).	• May repeat some words and sounds.
• Identifies objects by function (e.g., "What do you wear on your feet?" "What do you use to cut?").	• Uses some plural words—initially those learned in plural form (e.g., shoes, eyes, and pants) and then others.

Sources: REEL (2020); LittlEARS (2004); ASHA Milestones; Integrated Scales of Development (2012); Zimmerman et al. (2011); http://zerotothree.com

Speech

The child with hearing loss who has good access to the auditory signal will move forward in their production of speech features. The child will demonstrate control of the suprasegmental aspects of speech (i.e., duration, intensity, and pitch [DIP]), which are carried by the production of the various emerging vowel sounds. Consonants begin to emerge and productions include some phonemes, demonstrating control and development of different manners, voicing, and places of production. These phonemes and speech features will be used in word approximations increasingly as expressive vocabulary expands.

As speech reflects both the auditory access and typical sequence of development, we expect phonemes to be typically correct by manner of production while place cues and some voicing discriminations remain incorrect. Old production habits might be evidenced. Though the child is discriminating more speech features, they may not yet correct their production. The child's auditory feedback loop continues to develop at this stage, resulting in improvements in approximations in babble, at the phonetic level, and in words at the phonologic level.

Goals for the Emerging Word Combinations Stage

Developing an Appropriate Therapy Plan by Addressing Strengths and Areas of Need

The typical sequence of development will be followed to develop listening skills and appropriate speech and language abilities. All previous goals will be used as the basis for expanding to the next skills. Some goals from the single-word stage might not be mastered and might be carried over initially in this stage. Goals for the emerging word combinations stage focus on:

- facilitating listening abilities for longer auditory messages and for quieter sounds and structures (e.g., morphemes, word-final consonants);
- facilitating productions of phonemes with all different speech features;
- facilitating comprehension of sentences with a variety of grammatical morphemes; and
- facilitating use of word combinations and initial morphemes.

Select appropriate goals based on your assessment results that identify the child's strengths and needs (see Chapter 4). With the understanding of speech features and the acoustics parameters related to an audiogram, monitor for emerging skills. Based on the hearing loss, predict and prepare for areas of potential difficulty (Chapter 1).

Goals must be individualized within the stage to meet the child's needs. Consider, for example, when determining goals related to expressive use of language, you might target initially developed morphemes (Table 3–7). The child might attend to and show some understanding of the quieter sounds of unstressed morphemes for present progressive (i.e., *-ing*), prepositions (e.g., *in*), and/ or plural and possessives (e.g., /s/). Select goals that target expanding auditory attention and comprehension and that facilitate the use of morphemes (Goals 2, 4, 17, 21). In this situation, you can see the overlap or cookie dough effect on the selection of goals for auditory attention, comprehension, and expressive language. However, a child who is not able to hear the higher-frequency speech elements would likely not be able to develop comprehension, through audition alone, for morphemes such as /s/ and -*ed*. Auditory access and use of additional modalities need to be addressed so this child can develop these structures. Choose goals within the child's auditory abilities and limitations (see Chapter 1) for attention, comprehension, and expressive use of the morphemes, which include lower-frequency information such as vowels and nasals and question forms (Goals 2; 4; 17a, b, f; 21a, b). Determine appropriate strategies to address the lack of access and to allow the child to develop the morphemes.

Typical Goals for the Emerging Word Combinations Stage

Select goals to expand the listening and spoken language skills that you have assessed and address the child's strength and needs. Focus on auditory goals for the child to attend to, discriminate, and identify elements of the auditory signal that are less accessible in language and across all environments of daily life. Phonemes should be targeted to include all manners, voicing, and an emerging variety of places of production at the phonetic and phonologic levels.

Goals for continued expansion of the child's auditory memory will allow for an increase in the child's MLU and ability to sequence words and morphemes within their communicative contributions. Auditory access and developed auditory skills related to quieter aspects of speech are a focus at this stage to optimize the child's ability to catch language structures without structured teaching or drill. These abilities will provide the foundation skills for the next stage of communication, where the child has developed many but not all grammatical structures and has errors.

Typical recommended goals for children with hearing loss at the emerging word combinations level are included in Tables 8–3 to 8–6. Goals are organized based upon defined skills related to the brain functions necessary for learning to use audition for language development (see Chapter 3, Table 3–5). The goals included in these tables should not be considered the definitive set of goals for all children at this stage. Neither should they be considered an exhaustive list of possible audition goals for the child with hearing loss at the emerging word combinations stage of language development. Goals must address the specific errors and needs determined during comprehensive assessment as well as from observation and informal diagnostic work.

How Do We Work on These Goals?

Professionals must have a knowledge base and multiple appropriate strategies applicable to the child in the emerging word combinations stage to accomplish the recommended goals. The knowledge and strategies, included in these tables, are the basis for you to guide and coach the parent as the primary person to develop their child's listening and spoken language abilities. Knowledge areas and strategies applicable to the child at the emerging word combinations stage are identified in Tables 8–7 and 8–8 (see p. 188).

Table 8–3. Auditory Goals for Understanding Sound as Meaningful in the Emerging Word Combinations Stage

Auditory Goals for Auditory Attention, Detection, Discrimination, and Memory

1. Expand attention, responses, discrimination, and imitation in variety of speech features with normal presentation levels and with decreased intensity at phonetic and phonological levels:
   a. suprasegmentals: duration, intensity, pitch (DIP)
   b. vowels and diphthongs
   c. oral versus nasal resonances
   d. manners of consonant production
   e. places of consonant production
   f. voicing of consonant production
2. Develop awareness of low-intensity morphemes in conversational speech.
3. Facilitate ability to attend through audition only to sentences of three to six words.
4. Reinforce and expand auditory memory to three to six critical items in short phrases and compound sentences using nouns, prepositions, pronouns, and verbs.
5. Expand auditory memory for rhymes, verbal interactive games, songs, and emerging rote tasks such as numbers and short phrases in books or songs.
6. Develop and reinforce auditory attention and discrimination for consonants in word-final position.
7. Discriminate minor differences of prepositions, plurals, possessives, negatives, and pronouns within phrases.
8. Facilitate ability to attend to auditory signal while engaged in a motor task or when visually engaged in an activity.
9. Facilitate singing (i.e., vocalizing) songs with accompanying actions and hand gestures.
10. Facilitate ability to comprehend simple phrases with key words through audition only while engaged in a play activity.

The parents will be learning strategies and implementing them during therapy sessions. At the stage of emerging word combinations, you will talk in conversations, expand the child's language, and use complete sentences and phrases with morphemes.

You will support parents in using these strategies (see Table 8–8). The parent who began with these strategies in the previous language stages should be using them consistently. As their child reaches the emerging word combinations stage, you will introduce the parents to some new strategies. When the parent is new to listening and language intervention, they might not be familiar with strategies and will require you to guide them in any strategies that they are not familiar with implementing. You will help parents to understand knowledge related to the next skills in listening and spoken language development with their child with hearing loss (see Table 8–7).

Table 8–4. Auditory Feedback and Speech Production Goals in the Emerging Word Combinations Stage

Auditory Goals for Development of the Speech Production System

11. Develop and expand control in babbling (at phonetic level) and words (at phonologic level) for:
    a. suprasegmentals: duration, intensity, pitch (DIP)
    b. vowels and diphthongs: to include a variety of low-, mid-, and high-frequency vowels and diphthongs
    c. manners of consonant production
    d. fricative and affricate manners of production including initially, but not limited to, /h/, /ʃ/, /s/, and /tʃ/ with vowel variety
    e. places of consonant production within different manners of production
    f. voicing of consonant production within different manners of production
12. Facilitate and reinforce emerging phonemes and their discrimination by manner and place of production, as well as voicing cues at phonetic and phonological levels in an appropriate developmental sequence.
13. Facilitate correct productions for consonants in word-final position at phonological level.

Table 8–5. Auditory Goals for Language Comprehension in the Emerging Word Combinations Stage

Auditory Recognition, Sequencing, and Comprehension

14. Expand recognition and comprehension with emergence of receptive vocabulary.
15. Facilitate and expand recognition of key words when embedded within three- to six-word phrases.
16. Expand and facilitate sequencing of word order for three to six familiar words.
17. Expand and facilitate sequencing and comprehension of sentences, including increased variety of grammatical morphemes beginning with but not limited to (Table 3–7, Morpheme Development):
    a. present-tense progressive
    b. prepositions
    c. plural forms
    d. possessive forms
    e. verb tenses including past and future tenses, and past-tense verb forms beginning with irregular forms and facilitating *-ed* endings
    f. a variety of question forms beginning with *who*, *what*, and *where*
18. Facilitate auditory comprehension of simple phrases with three to six critical items.

Table 8–6. Auditory Goals for Developing Expressive Language in the Emerging Word Combinations Stage

Auditory Retrieval and Expressive Communication
19. Facilitate emergence and consistent use of expressive vocabulary.
20. Facilitate and reinforce consistent use of three- to six-word sentences and phrases.

21. Facilitate and elicit expressive use of morphemes (Table 3–7, Morpheme Development):
    a. present-tense progressive
    b. prepositions
    c. plural forms
    d. possessive forms

22. Facilitate and reinforce auditory retrieval of several sentences to tell a simple story.
23. Facilitate and elicit spontaneous auditory retrieval of a variety of simple question forms.
24. Reinforce and expand use of grammatical morphemes to produce some correct phrases and sentences spontaneously and through use of modeling and expansion.

Table 8–7. Knowledge Areas in the Emerging Word Combinations Stage

- Hearing technologies being used
- Effective troubleshooting of technology
- Speech acoustics related to emerging speech and morpheme development (Chapter 1)
- Ling six sounds
- Sequence of development of speech phonemes
- Stages of development of receptive language
- Stages of development of expressive language
- Sequence of developmental of initial morphemes
- Reading and the stages of literacy

Table 8–8. Optimal Strategies to Implement in the Emerging Word Combinations Stage

Chocolate chip cookie theory
24/7 and ADL
Three-act play
Expansion
Auditory sandwich
Acoustic highlighting
Auditory closure
Reading
Vocabulary enrichment
Teach the unknown concept by connecting to the known
Incorporate sequence stories from personal life and books
Incorporate thinking words for Theory of Mind

You and the parent will talk to the child with hearing loss in conversational turns using short sentences that are longer than in the previous stage and that will model correct usage of morphemes and grammatical structures. Basic principles as used at the prelinguistic and single word stage continue to be the foundation of interaction and facilitate the listening and spoken language skills as the child begins to use morphemes in longer strings of word combinations. This interaction style will prepare the child for conversations, expressive use of morphemes by facilitating auditory attention and memory beyond key words for language that is potentially less accessible. You should remember the chocolate chip cookie theory so that you and the parent are integrating all of the child's listening and spoken language skills in all of their interactions. Talking when engaged in activities promotes auditory integrations and natural interactions.

Additional suggested activities for you to use and to guide and coach the parents are included in Table 8–9.

Targeting and Incorporating Goals

Auditory Attention, Detection, Memory, Discrimination, Auditory Recognition, Sequencing, and Comprehension
(Tables 8–3 and 8–5)

Activities explained in the following text will illustrate goal areas but will also indicate how to use these goals for other areas of listening and spoken language development.

Activities of Daily Living (ADL)

Exploiting the activities that are happening anyway for listening and spoken language is a foolproof way to meet goals for the child. Among the first morphemes to develop are prepositions, plurals, possessives, and the *-ing* form of the present progressive verb. There are limitless opportunities for short phrases and complete sentences. As always, remember the chocolate chip cookie theory—we are always integrating all of the child's listening and spoken language skills in our interactions.

Talking about what you are doing naturally incorporates the appropriate verbs and actions for what will be done. With the toy or item, you will be cleaning, helping, working, getting, picking up, holding, finding, putting, and placing. Using the three-act play (see Chapter 5) allows for good, repeated exposure to the verb structure targeted.

Reinforce the singular and plural forms for the items (e.g., *car* versus *cars*, *shoe* versus *shoes*, *block* versus *blocks*, *marker* versus *markers*). Don't forget the possessive. Who owns the item? Those are Daddy's shoes, the dog's toy, Jessica's doll. Be sure to pause and take turns providing the child with opportunities to understand and to use the modelled structures.

Regardless of the activity, cleaning up is almost always the final act! Introduce clean up with the stereotypic phrase that the family uses or the "clean up" song so commonly used in school settings. Talk about where the item is to incorporate the prepositions. That book is on the floor, under the chair, in the corner. Where is the item supposed to be? Put it in the bucket, on the shelf, in the closet, or on your bed. For example, when cleaning up, "I'm looking for all the cars. There's a car under the chair. I'm walking to the chair. I'm reaching for the car. I'm walking to the box. The car goes in the box. You are cleaning up the balls. There's a ball on the bed. You're looking for all the balls. You are putting the ball away in the basket. I'm tossing balls into the basket."

Table 8–9. Guide and Coach Parents To:

Implement optimal strategies for the emerging word combinations stage (Table 8–8)

Listen! Talk, talk, talk!
- Speak in the language that is natural in the home.
- Have a conversation.
- Ask questions with a choice instead of yes/no questions (e.g., rather than asking, "Do you want milk?" ask, "Would you like milk or water?").
- Wait for a verbal answer to questions rather than anticipating the response.
- Reinforce verbal responses and requests (e.g., "Thank you for telling me what you want. I can get you a glass of milk").
- Use concept words related to spatial relations (e.g., *behind, corner, middle, next to*), time sequence (e.g., *first, after, then*), and quantity (e.g., *some, more, all*).
- Use specific words (e.g., instead of "here" say "beside me"; instead of "there" say "on the shelf"; say the actual name of the object instead of "this" or "thing").
- Talk about attributes such as colors, shapes, size, and texture.
- Expand what the child says (e.g., if child says, "big dog," reply, "That is a big dog. The dog is brown with spots. He is soft. Do you want to pat the dog?").
- Let the child know that their communication is important. Ask them to repeat things that you do not understand (e.g., "I know you want a block. Tell me which block you want").
- Use short, grammatically correct sentences.
- Use words that are similar in meaning (e.g., *child, kid, baby, infant, toddler, boy, girl, son, daughter*).
- Use new words in sentences to help your child learn the meaning.
- Incorporate the three-act play to talk about the child's experiences: that happened, is about to happen, or will happen.
- Repeat what the child says and add to it.
- Help categorize objects into like items (e.g., clothes, food, animals).
- Teach the child new words.
- Look at family photos and name the people and the relationship. Talk about what they are doing in the picture.

Play, play, play!
- Place objects into a bucket and have child remove them. Name them. Talk about them. Put them in, on, under, next to, and out.
- Cut out pictures from magazines and make a scrapbook. Help your child glue the pictures into the scrapbook.
- Pretend play and role-play.
- Practice counting. Count toes and fingers. Count steps. Count crackers.
- Name pictures of objects and talk about how you use them.

Sing
- Sing songs, play finger games, and tell nursery rhymes. These songs and games teach your child about the rhythm and sounds of language.

Table 8–9. *continued*

Read
- Read every day.
- Read books with short sentences on each page.
- Read to find and teach new words.
- Do not simplify the rich language.
- Read with animation to indicate different emotional states.
- Read books with rhymes and rhythms.
- Read books with repeated patterns and use auditory closure so the child completes the last word or words.
- Use specific book language (e.g., the title, turn the page, the end, and read it again!).
- Name objects and talk about the picture on each page of a book.

Theory of Mind
- Use thinking language that expresses state of mind vocabulary and discuss a variety of emotions of others throughout the day and when reading books.
- Pretend play and role-play to encourage Theory of Mind and different perspectives. Pretend to be the mommy with a baby doll, have an imaginary tea party, and feed guests the foods they like.
- Explain how you know things (e.g., "I know you are hungry because you are going to the kitchen," "I know Daddy is home because I heard the door open," "I know the dog wants to go out because he barked").

Sources: Compiled from ASHA https://www.asha.org/public/speech/development/01/; and http://www.hanen.org/helpful-info/articles/tuning-in-to-others-how-young-children-develop.aspx

Sequencing Life!

Everything has an order. Favorite books and life stories are familiar and effective, and provide perfect opportunities for the child to remember and anticipate what will happen in activities they are doing or in books. Simple steps that are the sequences of daily routines or stories can be taken advantage of for building auditory memory, sequencing steps and, of course, facilitating verbs and other activity-specific vocabulary. It is very easy to add the three-act play with simple explanations such as "We are going to walk to the kitchen. We are walking to the kitchen. We walked to the kitchen." The next time, you can hop, march, or run to the kitchen! Requests or explanations that are naturally incorporated into the narrative or conversation between the adult and child can be built from these routines. These routines easily become some of the child's first simple sequence stories that are personal, meaningful, and repeated in life.

During intervention, we can build a sequence by stringing together stereotypic phrases that have emerged and expanded in the previous stage. Mom can say "All done eating! Wash those dirty hands. I'll pick you up, up, up." Using combinations of familiar phrases builds on the child's ability to follow multistep tasks and expands their auditory memory. When giving the child a multistep request or direction, there are critical steps to accomplish the task that we do not necessarily say. Think of it as the default action. By adding the default action, the unspoken yet understood step, we will work toward the goals related to expanding auditory memory, sequencing, and comprehension. Consider throwing a dirty tissue in the trash. Rather than just saying "Throw it in the trash," we can add the other related and necessary steps. Tell the child to stand up, then walk to the trash and throw out the dirty tissue and come back. Many tasks can be broken down into simple steps and components. This strategy can be applied to many if not most activities and requests. These activities are the perfect opportunity to playfully play dumb.

Sabotage the Task

Be silly. When the child says "shoe," you can respond, "Yes, there's a shoe. Should I put it on my head or do you want it? Where should I put it (on, in, etc.)?" Facilitate expressive communicative attempts to express wants and needs instead of anticipating. With the child's limited ability to communicate verbally, adults need to anticipate the child's needs, but at this stage of development, this is changing. Anticipate less, but be certain not to foster frustration.

As the professional, you can help the parents to look at how to optimize everyday tasks. For example, consider brushing teeth. This is a task that is happening more than once a day. Explore the stereotypic phrases and key words that the child knows around this activity. The parent can begin by combining stereotypic phrases such as "Let's go brush your teeth. You have dirty teeth. Head out to the bathroom and find your toothbrush." Encourage the parent to use explanations to help the child to learn. Talk about the what, where, why, and how of the activity. "We have to clean your teeth so they stay healthy. We have to get rid of the teeth germs. Should we march or tiptoe to the bathroom?" We can do a task analysis of many more steps, some of which are necessary, to include in the language narration and instructions. For example, "We have to wet the toothbrush. Hold the toothbrush in your fist. Now we will turn on the water. Great job turning on the water. Is the water hot? or cold? or warm? Hold the toothbrush bristles in the stream of water."

Receptive elements are incorporated as the child listens to the steps and follows the series that is being presented. Expressive language elements are incorporated when the child tells the adult the steps. When the child says "put on toothpaste," you can suggest the parent be silly and put the tube on their head or their shoulders. Encourage the child to be precise with their language. "On the toothbrush" can result in the whole tube being placed on the toothbrush. "Oh no! We can't put the toothpaste on the toothbrush. We need to screw off the cap of the tube. Squeeze the toothpaste. It's coming out of the tube onto the bristles. Just a little bit."

Words! Words! Words!

Use an abundance of words—different words and words in grammatically correct short sentences. Be certain to use them in meaningful interactions. At this stage the child is rapidly learning new words with limited exposure. Do not get stuck using the same vocabulary just because the child knows those words. Use known words and new words embedded within phrases. Expand vocabulary by using different words to convey the concept or item (e.g., *big, large, huge, gigantic, enor-*

mous or *doggie, puppy, dog, pet, pooch, animal, Rover*). Use different words and the appropriate word. We peel the banana, we do not open it. Expand vocabulary by using descriptive words such as the long rough rope, the crunchy twisted salty pretzel, and the long-sleeved T-shirt with blue stripes. Move rapidly away from baby talk and pair known words with new unknown words to teach advance receptive and expressive vocabulary. Instead of "night-night," "The boy was sleeping. He was having a good snooze. He is dreaming. He is snoring while he takes his nap." Help the child with discrimination of sounds in known words that might have old misarticulations and also with correct speech features when learning new words. Acoustic highlighting can be used for the appropriate number of key words as appropriate for the child's language level.

Read! Read! Read!

Read with enthusiasm. Have a fun stereotypic phrase to announce reading time (e.g., "reading magic time, let's travel with a book"). Use and reinforce book-related words phrases (e.g., "open the cover," "turn the page"). Use the vocabulary and expressions that are specifically related to books and stories (e.g., front of the book, back of the book, cover, title, author, illustrations, once upon a time, they all lived happily ever after, the end and let's read it again!).

Books are an amazing way to expose the child to rich language and new vocabulary. Books remind us to use new and different vocabulary and language structures. In *The Napping House* by Wood and Wood (1964), the characters are not just sleeping. They are napping, dozing, dreaming, snoring, snoozing. This is rich language all related to sleeping. This reminds parents interacting with the child to not to get stuck with "shh, night-night." Books are a great way to introduce new vocabulary and to remind parents to get past the first, simple words.

Let the child be engaged by the different elements of the book and do not just simplify the language in the book. Find books of interest to the child that include rhymes, rhythms, and repeated patterns that lend themselves readily to auditory closure (e.g., *Hands, Hands, Fingers, Thumb* [1988], *Jamberry* [1994], and *Chicka Chicka Boom Boom* [1989]). The child will develop their memory by reciting the short, repeated phrases through the book (e.g., *The Hungry Caterpillar* [1969] and *The Napping House*). Look at the pictures while naming and pointing and encouraging the child to doing so as well.

Targeting and Meeting Goals for Development of the Speech Production System: Auditory Retrieval and Expressive Communication (Tables 8–4 and 8–6)

Let's Talk About It!

Everything we do has language. Let's take advantage of what is already occurring. It does not matter what you are doing, be sure to be conversing about it with the child. This way, you are engaged and interested in the content of the communication. Accept the communicative intent first. We can then respond or explain to the child to indicate what we think they said. In this way, the child knows they were able to communicate and gets validation through your response. This provides an opportunity to correct, clarify, and expand the communication.

Correcting the communication might address the language or the production. We encourage the use of specific words as names of items and actions that are meaningful and relevant in the situation. We might be encouraging the use of a new word expressively when we know the child understands it receptively. We want to encourage the use of the word by expanding the contribution and adding the specific word. For example, when playing with Play-Doh the child might say "Cut, cut please" and the parent could respond, "Oh, cut. I think you want a knife. The knife cuts." The child might shake their head and respond, "Yes cut, cut." We can acoustically highlight the word *knife* and say it a few times to naturally encourage the child to say it. Use some combinations of phrases such as "I have a knife," "The knife is for cutting," "Do you want a knife or should I cut?" and "I can share the knife."

If the issue in the communication is production, we go back to enhance the perception. Match the known sounds and words and with the new word. You could highlight the specific speech feature or contrast different speech features when appropriate. Another example could be when the child says "Pour please." The adult might respond saying "I think you want four cars." And the child shakes their head to indicate "Yes." You could say, "OK, let's get you four. Listen: *ffffff*. You want four. Here are four cars." In this case, the child might not be able to produce the /f/ phoneme, but we want to facilitate the discrimination of the different sounds. We could also contrast and let the child know that *pour* means something else. "I don't think you mean *pour*. You don't want me to pour water. I think you mean you want four."

Toys for Learning

Puzzles, shape sorters, stacking rings and cups, play putty (e.g., Play-Doh), building blocks or tiles, baby dolls, favorite stuffed animals, and dishes with pretend food are all equally magical to facilitate language. Look for the language that is intrinsic in the toy and the way we play with it. Talk about the interaction and encourage serve and return. This is the ideal time to follow the child's lead while immersing them in language and conversation (Schwartz, & Miller, 1988). Remember, Piaget (1962) notes, "Play is the work of childhood."

Use imagination and set up scenarios. Set up tea parties or pretend to go to a restaurant. Name the toy. Determine the relevant category for the puzzle: wild animals, fruits, vehicles. Describe the toy's attributes. Use verbs related to the action of the toy. Narrate what is happening. Engage in conversation about the play. For example, when playing with blocks, there are a variety of shapes, colors, sizes, and materials. What we are going to construct or build? How do we build it? Who lives or works in that building? Should we knock it over? How will you feel if it falls over? When using Play-Doh, we roll it, flatten it, shape a ball, cut it, create, destroy, squeeze, and squash it. Don't forget to clean up!

Up the Ante!

The ongoing conversation is natural, but with children at a simple language level, sometimes the best opportunities to talk are related to an activity, craft, game, toy, or specific event. Prior to this stage with more emerging expressive language, adults typically anticipated the child's needs. At this stage, we must transition with the child so they understand that we cannot always anticipate their more complex thoughts. Encourage them to communicate more clearly. We let the child know we really want to know what they are trying to tell us, but sometimes, we are not certain—all the while balancing the situation to be certain not to foster frustration, a battle of wills, or break down to insisting on the imitation of a word.

We must remember at this time the goal is to facilitate communication rather than imitation (see Chapter 5). Virtually any situation can be manipulated into the perfect opportunity to playfully play dumb. Sabotage the task. Be silly. You can also remember that, at this stage, we are facilitating initial morphemes (both receptively and expressively) such as prepositions *in* and *on*, *-ing* verb structure, plurals, and possessives (Chapter 3, Table 3–7).

Many scenarios can effectively facilitate word combinations or the use of morphemes. We can facilitate expressive communicative attempts by providing some models and choices and encouraging the child to more precisely express their wants and needs. When the child says "shoe," this scenario makes it clear to the child you understand they want to talk about the shoe. However, there are many possible things you might be trying to communicate. What about the shoe? Encourage the child to respond with more than a single word. You can pick a response or two as models: "That's a shoe. We need two shoes. Should I put it on my head? I'm putting my foot in the shoe. Do you want the shoe? That's Suzie's shoe." A variety of playful interactions can result: "Put the shoe on my foot. Too small! Give you the shoe? Smell the shoe? Pee-yooo! Stinky shoe!" And yes, we understand that sometimes, we just need to get the shoes on the child!

Questions: Your Choice . . . Yes! No!

Do ask questions. Do expect answers. Do give choices. Do move through different basic types of questions as soon as you can. Do you want . . . ? Is it . . . ? When to start with questions? Essentially when the child can be successful at understanding and beginning to respond. The child at this stage will have the auditory skills that allow them to understand the difference between a question and a statement (see Table 8–1). We must be careful to reinforce a question that requires a response. If the child is not vocalizing or responding to the intonation of a question, this is an indication that questions are not yet successful for this child.

If the child does not yet understand that a question requires a response, be careful not to overuse questions. This means we should be providing more statements and narrating and using fewer questions. Among the earliest questions that children master is the basic yes/no question. It is a great way to get clarification from the child with hearing loss as to what they want or are really expressing. Initially the child may just shake their head as an indication. You should facilitate the expressive use of yes or no by modeling and expanding with it. We might see this when the adult asks, "Do you want more?" and the child shakes their head to indicate "no." We can respond, "No. No more grapes. Do you want crackers? Do you want me to pick you up? Should we go outside?"

Facilitate the use of questions in daily interactions to promote successful communication. This will foster more communication. Once this is mastered, keep moving on. Do not let parents get stuck and overuse a specific form of question. The professional should help monitor the parent's language and strategies and make that observation. It is not unusual to see parents overusing the yes/no question form. This happens for a very good reason: It results in a successful communication. When they are trying to use a variety of questions, you must help them to be aware of that overuse. A great strategy is to go for the choice. Add a choice by using the "or" option (e.g., "Do you want something to eat or drink? Should I pick you up or wipe your hands?"). These choices are a great next step in moving to open-ended questions. Asking the child, "So you want to drink milk or water?" will transition to "What do you want to drink?" Asking the child, "Do you want to read a book or do a puzzle?" will transition to "What do you want to play?" We must avoid questions where only one specific, often adult-predetermined response, is correct. The nature of the open-ended question allows for multiple correct responses.

Let the Games Begin

Language of games is not to be missed! This language level is a great time to introduce beginning games. Board games, matching games, word games, and movement games all have fun and language built in and ready to be introduced and mastered. Games inherently are structured based on turn taking, which is being reinforced in language and conversing or is showing some level of mastery.

Board games allow further development of sequencing steps as we teach the child to follow rules. Do not forget to examine the illustrations on the box and talk about the different pieces or objects used in the game. There could be pawns to move, a spinner to spin, dice to roll, or cards to draw from the pile. The child learns what you are supposed to do to win or complete the game, what you do on your turn, how to decide who goes next, and how we have to wait for our turn. "My turn," "your turn," "take a card," "move one space," and "lose a turn" are all game-specific language that should be used as we play the game.

Good old-fashioned word games focus on language. Guessing games such as I Spy or variations require the child or adult to guess what the other person is "spying with their little eyes." We love that it uses Theory of Mind principles. We love that the child gets to repeat and practice a short rote phrase, allowing for expanding memory or auditory closure and reinforcing their speech for what might be new words in an interesting language structure using a rhyme. This is often introduced with colors (e.g., "I spy with my little eye something that is blue"). We can modify to introduce and reinforce new vocabulary and concepts, or decide to use other attributes or functions or categories: "I spy with my little eye something that is small" or "I spy with my little eye something that bumps (or something round or soft)." Make up your own variation of the game, changing the phrase used or the descriptor, or providing additional clues. You can modify to, "I'm thinking of something you eat" or give several features and have the child guess an animal that lives on a farm and gives milk and (maybe to help initially) says "moo."

Matching games or sorting games introduce and explore a variety of concepts such as same or different, similar, matching, a pair (but not a pear!), and negative forms such as not the same and not a match. Using a collection of cards with matching pairs, the child might be required to remember where items were. Was it at the top? In the corner? At the bottom?

Movement games, sensory paths, obstacle courses, and songs engage the child physically while relying on language and instructions. These simple and fun games have wonderful elements to work on goals at this stage of listening and spoken language. Other cultures might have many similar games.

- Obstacle course: Set up a route using prepositions to describe where to go and have the child take a turn telling others where to go next.
- Sensory path: Create a walk with stops where they have to complete different actions. Move between stops in different ways (e.g., giant steps, skipping, marching). When they get to each space, they have to follow the instructions (e.g., jump three times and touch their toes on one space and then turn around holding their arms out like an airplane on another).
- Scavenger hunt: Find a list of items. Find unusual or interesting items or use descriptions of an item, such as something that is long or round, or any other variations on games to find hidden objects or people.
- Hot and cold: Use *hot* and *cold* as hints to where to find the item. *Hot* when close to the item, *cold* as you get farther away, having the child listen to and discriminate those words from varying distances and intensities. As the child learns to listen to the morphemic endings, you can modify to *hotter*, *hottest*, *colder*, and *coldest*. You can use different voice qualities, such as volume or pitch, as variations. Use a loud voice or high-pitch voice as the child gets closer, and a quieter voice or lower pitch as they get farther away.
- Simon Says requires the child to attend to several critical items, such as specific verbs and descriptions, and listen for the key phrase "Simon says" to carry out the action. Otherwise, they are out when they complete an action without the critical phrase. The child listens to and carries out the instructions: "Simon says touch your elbow." "Simon says turn around." "Simon says hop on one foot." The child then becomes Simon and gives the commands to the other players.

Here is a short list of some games to try. Parents, professionals and children can make up their own.

Mother, May I Take a Step?

Red Light, Green Light

Chicken Dance

Musical Chairs

Duck, Duck, Goose

Balancing (walking on a line)

Keep the Balloon Up

Hide and Seek

Pop the Bubbles

Freeze Dance

Hokey Pokey

Ring Around the Rosy

Head, Shoulders, Knees, and Toes

Jump the Candlestick

Putting It All Together: Case History

Suzie was referred for auditory brainstem response (ABR) testing as she failed her newborn screening twice. There is no family history of hearing loss and her mother's pregnancy was unremarkable. She has two older siblings with normal hearing.

She underwent two ABR testing sessions at ages 2 weeks and 5 weeks, which determined that she had a profound bilateral sensorineural hearing loss (SNHL) During repeat testing at 10 weeks, Suzie had no responses at the limit of the equipment in the right ear and a probable response at 100 dB at 1000 Hz and a response at 2000 Hz. The family was referred for auditory-verbal therapy (AVT) by another family. Suzie's parents are choosing to raise her to use listening and spoken English. They aggressively pursued cochlear implants and met with several doctors. Suzie had a CT scan at 7 months of age and was scheduled to be bilaterally implanted. Surgery was postponed several times due to illness and ear infections. Suzie was bilaterally implanted at 8 months and initially mapped at 9 months. She wears her cochlear implants during all her waking hours. Her current hearing age with her cochlear implants is 1 year 4 months (Rotfleisch, 2009).

Auditory Processes for Using Sound Meaningfully

Auditory Attention, Discrimination, and Integration

Suzie is able to listen and generally comprehend when adults speak to her in normal language. She is demonstrating the emergence of overhearing of key words in others' conversations that were not directed at her.

LittlEARS (2004) is an auditory questionnaire administered to parents to evaluate the auditory development of young children with normal hearing and with hearing loss who are using technology such as cochlear implants or hearing aids to access auditory information. Per the publishers, "it covers auditory development in the first 2 years after CI or HA fitting." She has reached the ceiling on this evaluation (Table 8–10).

Table 8–10. LittlEARS Scores

Score	Hearing Age	Chronologic Age
29/35	6 months	15 months
34/35	22 months	25 months

Auditory Memory

Suzie is able to follow three related commands and two requests that are unrelated.

Auditory Processes for Learning to Talk

Auditory Feedback

Suzie is beginning to show an increase in the variety of consonants that she will use spontaneously. The phonemes are of varying manners and places of production. She most frequently uses:

Plosives:

/b/ as in <u>b</u>ee

/p/ as in <u>p</u>ea

/d/ as in <u>d</u>o

/t/ as in <u>t</u>ea—in word final

/k/as in <u>k</u>ey

/g/ as in <u>g</u>o

Fricatives:

/h/ as in <u>h</u>op—primarily in isolation

/ʃ/ as in <u>sh</u>e

/s/ as in <u>s</u>o—primarily in isolation

/v/ as in <u>v</u>ery—emerging

Nasals:

/m/ as in *my*

/n/ as in *no*

Semivowels:

/w/ as in *we*

Laterals:

/r/ as in *red*—emerging

/l/ as in *look*—inconsistent

Auditory Processes for Learning Language

Auditory Recognition

Suzie is recognizing the meaning of new words on a daily basis and is saying at least two new words per week.

Auditory Sequencing

Suzie will imitate longer phrases that she hears her mother or sisters say in the correct order, such as "Jenny, wanna go outside?" She has a variety of expressions indicating good sequencing (e.g., "oh my God," "1 2 3 go," "love you").

Auditory Comprehension and Auditory Retrieval

The Receptive-Expressive Emergent Language Scale (REEL) (2020) was initially administered at 3 months and readministered repeatedly. It was most recently administered at 2 years old. This evaluation is an informal test in which the mother reports on the child's abilities. The REEL shows Suzie scoring 22 months in receptive language and expressive language. This shows age-appropriate comprehension abilities and expressive skills. Scores over time are indicated in Table 8–11. The testing over time indicates change over 6 months as 4 months' growth in receptive abilities and 8 months' growth in expressive abilities. In the 13-month interval, from 11 months of age to 24 months, she showed 16 months' improvement in receptive and expressive language abilities.

Suzie's language skills were also assessed at 2 years of age using the Preschool Language Scale–4 (PLS-4) by Zimmerman et al.

Table 8–11. Receptive-Expressive Emergent Language Scale-3 (REEL-3) Scores

Age	Receptive Language Age	Lag	Expressive Language Age	Lag	Hearing Age
3 m	0 m	3 m	0 m	3 m	2 m
Cochlear Implantation					HA With CI
9 m	0 m	7 m	4 m	5 m	0 m
11 m	6 m	5 m	6 m	5 m	2 m
14 m	11 m	3 m	9 m	5 m	5 m
18 m	18 m	none	14 m	4 m	9 m
21 m	19 m	2 m	17 m	4 m	1 y
24 m	22 m	2 m	22 m	2 m	1 y 3 m

(2011). This evaluation assesses auditory comprehension and verbal ability of language and provides an age-equivalent score compared to normal-hearing children. (Suzie's auditory comprehension score yielded an age equivalent of 1 year 10 months. Her expressive communication score yielded an age equivalent of 2 years (Table 8–12).

As assessed by the PLS-4, Suzie is able to understand verbs in context, identify clothing and body parts, and understand some spatial concepts. Expressively, she uses words more often to communicate, asks questions using a rising intonation, has a variety of pragmatic functions, and combines two words together and occasionally three to four words using known two-word expressions combined with other words. She is not demonstrating comprehension of a variety of verbs in pictures, and shows limited comprehension of pronouns. In the testing situation, Suzie was unable to use plural forms, answer questions other than yes/no forms, and use the verb form -ing; she also has limited three- to four-word combinations.

Suzie comprehends yes/no questions and other common everyday questions such as "What's your name?" and "How old are you?" Suzie will typically speak with a combination of jargon, real words, and two-word expressions along with some gestures and motions. She will embed words within her canonical babble. She has approximately 70 words that she uses spontaneously and will say one to two new words weekly. She refers to herself by name and is beginning to use some pronouns such as *me* and *mine*. She uses *no* when she doesn't want something. She is using a variety of two- to three-word expressions. Some of her multiword phrases are:

love you	*sit down*
bless you	*thank you*
are you OK?	*what is that?*
how are you?	*get me out*
want that back	*oh my God*
goes back	*I want* ____

She is not yet using the morphemes -*ing* or /s/ for plural or possessive. She will ask for help with personal needs and typically answers yes/no questions appropriately. She will greet somebody when asked to and also will spontaneously greet and say goodbye to people appropriately. Suzie will produce a variety of two-word combinations. She is showing an increased number of three- and four-word combinations, per her mother. Samples of some of spontaneous combinations are:

hi mama	*no car*
I want more, mama	*make car go*

Table 8–12. Pre-School Language Scale-4 (PLS-4) Scores

	Auditory Comprehension	Expressive Communication	Language Age
Age Equivalent	1 year, 10 months	2 years	1 year, 11 months
Standard Score	84	91	86
Percentile Rank	14	27	18

mama look
watch Suzie
Benny stop
hi guys
goes there
goes back here
no mine
Suzie have phone

Summary

Suzie shows good development of auditory abilities, which is reflected in improvement in the areas of speech and language skills as measured by informal and standardized assessments. These assessments show excellent progress in the areas of audition, speech, and language abilities. Her current testing indicates that she has a receptive language level of 1 year 10 months per the REEL, which agrees with the results from the PLS-4. Her expressive skill scores are 22 months per the REEL and 2 years per the PLS-4. This indicates that she is demonstrating age-appropriate skills. These assessments indicate that she has made more than 1 year of growth in the past year and in the time since she was activated with her cochlear implants.

The Intervention Session

In this session, we use play as the natural way that children learn everyday routine interactions. In this scenario, most of Suzie's productions remain approximations, and production of some of the phonemes is not always accurate. The /s/ and /ʃ/ perception and its production are briefly addressed in this scenario, and Suzie's production for that word is indicated in quotation marks. However, many other words are written out correctly, though she doesn't necessarily pronounce them correctly. The end of the session takes advantage of some basic routines to reinforce listening and language through basic ADL and routines.

Suzie (pointing at the boxes of Play-Doh): Two bok

Professional: Oh, do you want two box or two boxes?

Suzie: Two bok

Professional: You want two boxes?

Suzie: Want bokeh

Professional: Your mom wanted you to ask me if you can have two.

Suzie: Want. Want two bokeh

Professional: You want two boxes.

Suzie: Two bokeh

Professional: Oh, you want two boxes. Look, I have three boxes. You can have two boxes or three boxes.

Suzie: Want bokeh

Professional: I know, you want boxes. Do you want two boxes or three boxes?

Suzie: Want three bokeh

Professional: OK.

Suzie: Want three bokeh

Professional: Listen: *ssssssss*.

Suzie: Sss

Professional: Good listening, I heard you say *ssss*. You are going to get three boxes (gives the boxes to the child and turns to mother). We have talked about plurals as being one of the first morphemes and that we want to be sure you are using the first morphemes and exposing her to them. Did you notice what was happening with the plurals?

Mother: Not sure when or what you mean. She isn't using any plurals.

Professional: Do you remember when you first got out the boxes of Play-Doh?

Mother: She didn't use the /s/ for *boxes*. She was counting and said "two box."

Professional: Yes, but what did I do? I contrasted the words *box* and *boxes* and asked if she wanted one box or two boxes. I let her know the word is different for plural and let her hear them, and acoustically highlighted the second syllable. It is easy to do that for *boxes* because as an irregular plural we add the syllable *-ez*. For regular plurals we just add the /s/ or /z/. She isn't doing that, but with her emerging auditory skills, she showed us that she is tuning into the extra syllable and said "box eh." That should not be difficult for her to do, since the number of syllables—in this case, two—is the suprasegmental duration. We know she is great with duration and how it transfers into words by the number of syllables. So that is a nice start. She does realize the word was different—plural form—for two or three of the items.

I know you are concerned about the /s/. We know she is hearing it and she will do it in isolation, like "sssss" for a snake. Since it is a continuant sound, it is easy for her to make it long and do it first in isolation. But that also brings us to the conversation about plurals. I also had her listen to the /s/ and repeat it but only in isolation, because we still can't get her to consistently use the /s/. So what I did was enhance her hearing, not correct her speech. I had her listen to the fricative. Now technically in *boxes* it is a /z/, but producing an /s/ is understandable as the plural marker to anybody who would hear it. So, we are helping her to listen to the word-final sound. I had her involved in a complete and correct auditory feedback loop. I had her listen to the sound and produce the sound, and then I put the sound back in the word. This will be the foundation for her developing and improving her auditory feedback loop to monitor her own speech sounds as she progresses.

Mother: So, should I start doing that?

Professional: I think highlighting the fricative /s/, especially in words that she knows or for the snake, is a great place to enhance her hearing and get her to attend to the fricative quality and practice it and set it up in her own auditory feedback loop. Remember, correct in and out. In her ears to her brain and out her mouth. But remember to be sure that the last production of the sound that she says and the last thing she hears you say are both correct and match. Then you have a complete and correct auditory feedback loop. The other thing is to contrast the singular and the plural forms for her to be paying more attention to them.

Mother: OK, great! Got it. So, you need how many more?

Suzie: 1 2 3

Mother: 1 2 3; you needed one more box.

Mother: You needed one more box. There you go, you got it.

Mother: Move it over, so it fits. Let's put it on the table.

Suzie: Table

Mother: Should we put it on the table or should we put it on the bench back here?

Suzie: Three bokeh

Mother: We should move it so you have a place to play. I'm going to move it, OK?

Mother: Wow, you got three boxes out!

Suzie: Wow three bokeh

Mother: You got three boxes out!

Suzie: Three bokeh

Mother: What color Play-Doh do you want?

Suzie: I want boo.

Suzie: I want boo. I want two.

Suzie: One two

Mother: Go sit down and ask me for what you want.

Suzie: I want Mickey Mou

Mother: Here you go. I am giving you Mickey Mouse.

Suzie: Thank you.

Mother: I have blue Play-Doh.

Suzie: Want more

Mother: You have more on the table

Mother: You want the red toy? But the purple works better.

Suzie: Want ed (red)

Mother: OK, we can try, but if it doesn't work we can change to purple.

Suzie: Moh

Mother: More what? I don't know what you want. (Points to the Play-Doh)

Mother: That's the Play-Doh. You want more Play-Doh?

Suzie (reaching for the blue Play-Doh): Want moo

Mother: You want the blue? Here you go.

Suzie: I want two boo.

Mother: OK. You have a small one and a big one.

Professional: So, mom, how do you feel about that interaction?

Mother: I felt like there were times she really wasn't listening to me.

Professional: I agree, some of the time she was very engaged with the activity. But what else was happening?

Mother: She did a lot of word combinations. Even some three and four words, I think.

Professional: Yes, she did! Like "I want two blue." We have to remember that for her, "I want" is a unit, so though we can count it as four words or morphemes, we know it is really a combination of three. But still lovely and in the right order, starting with *I want* and with *two* before the word *blue*. Nice. What else?

Mother: I don't know. Her speech isn't good with the /s/ and no /r/ for *roll*.

Professional: Yes, true, but let's get to that in a minute. One of the big goals has been to be moving her to consistent use of two-word combinations and beyond. How do you think that went?

Mother: Seems more natural to get her to say two words.

Professional: Well, more natural, also because you are setting her up for success. You are acoustically highlighting two to three key words in phrases. So, you are expanding her auditory memory and giving her combinations with words that she knows.

We can keep facilitating her attention to the word endings for the plurals, since we know she hears the sound. I also loved that you were using the *-ing* and trying to incorporate the three-act play to give her lots of opportunities to hear that morpheme! Do you remember the first morphemes that develop and that you should be incorporating into your language with her?

Mother: Yes: plurals, *-ing* ending, and *in* and *on*.

Professional: Perfect. How do you feel it is going remembering to include them?

Mother: Feeling OK with the *-ing*, using the three-act play pretty often at home. I'm not doing the plurals and just starting to use the *on* and *in* more at home.

Professional: Great. Keep in mind that we don't expect her to be saying those yet, and expressively the main focus is the word combinations and that also works on the auditory memory! So as long as you are keeping them in mind to be adding to your language so she can develop the comprehension, that is great.

Suzie: Help, help

Mother: I can help you.

Suzie: Big one

Mother: You have the big one.

Suzie (gets out toy knife with opener): Mama, mama help

Mother: Do you need help?

Suzie: Mama, mama knife

Mother: Not that one, you asked for the knife. That's not the knife.

Suzie: Mama, mama knife

Mother: This is the red one.

Suzie (pulls open toy): Mama, mama knife

Mother: Oh! Not the knife. You want the opener.

Suzie: Wee-oh

Mother: I think you want to open the Play-Doh.

Suzie: Open

Mother: Open? Open my mouth? Open the Play-Doh?

Suzie: Open Ay-Doh

Mother: Oh! Let's open the Play-Doh!

Suzie: Help open

Mother: OK, I'm helping you.

Suzie: Open

Mother: We need to put the opener on the lid.

Suzie: Open

Mother: Yes. We are opening the Play-Doh.

Suzie: Open

Mother: We are opening, opening, opening.

Suzie: Openih

Mother: Help me. We are opening the Play-Doh.

Suzie: Want more

Mother: You have more on the table.

Suzie: Want more

Mother: You want more what? More Play-Doh?

Suzie: I want more.

Mother: More what? Use your words.

Suzie: More

Mother: You want more what?

Suzie: I want

Mother: I don't know what you want.

Suzie: O

Mother: Oh, you want the roller! I'm giving you the roller.

Suzie: Thank you.

Mother: I gave you the roller.

Mother: Now you are going to roll it flat.

Mother: Roll and roll and roll the Play-Doh. Roll and roll and roll the Play-Doh.

Suzie: Help you

Mother: You want me to help you?

Suzie: Help you

Mother: I can help you. Can you help me?

Suzie: Help

Mother: Help me please. Let's do it together.

Suzie: Puh

Mother: Yes, we need to push.

Suzie: Puh

Professional: OK, so you gave her the right model for push when she left off the *-sh* at the end of the word, but she didn't do it when she repeated it. Remember what we did with the /s/ when we wanted to enhance her perception? She didn't do the *-sh*, and we know she can, particularly in that word. Take it out in isolation and have her imitate it and then put it back in the word. If she says it right, you can try to have her say it in the word, because we know she can do that. So, start with having her perceive and then produce the *-sh*.

Mother: OK, Suzie, listen. Tell me *shhhh*.

Suzie: Shhh

Mother: Good listening. We need to push, push push.

Suzie: Push

Mother: Yes! Push, push, push!!

Professional: Perfect!

Mother: I think you need to push harder.

Suzie: Push

Mother: Push down, make it flat.

Suzie: Oh, roh, oh

Mother: Good rolling and rolling.

Professional: You aren't making her imitate directly, just providing sentences with some key words that she can pick and use. Sometimes she has something else in mind, like when she suddenly decided that she wanted the rolling pin toy. But you went with it and figured it out. She was good, she pointed but also did her approximation for *roll* which, as you said, wasn't very good. Just the "o," but she isn't consistent with the /r/ or /l/, so that is probably the best we can expect right now. I think there was one /r/ in her approximation for *roll*. Good language and using the *-ing* verb ending. Another place you can use it is when you say "good job" to her. You can add a verb with the *-ing* ending. "Good job pushing" or "Good job cleaning up," which is what we need to do. So, without showing her, let her know it is time to clean up and put on her shoes that she took off and leave.

Mother: Suzie, we have to clean up. Time to go home for lunch.

Suzie: Clean up?

Mother: Time to clean up and go home for lunch.

Suzie: Clean up bye-bye.

Mother: We will clean up and go home. You need to put on your shoes and say "Bye bye."

Suzie: Clean up shoe

Mother: Good job cleaning up.

Professional: Good job adding the *-ing* verb. (Quietly to mother and then picks up the shoes.) Suzie, we cleaned up. Now put your shoes on. Here are your shoes.

Suzie: Shoe

Professional: I have two shoes. I can give you a shoe or both shoes. Listen: *ssss*.

Suzie: Ssss

Mother: I think we need your shoes.

Suzie: Shoe

Mother: You need both shoes. Listen: *ssss*.

Suzie: *Ssss*

Mother: Yes, let's get your shoes.

Suzie: Shoes

Mother: Yes!! Shoes. Let's put on your shoes.

Suzie: Shoe on

Mother: Let's put one shoe on and then the other shoe on.

Suzie: Shoe on

Mother: Put your foot in the shoe.

Suzie: Shoe on

Mother: We put your shoe on.

Suzie: More shoe

Mother: Yes, I will put your other shoe on.

Suzie: More shoe on

Mother: There, we put your shoes on. See two shoes.

Suzie: Shoes

Mother: Yay! Shoes! We put on your shoes. That was so good Suzie.

Professional: That was so good, mom!!!

Mother: I didn't expect her to say that.

Professional: Actually, that makes sense that *shoes* would be one of her first plurals. We don't usually talk about *shoe* since we rarely wear one shoe. Though you did a nice job contrasting, putting on a shoe and then both shoes. And we know she is starting to pay attention to the sounds at the ends of words. That is the way to do it! Think about other words that we more typically use in plural form like *eyes*, *pants*, *hands*. Like "wash your hands."

Mother: That's a good thing to do this week.

Professional: Yup! So, time to leave. Give her two to three things to listen to together, like you did with clean up and going home.

Mother: OK, Suzie, say "bye-bye" and then we can open the door.

Suzie: Bye-bye

Mother: Bye-bye, let's open the door!

Professional: Bye! Nice job repeating the two commands even after she had said "bye," because it reinforces that auditory memory.

Analysis of Session

In discussion of the therapy session, we can analyze which goals are being addressed in the described interval of therapy. The goals are indicated by number and refer to Tables 8–3 to 8–6. This scenario helps to show the integration and overlap of multiple goals in the natural interactions, just like the cookie dough theory (see Chapter 5). Suzie listens throughout this play activity; as she is engaged in an activity with joint attention, she is naturally integrating listening into her interaction style as structured by her mother and the professional. By virtue of embedding listening into this activity, many of her auditory goals for auditory attention, detection, and discrimination (Table 8–3) are being addressed as she is engaged in a play activity while she listens and demonstrates excellent conversational turn taking (Goals 1a–f, 2, 3, 4, 7, 8, 10). The mother models expanded phrases she is using based on the activity, incorporating a closed set and allowing Suzie to develop her listening and spoken language (Goals 1, 2, 3, 4, 7, 10, 14, 15, 17, 18).

Suzie attends to and discriminates a variety of suprasegmental features, vowels, and consonants (Goals 1a-d, 2). Her mother and professional stimulate her hearing and comprehension by using grammatically correct, short phrases with two to four key words that are supported strongly through context and the physical toys (Goals 2, 3, 4, 14, 15, 16, 17). We can monitor her auditory feedback with her many spontaneous productions. We facilitate her speech and enhance her perception in having her listen to and repeat the /s/ phoneme (Goals 1d, 2, 6, 7, 11c–d, 12, 13, 16c). There is clearly an established conversational interaction in which she participates as a communicative partner in both listening and speaking. She listens to her mother and the professional and responds, indicating she is attending and comprehending what is being said (Goals 2, 3, 4, 7, 10, 14, 16, 17). Suzie uses her spoken language and vocabulary in a functional interaction to communicate her needs and wants with a variety of pragmatic functions (Goals 18, 19). Suzie is showing a variety of emerging word combinations used spontaneously and easily combines two words together.

Summary

The professional's knowledge base and work guide and coach the parent to understand relevant elements of auditory,

Table 8–13. By the End of the Emerging Word Combinations Stage, the Child Should:

> Combine three to four words.
>
> Show comprehension of a variety of grammatical structures including pronouns, negatives, and prepositions.
>
> Use some grammatical morphemes; e.g., *-ing* verb endings, prepositions (e.g., *in, on*), plural and possessive /s/ functions.
>
> Rapidly learn receptive and expressive vocabulary with early concepts emerging.

speech, and language skills and strategies to promote development in these areas at the stage of emerging word combinations. This will help the child to achieve the skills outlined in Tables 8–1 and 8–2 and the outlined goals from this stage of language development. The achievement of these goals will provide a strong basis for the child with hearing loss to progress to the next level of listening and spoken language abilities. Behaviors that are indicative of the child emerging into the next stage of development are indicated in Table 8–13.

Discussion Questions

1. How do you determine if a child is at this stage?
2. How would you illustrate the chocolate chip cookie dough analogy to the parents of a child with hearing loss at this stage?
3. Select a goal from one of the Tables 8–3 through 8–6. How would you explain to a parent to use a specific activity of daily living to target the goal? Consider and identify other goals would be naturally included in that selected ADL.
4. What activities could you do with an older child to work on the goals at this level?
5. Consider a child with additional disabilities or needs and discuss an activity that you could work on to target a selected goal at this level.

References

American Speech-Language-Hearing Association. (1997–2021). *Developmental norms for speech and language.* https://www.asha.org/public/speech/development/chart/

Brown, V. L., Bzoch, D. R., & League, R. (2020). *Receptive-Expressive Emergent Language Test* (4th ed.). Western Psychological Services.

Carle, E. (1969). *The hungry caterpillar.* World Publishing.

Degen, B. (1994). *Jamberry.* HarperCollins.

Cochlear Corporation. (2010). Integrated scales of development. In *Listen, learn, talk* (pp. 16–31). Cochlear Limited.

Ling, D. (2003). The Ling Six-Sound Test. *The Listener,* 52–53.

Madell, J. R., Hewitt, J. G., & Rotfleisch, S. (2018). Chapter 25: Red flags: Identifying and managing barriers to the child's optimal auditory development. In J. R. Madell, C. Flexer, J. Wolfe, & E. C. Schafer (Eds.). *Pediatric audiology: Diagnosis, technology and management* (3rd ed., pp. 267–276). Thieme.

Martin, B., & Archambault, J. (1989). *Chicka chicka boom boom.* Simon & Schuster.

Perkins, A., & Gurney, E. (1988). *Hands, hands, fingers, thumb.* Random House.

Piaget, J. (1962). *Play, dreams, and imitation in childhood.* W. W. Norton & Co.

Rotfleisch, S. (2009). Auditory verbal therapy and babies. In L. Eisenberg (Ed.), *Clinical management of children with cochlear implants* (pp. 435–493). Plural Publishing.

Schwartz, S., & Miller, J. (1988). *The new language of toys: Teaching communication skills to children with special needs: A guide for parents and teachers*. Woodbine House.

Tsiakpini, L., Weichbold, V., Kuehn-Inacker, H., Coninx, F., D'Haese, P., & Almadin, S. (2004). *LittlEARS Auditory Questionnaire*. MED-EL.

Vickers, J., & Vickers, N. (1956). *Play-Doh*. Rainbow Craft.

Wood, A., & Wood, D. (1984). *The napping house*. Houghton Mifflin Hardcore.

Zimmerman, I. L., Steiner, V. G., & Pond, R. E. (2011). *Preschool Language Scales* (4th ed.). Pearson.

Chapter 9

Communication With Typical Childlike Errors Stage

Sylvia Rotfleisch

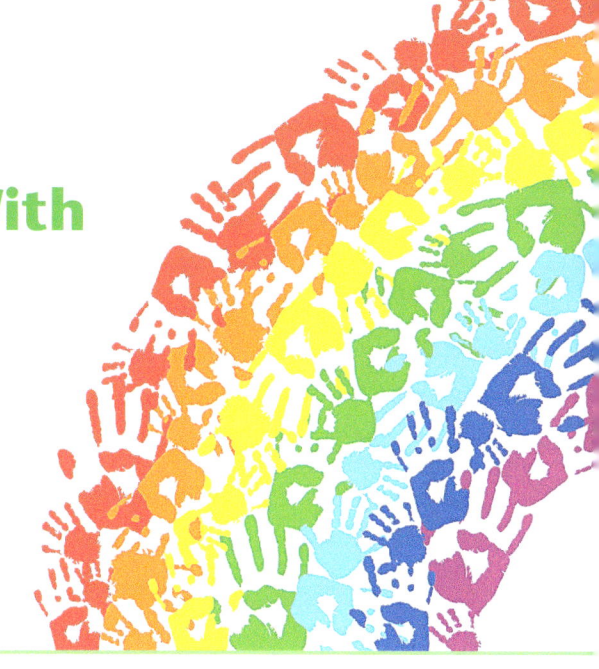

Key Points

- The child at the communication with childlike errors stage is typically very successful at communicating with listening and spoken language.
- At this stage, the child will learn to listen to and understand more complex language across a variety of their daily life environments.
- Grammatically complete and correct sentences will be produced as the child masters a variety of more advanced morphemes.
- The family should include goals that incorporate the family culture in their activities of daily living.
- Goals should be incorporated into the child's play, interactions, and various settings. We continue to adapt to the child's age, cognitive and developmental stages, and interests.

Basic Characteristics of the Child Who Communicates With Typical Childlike Errors

Listening

The child with hearing loss has developed some advanced auditory abilities that are naturally integrated into their personality, daily functioning, and interactions with others in different environments. Technology is seen as a natural part of themselves, as is listening and interacting using spoken language. The child with hearing loss is able to understand most language from daily experiences and typical routines. The child is now able to understand language from less-familiar adults (e.g., neighbors, other parents, teachers). However, listening in acoustically challenging situations, such as with background or competing noise (e.g., playground, TV, or radio in the background; noisy classroom; distance) is still difficult (Klatte et al., 2010). Errors in comprehension will happen due to not accessing some sounds or misperception of unstressed and quieter words (e.g., *crayon* versus *crayons*, *can* versus *can't*).

A child at this stage is able to listen to longer sentences with multiple elements and retain the details. We see the development of grammatical morphemes as the child learns to attend to and comprehend these structures (see Table 3–7). The intermediate auditory skills are demonstrated by attending to and comprehending advanced language structures such as a variety of verb tenses (e.g., past tense verbs such as *jump* versus *jumped* or *pull* versus *pulled*). Listening to longer messages, including personal stories, explanations of how and what, and books, is evidenced throughout the child's day. There is clear evidence that the child is learning new information from this auditory input. The child demonstrates "thinking while listening" abilities. After listening, comprehension is demonstrated by responding to a question with new information not contained in the auditory message but possibly implied (e.g., "Would you like something to drink that comes from a cow or that comes from fruit?"). These intermediate auditory abilities typically evident and/or emerging in the communication with errors stage are indicated in Table 9–1. Skills listed are not sequential.

Language

At this stage of language development, the child with hearing loss is becoming a competent conversational partner. Full sentences are used to communicate and are understood by most people, including unfamiliar adults. Comprehension

Table 9–1. Auditory Abilities Evidenced in the Communication With Childlike Errors Stage

- Demonstrates auditory memory and comprehension for sentences of four to six elements/words (e.g., "Put the bumpy red ball in the empty cup," "Give Daddy your boots and jacket with the hood").
- Demonstrates understanding of sentences with multiple elements, including unstressed grammatical morphemes (e.g., "She is playing with the little boy under the tree").
- Attends to and processes complex language structures. (e.g., "The boy, wearing the hat, gave a book to the girl sitting in the corner").
- Listens to longer stories and remembers details.
- Demonstrates auditory memory for a short story and can retell events in sequence in several stories.
- Attends to and discriminates word-final differences in sounds (minimal differences such as *cat, cap, tap, bat*) and morphemes (e.g., *jumps, jumpy, jumper, jumping, jumped*).
- Demonstrates thinking while listening (e.g., responds with new information by attending to and integrating information, "It's an animal that is green and eats flies").
- Identifies initial sounds.
- Understands and tells rhyming words.

Sources: Brown (2020); LittlEARS (2004); ASHA Milestones; Integrated Scales of Development (2012).

has increased significantly and the child is able to answer a variety of questions. Expressive language continues to evolve rapidly in this stage and the child typically uses four-word utterances. Longer utterances incorporate a variety of grammatical morphemes including, but not limited to, pronouns, plurals, and a variety of verb tense markers (see Morphemes, Table 3–7).

There is an ease in the acquisition of new vocabulary including words from Tier 2, which includes high-frequency words, function words, and words with multiple meanings. At this stage it is typical that a child will have between 1,000 and 2,000 words expressively (see Chapter 3, Vocabulary). It is expected that there will be multiple grammatical errors that reflect an emerging language system.

Receptive and expressive language abilities evidenced or expected to emerge in this stage are included in Table 9–2. Skills listed are not sequential.

Speech

A child with hearing loss will produce phonemes that reflect auditory access, speech perception abilities, and hearing and listening experience. The child with hearing loss who has appropriate auditory access will be developing phonemes, both vowels and consonants, in the expected sequence. We expect emerging mastery at this stage, but we must keep in mind that with typically developing children, mastery of speech sounds continues until the age of 8 years and beyond (see Chapter 3).

Table 9–2. Language and Speech Skills Evidenced in the Communication With Childlike Errors Stage

Audition and Auditory Comprehension of Language	Expressive Language/Vocalization and Communication
• Responds when you call from another room. • Understands words for different concepts and attributes; e.g., color, shapes, sizes, positions, categories. • Understands words for family relations; e.g., *brother*, *grandmother*, and *aunt*. • Understands time concepts such as *day*, *night*, and *tomorrow*, as evidenced in verb tenses (past, present, and future). • Understands derivational suffixes; e.g., *bigger*, *biggest*, *farm*, *farmer*.	• Answers simple *who*, *what*, and *where* questions. • Says rhyming words; e.g., *hat—cat*. • Uses pronouns; e.g., *I*, *you*, *me*, *we*, and *they*. • Uses plural words; e.g., *books*, *dogs*, and *cars* and some irregulars such as *feet*. • Most people understand what the child says. • Asks *when* and *how* questions. • Puts four words together. • Makes some grammatical mistakes; e.g., "I goed to school," "I want eat cracker." • Talks about what happened during the day. • Combines several sentences at a time to convey more information.

Sources: Brown (2020); LittlEARS (2004); ASHA Milestones; Integrated Scales of Development (2012).

Goals for the Stage of Communication With Errors

Developing an Appropriate Therapy Plan by Addressing Strengths and Areas of Need

The typical sequence of development will be followed to develop listening skills and appropriate speech and language abilities. All previous goals will be used as the basis for expanding to the next skills. Some goals from the emerging word combination stage might not be mastered and might be carried over initially in this stage. Goals for the communication with errors stage focus on:

- facilitating listening abilities for longer and more complex auditory information across all acoustic environments in the child's daily life;
- reinforcing the auditory feedback loop for consistent use and self-monitoring of all appropriate phonemes;
- facilitating comprehension of language with a variety of grammatical morphemes in a variety of formats (e.g., conversations, stories, books); and
- facilitating use of grammatically complete sentences to communicate clearly.

Select appropriate goals based on your assessment results that identify the child's strengths and needs (see Chapter 4). With the understanding of speech features and the acoustics parameters related to an audiogram, monitor for emerging skills. Based on the hearing loss, predict and prepare for areas of potential difficulty (see Chapter 1).

Goals must be individualized within the stage to meet the child's needs. Consider, for example, when determining goals related to comprehension. One child might be able to listen to short chapter books with limited pictures and be able to answer some basic questions that demonstrate comprehension. Goals for this child could facilitate responses to a greater variety of questions, including prediction or inference, and expand to expressive language by retelling portions of the story (Goals 10, 11, 12, 15, 16, 17, 18). However, another child might be able to listen to a few sentences on a page from a picture book with a story based on a familiar topic. For this child, target goals that will expand the auditory memory for longer auditory input. The goals should address increased length of sentences, increased number of sentences, more complex language and morphemes, new vocabulary, and listening to several sentences in a conversational turn (Goals 2, 3, 4, 9, 11).

Typical Goals for the Communication With Errors Stage

Your selected goals should continue to focus on expanding complex auditory skills for attending to, comprehending, and responding to increasingly complex language and messages. Goals will support the mastery of linguistic competence in this stage. The child will learn to apply those linguistic competencies in more difficult acoustic environments in their daily life. Use of the expanding auditory memory and auditory feedback loop will be the basis for developing self-monitoring and self-correcting both speech phonemes and language structures. These abilities will provide the foundational skills for competent communicator stage.

Typical recommended goals for children with hearing loss at the communication with errors level are included in Tables 9–3 to 9–6. Goals are organized based upon defined skills related to the brain functions necessary for learning to use audition for language development (see Chapter 3). The goals included in these tables should not be considered the definitive set of goals for all children at this stage, neither should they be considered an exhaustive list of possible audition goals for the child with hearing loss at the communication with errors stage of language development. Goals must address the specific errors and needs determined during comprehensive assessment as well as from observation and informal diagnostic work.

How Do We Work on These Goals?

Professionals must have a knowledge base and multiple appropriate strategies applicable to the child at the stage of communication with errors to accomplish the recommended goals. Knowledge areas and strategies applicable to the child at the communication with errors stage are identified in Tables 9–7 and 9–8 (see p. 217). The knowledge and strategies included in these tables are the basis for you to guide

Table 9–3. Auditory Goals for Understanding Sound as Meaningful in the Communication With Childlike Errors Stage

Auditory Attention, Detection, Discrimination, and Memory

1. Reinforce and expand discrimination and production of speech features at phonetic and phonological levels in variety of listening environments:
   a. suprasegmentals—duration, intensity, pitch (DIP)
   b. vowels and diphthongs
   c. manners of consonant production
   d. places of consonant production
   e. voicing for consonant production
2. Facilitate expanded awareness and discrimination of minor differences of morphemes (see Table 3–7, *Morpheme Development*) of negatives, conjunctions, prepositions, pronouns, and articles in conversational speech.
3. Facilitate ability to attend through audition only to sentences of six to ten words, including four to eight elements or requests.
4. Reinforce and expand auditory memory to four to eight critical items in short phrases and compound sentences using closed set, familiar and new vocabulary including nouns, prepositions, pronouns, and verbs.
5. Expand auditory memory for rhymes, songs, and other tasks (e.g., numbers, days of the week, and months).
6. Facilitate and expand ability to attend to language and converse while engaged visually or in a motor task.

Table 9–4. Auditory Feedback and Speech Production Goals in the Communication With Childlike Errors Stage

Auditory Goals for Development of the Speech Production System

7. Reinforce and expand consistent control and productions of all speech features at phonologic level in longer sentences and phrases to improve levels of speech intelligibility:
   a. suprasegmentals—duration, intensity, pitch (DIP)
   b. vowels and diphthongs
   c. manners of consonant production
   d. places of consonant production
   e. voicing for consonant production
8. Reinforce and monitor emergence of auditory feedback loop to monitor and self-correct productions of words, including word-final consonants and words with errors determined to be old habits.

Table 9–5. Auditory Goals for Language Comprehension in the Communication With Childlike Errors Stage

Auditory Recognition, Sequencing, and Comprehension
9. Facilitate and expand recognition of familiar key words and morphemes when embedded within six- to ten-word descriptive and complex phrases.
10. Facilitate and expand consistent comprehension of morphemes and sequencing within sentences, beginning with those assessed as inconsistent.
11. Expand auditory comprehension of multiple sentences of six to ten familiar words, each with new vocabulary in closed set material (e.g., books, conversations).
12. Expand and reinforce auditory comprehension of a variety of question forms, including *why*.
13. Expand auditory comprehension of verb tenses, including past, present, and future tenses.

14. Reinforce and expand auditory comprehension of all morphemes (see Table 3–7, *Morpheme Development*):
   a. present progressive tense
   b. prepositions
   c. plural forms including /s/, /z/, /es/, and irregular forms
   d. possessive forms
   e. pronouns
   f. past tense
   g. negatives

Table 9–6. Auditory Goals for Developing Expressive Language in the Communication With Childlike Errors Stage

Auditory Retrieval and Expressive Communication

15. Facilitate consistent use of emerging and inconsistent morphemic functions (see Table 3–7, morpheme development) in conversational speech as identified through assessments:
    a. present tense progressive
    b. prepositions
    c. plural forms including /s/, /z/, /es/, and irregular forms
    d. possessive forms
    e. pronouns
    f. past tense
    g. negatives
16. Facilitate use of six- to ten-word sentences for a variety of complex pragmatic functions (e.g., persuading, negotiating, arguing).
17. Facilitate and reinforce auditory retrieval of several sentences to tell a simple story that includes newly emerging vocabulary.
18. Facilitate and expand spontaneous auditory retrieval of a variety of question forms.

Table 9–7. Knowledge Areas in the Communication With Childlike Errors Stage

- Hearing technologies being used
- Effective troubleshooting of technology
- Speech acoustics related to speech development
- Speech acoustics related to language development
- Ling six sounds
- Sequence of development of speech phonemes
- Development of complex receptive language
- Development of complex expressive language
- Reading and fostering emerging foundations in literacy

Table 9–8. Optimal Strategies to Implement in the Communication With Childlike Errors Stage

- Chocolate chip cookie theory
- Activities of daily living
- Three-act play
- Acoustic highlighting
- Enhancing perception
- Natural correcting strategies
- Vocabulary enrichment
- Preteaching vocabulary for new experiences
- Teaching the unknown connected to the known
- Expanding world knowledge and the related language
- Elicit multiple events from stories and multistep instructions from personal experiences
- Reading
- Thinking words for Theory of Mind

and coach the caregiver as the primary person to develop their child's listening and spoken language abilities.

Parents will be learning strategies and implementing them in therapy sessions. At the stage of communication with errors, you will talk in conversations, expand the child's language with corrected use of morphemes, engage the child in a variety of topics with new vocabulary, and use complete sentences and phrases with morphemes.

Support parents to successfully use these strategies (see Table 9–8). At this stage, the parents should consistently use previously learned strategies. As their child reaches the communication with errors stage, introduce the parents to some new strategies. It is always important that strategies rapidly carry over into natural daily interactions. If the parent is new to listening and language intervention, they might not be familiar with strategies used at the earlier stages of listening and spoken language development. Guide and coach them to understand optimal strategies and support their ability to rapidly carry them over into natural daily interactions with their child. Parents should sound like the professional. Help parents to understand knowledge related to listening and spoken language development so they can find natural activities and situations that facilitate the next skills for their child's continued development.

The parent and professional will talk to the child with hearing loss in conversations and will model correct use of morphemes and grammatical structures. At this stage, the child is communicative and conversational, and has developed interests. The child is easily engaged in preferred activities using natural interactions where it is easy to integrate all of the child's listening and spoken language goals. You will find that at this stage you can easily and actively engage the child in their own progress through listening and spoken language. You can introduce other things that might be of interest, such as tongue twisters, memorizing funny poems, or rote lists. These can also be used to practice their speech production in a fun way.

The child will talk about what is of interest to them, or play with preferred toys and games. The adults will incorporate new words and concepts in their interactions with the child. Point out new words or irregular grammatical structures as unusual ways to say things. Using this positive natural interaction style will help the child understand that you and the parent care about the communicative interaction, though you are also helping them to learn more skills. This will help to establish your relationship with the child with hearing loss who still has listening and language skills to develop.

You can accept and validate their communication by restating what was said, and nonchalantly correct errors by modeling the correct language structure. For example, when the child says "I goed so fast!" you can opt to say, "I saw that you went so fast!" This is not a stage for correcting and drilling. Adults can take the same strategy for modeling proper pronunciation. For example, when the child says, "I learned how cars are made in the *faptory*," you can respond, "I know you are telling me about factories. That's a new word for you. It has a /k/ sound, *factory*" or "That's exciting! Cars are made in factories, so I know that is what you mean. Tell me more about factories."

You will easily be able to incorporate the cookie dough theory at this stage. Goals from all areas of listening and spoken language (Tables 9–3 to 9–6) are interrelated and can be integrated in almost any appropriate activity or interaction that is engaging to the child. This allows you and the parent to focus on multiple goals when interacting with a child at this stage of listening and spoken language development.

Additional suggested activities for you to use and to guide and coach the parents are included in Table 9–9.

Targeting and Incorporating Goals

Auditory Attention, Detection, Memory, Discrimination, Auditory Recognition, Sequencing, and Comprehension
(Tables 9–3 and 9–5)

Auditory Retrieval and Expressive Communication
(Tables 9–4 and 9–6)

Activities of Daily Living (ADL)

At this stage of language development, exploiting the activities of daily living addresses more complex thinking and executive function (See Bloom's Taxonomy, Table 3–13). Grocery shopping, an outing to the farmers' market, and meal planning have a variety of elements that can be considered and can be part of a weeklong listening and language focus. With some creativity, you can help the parent to incorporate every goal targeted for the child. While planning dinner menus for the week or school lunches, the child can recite the days of the week and consider if there are dairy items, vegetables, and fruits planned for each day. These conversations allow the parent to introduce or reinforce vocabulary such as categories. Incorporate new concepts with conversation topics about balanced healthy meals, family members' favorite meals, budgeting, picking food items on sale, and cutting coupons. (Goals 4, 5, 11).

Consider an activity such as baking a special treat. In a therapy session, you could find a recipe and check if the family has all the ingredients. Discuss the steps of the recipe. The parent can continue the activity at home. This activity is a perfect opportunity for receptive and expressive use of more complex language and longer phrases with more critical items (Goals 2, 3, 4, 6, 9, 10, 11, 13, 14). After the child has asked to bake a specific item, there will be a conversation. Ask, "Can we bake today? Why do you want to bake?" If there is a missing item, can the child make some suggestions to problem solve? The adults' portion could include explanation and instructions such as: "If we have all the ingredients for the cupcakes, then we can bake them today. But if we don't, we will have to put them on the shopping list. We can bake after we get to the market. I need you to look for the ingredients while I read the recipe. Look for the baking soda on the bottom shelf in the pantry next to the salt. It's in a rectangular orange box with a picture of a flower on it" (Goals 12, 13, 15, 16, 17). Missing items can be put on a grocery list and a plan can be made for when there will be time for a trip to the grocery store (Goals 2, 3, 4, 6, 9, 10, 11, 12). A trip to the grocery store will allow for listening in a different acoustic environment (Goal 1). Do not forget to share the sequence story about baking, or not baking, with other family members.

Table 9–9. Guide and Coach Parents To:

Implement optimal strategies for the stage of communication with childlike errors (Table 9–8)

Listen! Talk, talk, talk!

- Speak in the language that is natural in the home.
- Talk about what is happening and where you go.
- Use rhyming words.
- Define words and help your child understand them (e.g., "This vehicle is on the highway. It is a car. A bus is another kind of vehicle. So are a train and an airplane").
- Help the child learn new words and sentences.
- Look at family pictures. Have the child tell a story about the picture.
- Optimize a routine like grocery shopping. Cut out pictures of foods, glue them on cards, and make "grocery lists" by listening to several items and remembering them. Have them sort the cards by areas of the store or categories (e.g., fruits, vegetables, snacks, produce, dairy, frozen, baking ingredients).
- Have the child plan a meal and figure out the ingredients.
- Use concepts related to spatial relations/locations (e.g., behind, corner, middle, next to), sequence (e.g., first, after, then), quantity modifiers (e.g., all, some), quality modifiers (e.g., similarities, differences), and attributes (e.g., shape, color, size, textures).
- Use clear and precise language (e.g., "Put the book on the bottom shelf next to the blocks").
- Use complex sentences with multiple elements and conjunctions to help expand what the child will understand (e.g., "After we go to the library, we can go to the grocery store to get fruit," "If you clean up then we can go for a walk," "We need to go to the kitchen for a snack because you are hungry").
- Encourage the child to ask questions about a book or event.

Play, play, play!

- Make silly pictures using old magazines and glue parts of different pictures together. For example, cut out a dog and a car. Glue the dog into the car as the driver. Help the child explain what is silly about the picture.
- Encourage pretend play dress-up and role-playing stories or experiences like cooking food or going to the doctor to help teach social skills and storytelling.
- Play "thinking while listening games"—"I am thinking of a fruit. It is crunchy. Its green on the outside and red on the inside."
- Sort pictures and objects into categories, like food, animals, or shapes. Ask your child to find the picture or object that does not belong. For example, a baby does not belong with the animals.

Sing

- Sing about actions and places.
- Sing songs from your culture.
- Sing songs that are age- and cognitively appropriate.

Table 9–9. *continued*

Read

- Read books with a simple story. Talk about the story with your child. Help them retell the story or act it out with props and dress-up clothes. Tell them your favorite part of the story. Ask for their favorite part.
- Read stories with animated voices that reflect the different emotional states in the book or of the characters.
- Read stories that are easy to follow. Help your child guess what will happen next in the story.
- Act out the stories or put on puppet shows.
- Have your child draw a picture of a scene from the story. You can do the same thing with videos, movies, and shows.
- Ask who, what, when, where, or why questions about the story.
- Encourage predictions and inferences when reading (e.g., "What do you think will happen next?" "How do you know the boy is hungry?")
- Help their child understand by asking questions.
- Have the child ask questions.

Theory of Mind

- Discuss how characters in books or people in different situations might feel and what they are thinking. What are their thought bubbles?
- Promote understanding false belief by using sabotage (e.g., put grapes in the empty bag of chips or a sock in the egg carton. Ask what is in the bag or carton).
- Discuss people's different preferences, likes and dislikes, favorite things, different thoughts, and ways of acting in situations.
- Support understanding different people's preferences (e.g., "What is your favorite color? What is your brother's favorite color? Since you know he likes blue, maybe he wants to play with the blue game pawn. Since he likes blue, maybe we should get him a blue shirt").

Sources: Compiled from ASHA https://www.asha.org/public/speech/development/01/; and http://www.hanen.org/helpful-info/articles/tuning-in-to-others-how-young-children-develop.aspx

The sequence story begins with the initial thought of wanting to bake cookies. Include the search for ingredients, the disappointment that there were missing ingredients for the recipe, the problem solving, or the plan to bake another day. All elements the child experienced are worthy of telling (Goals 1, 2, 3, 4, 6, 7, 8, 9, 10, 11, 14, 15, 16, 17).

Auditory memory can be reinforced by remembering an increasingly larger number of items that need to be bought. The location of specific items can be described using sentences with increased numbers of key and critical items such as, "The pasta noodles are on the bottom shelf between the cans of tomatoes and the jars of spaghetti sauce. After you get the pasta, we will need the largest pot from the middle drawer." Items to be bought can be described with several descriptors, such as, "I'm thinking we should eat a vegetable with dinner. I think one that is green. It should be something crunchy that we can eat raw, but we could also cook it." The closed set of language related to food has an abundance of vocabulary and concepts, and can elicit the correct productions of new words.

Encourage the parent to help the child learn several new items when preparing meals, going out to eat, or food shopping. The parent could pick a category such as produce, perishables, or canned goods and play an alphabet game, taking turns as they go through the letters in alphabetical order and naming an item for each letter. Consider introducing the word *paprika* and the closed set of words that belongs with it; for example, *seasoning*, *powdered*, *granules*, *shaker*, *spicy*, *hot*, and *salty*. Reinforce the correct perception, production, and pronunciation of *paprika*, as it is a new word, with the simple explanation that we want everyone to know what the child is saying when they use it in conversation (Goals 1, 7, 8, 11).

In food-related activities, we find multiple meanings, such as the word *hot* as in temperature, spicy, the latest popular item, or when we are keen on an idea. You can introduce the idiom that a person runs "hot and cold." Another multiple meaning presents as you beat the eggs. The word *beat* can be used different ways (e.g., "I beat you in the race," "A beet is a vegetable," or to pound something).

And the Games Go On

There are probably thousands of physical activities and movement games, and most require limited or no specific materials or equipment. All of these have language of the game, instructions, and interactions. Find games that are appropriate to the child's age, gross or fine motor level, and culture and environment. Children can learn games and rhymes related to fine motor skills, creating patterns with their hands and fingers, such as clapping games, classic string games such as such as cat's cradle, or various finger patterns for shadow puppets. Children can learn thumb wrestling, rock paper scissors, or hand-clapping games to rhymes and songs. Gross motor activities can include ball-bouncing games; hopscotch; jump rope; or riding a bike, skateboard, or scooter. Various circle games can be played with small groups of children (e.g., siblings, friends, neighbors, cousins) and can be accompanied by songs or verses. Variations on hide and seek or Sardines, where one person hides and all the others have to find the person and hide with them until the last person finds them, are fun at this stage. All these activities have rules or expressions (e.g., "Ready or not, here I come"), instructions, and specific vocabulary to help target goals for the child with hearing loss.

At this language level there are many commercially available board games that a child can play that will promote language, concepts, collaborations, problem solving, and good sportsmanship. Each game has specific language and vocabulary related to the theme of the game and game language that was introduced with beginning games, such as *my turn*, *your turn*, *roll the die*, and *spin the spinner*. Game-specific vocabulary should be expanded to include concepts and words such as *clockwise*, *object of the game*, *strategy*, *cheating*, *good sport*, *win*, *lose*, and *tie*. Some classic board games have junior versions, which will familiarize the child with the concepts before they transition to the regular version of the games. Repetition is inherent in these games. As the players take their turns, you can reinforce the expressive use of the verb tenses, pronouns, and repeat key phrases (e.g., "She is taking her turn. She took her turn. She moved four spaces and bumped me. It's my turn because he is finished moving").

Card games can begin with simple ones such as Go Fish (1984) and progress to more complex games. Commercial versions of games such as Go Fish use a special deck of cards, as does the popular game Uno. Use the correct vocabulary related to cards and the specific game. As we play with a deck of cards, we shuffle, cut, and deal. Cards have: suits (hearts, spades, clubs, diamonds); number cards; aces; and face cards such as jack, queen, and king. Take the time to explore the deck in simple games or by playing a memory game to find matching pairs of cards and define the feature to be matched. With young children and their little hands, you could use a card holder to prevent frustration in holding the cards, such as a wooden clothespin, chip clip, or an easy do-it-yourself one that could be a craft project.

As the child masters a game, you can introduce variations and new games, and incorporate other skills and language. Before you play a card in a game, give the child a clue and have them guess. You can use a variety of concepts appropriate for the child, such as, "This number is how old you are," "This number is even and less than 8," or "This number is the number of fingers you have on one hand," or "This is the number of points on a triangle." This strategy can be applied to any game that uses numbers (e.g., Uno, Sorry).

Good old-fashioned word games are classic. The wonderful thing is they don't require any particular equipment or items. They can be played indoors or outdoors. They can be used for a brief time, anytime, anywhere. Word games can be used to foster listening, Theory of Mind, and aspects of receptive and/or expressive language.

I Spy is a guessing game, often taught with colors, where one person begins by saying, for example, "I spy with my little eye something that is blue." The other person has to guess the specific item. The players then change roles. The players' roles and steps of the game include many listening and spoken language elements. The players think of an item; keep a secret; memorize and say the prompt phrase; provide an appropriate descriptor (in this example, color); listen to the clue; listen to determine if the guess was correct; and ask questions. This provides the child repeated opportunities to practice the different listening and language elements. This game, once taught and understood, can be modified to use a variety of descriptors to include other attributes or functions or categories or locations, such as "I spy with my little eye something that is: small; bumpy; round; made of wood; fragile" (Goals 1, 2, 3, 4, 5, 7, 8, 9, 10, 11, 16, 18).

Going on Vacation is a game that uses a prompt to elicit a list of items that all players must remember, in sequence, when it is their turn. The prompt is repeated by everyone to begin their turn and then they add an item. For example, the first person says, "I'm going on vacation and in my suitcase, I am packing..." and follows with an item such as a toothbrush. The next person would repeat what was said and add an item: "I'm going on vacation and in my suitcase, I am packing a toothbrush and my teddy bear." The last player to remember all the items wins. To initially teach the game, you can use a stack of picture cards that get piled onto each other. You can keep score by seeing how many items people can remember. This game, once taught and understood, can be modified to use a variety of different sentence prompts limited only by your imagination. Examples include "I went for a walk and I saw . . . "; "I went to the store and I bought . . . "; and "I drove/rode to the park (beach, zoo) and I saw . . . "

Create a prompt that reinforces the language structures or speech sounds that need to be reinforced. You and the parents can include new vocabulary, different verb tenses, irregular past-tense verbs, and irregular plurals. Add the silly factor by naming something ridiculous and then having a discussion why you cannot bring your bed or a shark in your suitcase. Other variations of the game could be: name items in alphabetical order, name items that begin with the letters in your name, or name items from a specified category. Use your creativity to focus on listening and spoken language as applicable to target goals for the child (Goals 1, 2, 3, 4, 5, 7, 8, 9, 10, 11, 12, 13, 14, 15, 16).

Twenty Questions (aka, Animal, Vegetable, or Mineral) is a guessing game in which a person thinks of something and lets the other players know if it is a person, place, or thing. The other players ask up to 20 yes/no questions to determine the answer. As with other word games, once taught and understood, you can modify the rules by starting from more specific clues to the item such as something in the house, a person you know, or a food.

Tic-Tac-Toe (aka, Xs and Os) is a classic but simple paper and pencil game. It provides the opportunity to teach a child the elements of a game. The child must know the object of the game; what to do on your turn; how to draw the grid; and the concept of three in a row horizontally, vertically, or diagonally, and when the game is tied. Keep score if you want by using tally marks grouping the tallies in groups of five or any other number. There are other games too—Hangman, Dots and Boxes, Battleship, and dozens more. Teach the game, have them learn it, and then explain or teach it to somebody else!

Initially teaching the game using pictures or toys can illustrate the object of the game using common categories such as food, clothes, animals. As the child understands the game, we can use only words to name the items and work toward more complexity in the categories and attributes such as fruits, striped animals, foods we eat hot, or items for a specific activity (e.g., going to the beach). The game can be played by determining the item that doesn't belong or by thinking of other items that could belong. You can begin the game by naming 1 item thinking of a specific category or attribute. The other player guesses another item that might go with it. If they are wrong then the first player names additional things for each turn until the opponent can figure out a correct item, e.g., Start with *frog*. The opponent says *lizard*, which is incorrect. Add a grasshopper. The person incorrectly guesses *snake*. We add *rabbit*. The person correctly guesses *kangaroo* as an animal that jumps.

Don't Stop Reading!

Read books with simple stories that will provide an opportunity to retell or act out the story in sequence. Use animated voices that will engage the child and help them to understand the characters. This is the stage to talk about the book and make it very interactive. Encourage the child to guess what might happen next in the story. Talk about the story and have the child retell the story with guided prompts and questions. Ask questions about the story including who, what, when, where, or why. Use props, stuffed animals, dolls, puppets, and dress-up clothes to act out the story. Many books have toys that go along with them, or you can use your own variation. Help the child to understand the emotions of the characters to promote Theory of Mind and empathy. Discuss your favorite and their favorite part of the story. Draw pictures. Discuss how the characters feel. Continue to use and expand the vocabulary terms and expressions that are specific to books and expand to, for example, cover, title page, book jacket, pictures, illustrator, and graphic novel.

Let's Get Busy

Children still want to play. Age-appropriate and cognitively appropriate toys and activities will engage them and provide a platform for listening and speaking. Children's interests vary from building toys, crafts, drawing, and dress-up to science experiments and imaginary play. Following the child's interests will set everyone up for being engaged and will foster successful interactions. Children enjoy imaginary play and want to play house, imitate what they see adults doing, and play the grown-up or the baby. Set up imaginary scenarios such as going to a restaurant or the doctor's office to provide an opportunity for play that is based on real experiences. This allows the child to role-play and practice conversations on specific topics.

Paper activities can be simple, imaginative, and creative. Drawing and painting are always fun and interactive. Ask questions about what they are drawing and provide narrative language. You can weave paper of different colors, fold it to make a fan, a book, or a paper airplane. Introduce origami to the child with projects that are simple or more complex as appropriate. Children love to make different paper creations such as water balloons or fortune tellers. Then they can give instructions to another person.

Simple science experiments are easy to find and foster curiosity while using listening and spoken language with a potentially new set of vocabulary to introduce. Baking soda and vinegar will create a volcano or do a good job cleaning dad's stained coffee mug or the dirty teapot. Using food coloring in water can teach about primary and secondary colors by mixing them. It is always fun to put celery in some water with food coloring and watch the color move up the stalk. You could transition into life sciences discussing plants, farmers, and food sources, and bring it back to a gardening project. You can cut off the bottom a few inches and grow a new celery in a shallow bowl of water. Before you know it, there could be a mini indoor garden in the kitchen with green onions, avocado pits, sweet potato vines, and a pineapple plant. Incorporate these and other topics to increase your child's world knowledge.

You Don't Say . . . Oh You Do!

These children are typically talking and talking and talking all the time. Engage the child in meaningful conversations that they initiate. Expand their language skills and general knowledge through these conversations. Any topic the child is interested in is a way to branch out to more complex language or a related topic and activity. While having a snack, we can discuss different types of snack foods and options. Topics branching from there could include taste and consistency of the food, if it is healthy, where it comes from, different favorite foods, what animal might eat that food or not, carnivores, and herbivores.

In conversations, continue to use language that is about thinking, and Theory of Mind. Deciding on a thoughtful gift or special meal for another person provides the opportunity to discuss their preferences likes and dislikes. Grandma probably does not want a superhero toy and might prefer something other than mac and cheese when she comes for dinner. Let the child think of false belief games, scenarios, or stories and discuss what happened and what people thought. You can put carrots in the box of cookies and talk about why people are surprised when they open it!

Putting It All Together: Case History

Jacob was identified with a hearing loss at age 2 years 3 months due to concerns of speech and language delays. He was bilaterally aided at 2 years 4 months with behind the ear (BTE) hearing aids. He currently is 4 years old and has a hearing age of 20 months. Jacob has a documented progressive hearing loss with changes evidenced when he was 2 years 3 months, 2 years 6 months, and 2 years 9 months. His parents report that Jacob was making good progress from the time he received hearing aids until about age 3. He was receiving intensive intervention from a private spoken language preschool and the local school district. His audiogram was completed at 3 years of age, and indicated a severe hearing loss bilaterally, which was poorer in the right than the left ear. The audiologist reported no change in hearing sensitivity at that time. Aided responses indicated responses between 35 dB and 45 dB binaurally. No speech perception testing was completed at that time.

Jacob attended an oral parent infant program until the age of 3 years. Per his mother, language assessment was performed at the time of completion of the program. The mother reports that testing showed language level from 24 months to 30 months, indicating that he was 6 months to 1 year delayed. Jacob then transitioned to the school district preschool program for children with language delays. The school district did a complete assessment for his individual education plan (IEP) at 3 years 5 months.

Jacob was seen for weekly auditory-verbal therapy (AVT) sessions beginning at the age of 3 years 5 months. No formal assessments were completed when he began AVT sessions, as school district professionals were assessing him extensively for his IEP. After Jacob's initial sessions in AVT it was recommended that he be seen for comprehensive audiological assessment including complete speech perception testing. It was observed in diagnostic therapy and explained at that time that his auditory skills as demonstrated in his language use, comprehension of language, and speech production and errors were not in agreement with his basic audiological testing results.

Jacob was seen for comprehensive audiological assessment at the age of 3 years 7 months. His test results were consistent with testing on 3 years 6 months. Speech perception testing was very poor, especially in his right ear, and he had little access to soft speech. The audiologist reported that when binaurally aided and listening at normal conversational level, without noise, using sentences, he scored 42% words correct and 0% for sentences. At normal conversational level, he scored 44% correct for words and 19% words correct in sentences aided in his right ear. At normal conversational level, he scored

64% correct for words and 36% words correct in sentences aided in his left ear. When listening to quiet speech aided, he scored 10% correct in his right ear and 15% correct in his left ear.

The audiologist stated that these results are consistent with very poor auditory access to speech and language, especially in a classroom environment. The audiologist felt strongly that his comprehension was an issue and not behavioral problems independent of the hearing loss. Medical referral was recommended for a cochlear implant evaluation. Subsequent testing at age 3 years 8 months indicated that he was a candidate for a cochlear implant and is waiting for insurance authorization to be able to schedule surgery and initial stimulation.

Auditory Processes for Using Sound Meaningfully

Auditory Attention, Auditory Discrimination

The Test for Auditory Comprehension of Language–3 (TACL) (Carrow-Woolfolk, 1999) was administered by the deaf and hard of hearing teacher as part of the IEP assessment. The TACL was administered to look at the specific receptive skills that it assesses: I. Vocabulary; II. Grammatical Morphemes; and III. Elaborated Sentences. This is a test of comprehension of a variety of grammatical structures and morphemes that is normed on hearing children. This evaluation was administered at the age of 3 years 6 months. This evaluation had not been previously administered (Table 9–10).

This assessment indicated difficulties comprehending sentences and phrases. His subtests on the TACL are a red flag, as typically children score poorest in the grammatical morphemes and best on phrases and sentences.

Auditory Memory and Comprehension

The Test of Auditory Processing Skills–3 (TAPS-3) (Martin & Brownell, 2005) was administered. This assessment is normed for ages 4 years through 18 years 11 months. Jacob was unable to follow the instructions for the phonologic subtests, which include word discrimination, phonological segmentation, and phonological blending. The subtests for auditory memory and auditory cohesion were administered to determine his auditory skills in these areas. Scaled scores between 7 and 13, and 85 and 115, are considered within the normal ranges. His scaled scores and percentile scores indicate that he is only

Table 9–10. Test for Auditory Comprehension of Language–3 (TACL-3) Age-Equivalent Test Scores

	Raw Score	Age Equivalent	Percentile Rank	Standard Score	Descriptive Rating
Vocabulary	16	3.6	50	10	Average
Grammatical Morphemes	15	4.6	84	13	Above average
Elaborated Sentences	4	<3	16	7	Below average

showing abilities in the average range for number memory forward and word memory, and below-average scores for number memory reversed, sentence memory, auditory comprehension, and auditory reasoning. His scaled score for auditory cohesion is below average. Table 9–11 indicates his scores, percentiles, and age equivalents for the subtests.

Auditory Processes for Learning to Talk

Auditory Feedback

Jacob demonstrates overall clear speech with some good word-final consonants (e.g., *look*), but his productions are very inconsistent. In addition, he demonstrates several speech errors that are indicative of a reliance on visual input, particularly for high-frequency speech sounds. These include production of /k/ for /h/ in *horse*, reduction of word-final blends, substitutions and additions of /d/ for /n/, addition of plosives in word-final positions (e.g., *airplanek, bowt*). He also demonstrates low-frequency errors, omitting /b/ in some words and showing poor voice/voiceless production (e.g., /s/ and /z/). He will typically use the unvoiced cognate. His productions and imitations are improved when presented in isolation and close to his technology.

Auditory Processes for Learning Language

Auditory Comprehension/ Receptive Language

Auditory Retrieval/ Expressive Language

The speech pathologist from the special day class reported that Jacob's language level was within the low average based on the Rosetti Language Scales (1990). He also reported that Jacob's expressive and pragmatic abilities were moderately delayed, which was commensurate with Jacob's articulation errors. He reported that echolalia was noted at the time of assessment and at various times in the

Table 9–11. Test of Auditory Processing Skills-3 (TAPS-3) Scores

Subtest	Raw Score	Scaled Score	Age Equivalent	Percentile
Auditory Memory		88		
Number Memory Forward	10	10	4 y 4 m	50
Number Memory Reversed	0	5	<3 y 9 m	5
Word Memory	8	8	<3 y 6 m	25
Sentence Memory	8	7	<3 y 6 m	16
Auditory Cohesion		78		
Auditory Comprehension	0	5	<3 y 6 m	5
Auditory Reasoning	1	6	3 y 6 m	9

classroom during Jacob's spontaneous speech. He reported that it was "a latent stage of language development as his echo has evidence of comprehension." Jacob's echolalia was evidenced by his repetition of partial or whole phrases and seemed to occur when he was excited or repeating something said to assist in his comprehension.

The Preschool Language Scale (PLS-4) by Zimmerman et al. (2011) was completed by the school district speech therapist as part of Jacob's IEP assessment. This evaluation assesses auditory comprehension and verbal ability of language and provides an age-equivalent score compared to normal-hearing children. His standard scores were in the average range, as indicated in Table 9–12. An average standard score is 100 and ranges from 85 to 115.

The Peabody Picture Vocabulary Test, fourth edition, Form B (2007) was administered by the school district speech professional as part of his IEP assessment. He received a standard score of 101, which is considered to be within the average range when compared to typically developing peers of the same age.

Diagnostic Therapy and Informal Assessment

When Jacob was initially seen for AVT, it was noted that his both comprehension and auditory skills were very poor. This was not as expected from assessments completed at the time of his IEP. His mother expressed concern about comprehension as seen in daily experiences and was not certain if this was related to vocabulary or language structures. During diagnostic therapy and informal assessment, these issues were also noted when interacting in one-on-one conversation in an acoustically treated room without ambient or background noise. In this situation, Jacob did not show comprehension when asked simple questions or when given a simple one-part request that was not part of his known routine. He would inconsistently respond when spoken to but typically not appropriately or on topic.

Jacob inconsistently heard and comprehended a key word but did not comprehend the complete sentence. He avoided responding to questions or staying on topic. He would typically control the conversation, often using strings of words without communicative intent that were not a clear communicative turn. He also demonstrated some echolalia. He responded inappropriately and used a variety of avoidance strategies that indicated he did not comprehend most of what was being said.

Auditory Processes for Learning Language

When Jacob was initially seen, his expressive language consisted of some two- and three-word utterances, but primarily single-word utterances. He used a few plurals in session, inconsistently used -*ing*, and

Table 9–12. Pre-School Language Scale-5 (PLS-5) Scores

Auditory Comprehension	Expressive Communication	Language Age
100	97	98

did not use the copula consistently. He did produce the contracted form *he's*, primarily in known formula phrases. He was unable to use the contracted *n't* negative form. He would say, "I see van" and "I can see van" (but he meant *can't*).

There had been a focus on /s/ morphemic functions in his other therapy session. His mother reported they had focused on plurals but they continued to be inconsistent. He continued to confuse *he* and *she*. He was able to answer questions that are structured around repeated events and familiar situations, such as "Where is mommy going?" and "What does he need in the van?" He was unable to respond to "why" questions logically, though he does often attempt a response that begins with "because." He used *because* inappropriately in spontaneous communicative contributions. Extensive modeling of questions has been used at home and in therapy, and he is beginning to ask some well-formulated questions with a prompt and spontaneously (e.g., "Mommy, can you read that book to me?") The following are some language samples produced spontaneously during this evaluation. They are typical of his productions and demonstrate his expressive language skills.

Daddy's tie	Look a books
I see book	A cookie and plate
Drinking milk	Take off all these stuff
He cleaning up	It red
It change color	He don't want it
Eat cookie	Drank it all

And this is the white ball

Your doggie is going to the chair

He sitting on a chair

Because he want wake up

Daddy say go put in room

Because he said only one

He is kicking a ball and reading

The girl and the boy playing outside

He is drinking a cup the juice

He wants to wake up see the window

He wants blow bubbles outside

Because he fall down the curb

The Structured Photographic Expressive Language Test–Preschool 2 (SPELT-P 2) (Dawson et al., 2003) was administered at 3 years 10 months. It is normed for age 3 years to 5 years 11 months. This is a test of expressive use of a variety of grammatical structures and morphemes, which is normed on hearing children. Jacob's score yielded a standard score of 96, a percentile rank of 41 and an age equivalent of 3 years to 3 years 5 months. Grammatical analysis of the test indicated development was not in the normal sequence of language structures and indicated inconsistent development of grammatical morphemes. He seemed to have some difficulty responding appropriately to some of the prompts for a presented image. When asked "Where is the dog?" he responded, "Your doggie is going." He would talk excessively to the prompt and then sometimes produce the targeted structure in a random string of language. It was also noted that he sometimes randomly produced a targeted structure for a different item. For an item targeting third-person present tense ("He sits"), he said "Sit on the chair," using the prepositional phrase, which he did not produce for the item assessing prepositions on the test.

Jacob demonstrated use of:

Possessive nouns

Possessive pronouns

Auxiliary—plural present

Present participle

Copula—plural present

Conjunctions

Jacob demonstrated errors or inconsistent use of the following structures:

Prepositions	Plural nouns
Present participle	Pronouns
Regular past	Irregular past
Third-person present	"wh" clause
Negative + verb	Infinitive + *to*
Question forms	
Copula—singular past	
Copula—singular present	

Jacob shows a pattern of language learning that is indicative of poor auditory access. It should be noted that, with the exception of irregular past-tense forms, these grammatical structures are acoustically difficult for children with hearing loss to access. It further supports his need for better auditory access through a cochlear implant.

Progress in AVT Sessions

Jacob showed improvement in his auditory memory for simple requests and commands with one to three critical items when using familiar language and everyday activities and routines. His mother reported that acoustic highlighting is an effective strategy for Jacob. The mother frequently used the strategy and feels comfortable with it, and finds that Jacob is occasionally correcting when provided with acoustic highlighting. The mother is also working on expanding and clarification strategies when Jacob uses short or unclear communications. He will produce a communicative contribution. Jacob has been very cooperative and is willing to attempt grammatical morphemes being structured including but not limited to plurals, possessives, and "is + ___ing" form of verbs.

As mentioned above, he is showing improvement receptively and expressively for question forms but is not able to respond or formulate "why" questions. In sessions and at home we are facilitating verb tenses by using the three-act play to elicit the present-progressive form. He will produce the *-ing* verb form with models but inconsistently. Jacob doesn't use *-ed* past-tense endings and it has not been possible to elicit those with several models and direct prompts.

Summary

Jacob's scores are mostly in the average range when compared to his hearing peers. This is above the skill level we would expect based on his hearing age, but as he had a progressive hearing loss we shouldn't only compare his skills to hearing age but also to his chronologic age. It should be noted that his performance indicates gaps in his language development over time due to his progressive hearing loss. In addition, at this time he has limited auditory access through hearing aids as he waits for cochlear implantation, which has been recommended and is pending insurance approval. Overall his performance indicates poor receptive and expressive abilities for the low-intensity acoustic information of morphemes. His areas of deficit reflect his lack of auditory access and are particularly apparent for the /s/ morphemic functions. Speech perception errors interfere with development of present progressive verb tense, past-tense -*ed* endings, irregular past tense, and pronouns. Additionally, at this time he demonstrates poor abilities in auditory memory and comprehension of sentences and phrases.

The Intervention Session

Listening and spoken language intervention is naturally integrated into this Jacob's activities of daily living, as noted by his mother's ease in the use of strategies when helping Jacob in washing his hands. Vocabulary expansion and morphemes are focused on in this session but there are teachable moments that are seized as opportunities for learning. Jacob is using basic sentence structure but is still working on consistency of some of the first acquired morphemes, particularly those that are dependent on high-frequency components. Mother and professional are particularly focusing on these typical grammatical errors that Jacob is making by expanding his contribution and acoustically highlighting the missing morphemes to facilitate his attention to and use of the specific morphemes. Mother uses natural interactions to expand auditory memory by giving strings of commands and multiple descriptions. She uses strategies to reinforce Theory of Mind by using thinking words for a guessing game.

The mother is using a variety of other strategies that she previously learned, such as auditory closure, expanding, avoiding vocabulary stagnation, three-act play, and slow motion within activities of daily living. She incorporates them in their interactions at home to address many of Jacob's goals and needs. The professional provides strength-based coaching strategies to reinforce the mother's abilities. The professional guides and coaches the mother to use the mastered strategies in new ways and also models new strategies to be implemented.

Mother: Your hands are very dirty! You need to wash them.

Jacob: I have paint on my hand.

Mother: I think you have paint on both hands. Look at your right hand and your left hand. Both of your hands are dirty.

Jacob: My hands very dirty.

Mother: Yes, your hands are filthy. We are going to wash your hands. Let's go to the bathroom, turn on the light, then you can stand on the stepstool so you can wash your hands in the sink.

Jacob: Wash my hand.

Mother: Your hands. We are going to wash your hands. We need to wash both of your hands. I'll help you.

Jacob: I am on the stepstool.

Mother: Right, the stepstool is because you can't reach the sink.

Jacob: I can reach.

Mother: No, but you can't reach on your own. But now you can reach because you are standing on the stepstool.

Jacob: I can wash my hands.

Mother: Great. Now what do we do?

Jacob: We have to wash.

Mother: We are going to wash your hands

Jacob: I gonna wash.

Mother: Yes. You are going to wash your hands.

Jacob: Was, wash, wash.

Mother: Yes, you are going to wash your hands.

Jacob: My hands.

Mother: I'm going to turn on the water. Here, I'm turning it, it's turned on.

Jacob: Wash my hands in the water,

Mother: Wait, what else do you need to wash your hands in the sink? You need to get some . . . ?

Jacob: Soap.

Mother: Yes. You wash your hands with soap and water. Here you go.

Jacob: I got enough soap.

Mother: What are you going to do with the soap?

Jacob: I have to wash my hands.

Mother: Yes. Take the soap and rub it. Scrub your hands.

Jacob: Rub. Rub. Rub.

Mother: Washing and washing. Scrubbing and scrubbing. Rubbing and rubbing. I am going to turn the water off while you . . . . . . *sssss*

Jacob: Soap.

Mother: Scrub.

Jacob: Scrub.

Mother: You are scrubbing. What happens when you scrub? You make . . .

Jacob: Bubbles. I make bubbles.

Mother: Ahhh! You are making bubbles. Did you make enough bubbles?

Jacob: Yeah. I making so much bubbles.

Mother: Lots of suds and bubbles. Ok, now what do we do?

Jacob: Turn the water off.

Mother: Wait, we have to rinse the suds.

Jacob: Yeah.

Mother: That's silly, we need the water.

Jacob: Need the water. Rinse my hands. I'm rinsing with water.

Mother: Rinse the bubbles! Good rinsing.

Jacob: Rinsing bubbles from my hands.

Mother: Are the suds all rinsed off? You have to rub, rub, rub when you are rinsing.

Jacob: Rinsing the soap all gone now.

Mother: The soap is all gone. Now what do we do?

Jacob: Dry!

Mother: First we turn off the. . .

Jacob: Water.

Mother: And then we . . .

Jacob: Dry!

Mother: You are going to dry your hands. Hmmm, how are you going to get your hands dry?

(Jacob points to the towels hanging on the towel rack)

Mother: Ah! (laughs)

Jacob: All wet from washing with water.

Mother: What is that?

Jacob: A towel for me!

Mother: It is a towel. OK. Can you reach it?

Jacob: I can reach it.

Mother: Oh, I don't think so. You cannot reach it. See, you can't reach it. There you go.

Jacob: Thank you.

Mother: Ok, you washed your hands and you dried your hands. Let's go play with something. We need to turn off the light in the bathroom, walk over to the table, sit down on our chairs, and see what toys there are for us today (as they walk from the bathroom to the table to sit down and play).

Professional: Nice job, mom, expanding vocabulary—I love *scrub* and *rub* and *rinse*. Nice auditory closure getting him to fill in the missing words. Also like the way you leaned in to his hearing aids when you turned on the water. You are getting very good at using the three-act play for facilitating the verb tenses. Jacob! I bought some new toys. They are inside the bag. Let's see if you can guess what I bought.

(Turning to mother) So he is using the plurals for the words he has learned in plural form. *Hands. Bubbles.* We don't usually talk about *hand* or *bubble*. But he isn't consistent and we want him to be using it for other plural forms. So, let's try to enhance his perception and understanding for the plurals.

Mother: I am still struggling with him at home with that. I can't get him to do it. I don't think he can.

Professional: I will pop in and model it for you when it is a natural situation and let's see if we can get him to do it.

Mother: But he doesn't hear it, so can we really do that? How should I do that?

Professional: He seems to get it from up close, when you were standing right behind him at the sink, just a few inches from his ears. And he has it in some words. Get the bag of toys and help him to guess what is inside.

Mother: Oh (peeking inside the bag but not letting Jacob see): Oh this is really fun!

Jacob: What inside the bag?

Mother: I see what is inside the bag. Here's a clue to help you think. When you come to play here, what do you like to play with?

Jacob: I don't know what inside.

Mother: I know. Listen to the clue. When we come here on other days, what do you like to play with?

Jacob: I don't know.

Professional: I know what's in the bag because I bought the toys. It has four wheels and it goes really fast. Sometimes we make it go through a loop.

Mother: And it goes on a track.

Jacob: That a car?

Mother: You think? A car? Is it? Is it a car? You can ask me.

Jacob: That a car inside?

Professional: Let me help, Jacob. I'll ask. Mom, is it a car?

Mother: Yes. But there are lots of them. Not just one. So, they are cars. Listen: *ssss*.

Jacob: *Ssss*

Mother: That's right, *ssss* for lots of cars. Try it. *Cars*.

Jacob: Cars.

Mother: Right! These are cars.

Jacob: These are cars.

Professional: Great, you got the idea of how to enhance his perception for the plurals. Make sure you don't let him say it again wrong or correct it again. What other morphemes should we be trying to facilitate with this? Which of the first morphemes?

Mother: He still isn't including *is*, probably because he isn't hearing it. Right?

Professional: Exactly, but you can use the same strategy as with the /s/ and also acoustically highlight the word. So, for some of the things he was just saying, you can expand and correct by acoustically highlighting the *IS* by making it louder or longer or playing with the pitch. You have been using that strategy for a long time! So you

can say, "That IS a car! I know what IS inside."

Mother: What kind of cars? Do you remember what they are called?

Jacob: Hot Wheel.

Mother: Just one wheel?

Jacob: Many wheel.

Mother: Right. Many wheels. Listen, remember *ssss*. *Wheels*.

Jacob: Wheels.

Mother: Good listening! So here are the Hot Wheels.

Jacob: Let me see.

Mother: Look.

Jacob: Wow!

Professional: But that's not cars. Look carefully. Do you what those are?

Jacob: Those are motorcycle!

Professional: Yes, listen tell me *ssss*.

Jacob: *Ssss*

Professional: *Ssss* . . . there are two motorcycles.

Jacob: There more toy in the bag?

Professional: Yeah mom, I want to know about the toys. Are there more toys in the bag? Jacob, can you ask her again?

Jacob: There more toys?

Professional: Yeah mom, are there more toys?

Mother: You both want to know. Are there more toys in the bag? There is another toy. I see one more toy in the bag. This one is the one for the cars.

With a loop. Because we had trouble with the loop last time.

Jacob: Can I see?

Mother: Wait. I can't see because it is upside down for me.

Jacob: What it?

Mother: I can't tell what it is.

Jacob: I don't know what that called.

Mother: You don't know what it is called? You can ask Sylvia what it is.

Jacob: What it is?

Professional: So, you are asking me, "what is it?"

Jacob: What is it?

Professional: I think that is another upside-down loop.

Jacob: There loop?

Professional: It's a double loop.

Mother: Double means there are two loops.

Jacob: There are two loop?

Mother: There are two loops. Try again for me. Remember? *Sss.*

Jacob: Double. Two of them.

Professional: Yes, listen, tell me *ssss.*

Jacob: *Ssss.*

Mother: Right. *Ssss.* We have two loops. Double loops.

Jacob: Two loops.

Mother: Right. Double loops.

Jacob: Double.

Professional (turning to mother): Good explaining the word *double*.

I wouldn't have known if he knew the word or not.

Mother: Which boy is winning in this picture?

Jacob: That boy he green one. That car going faster.

Mother: So, he has the green one and it is going faster. He is the boy that is winning. What do you think he is saying?

Jacob: He say, "Yeah."

Mother: Good thinking, he might be saying, "Yeah!"

Professional: I think he is saying, "I won!" How do you think the other boy feels?

Jacob: The other boy sad.

Mother: He might feel disappointed but he looks like he is having fun.

Jacob: Mommy, wow, look at that!

Mother: Wow. Pretty cool.

Jacob: That car going upside down.

Mother: The green car is! It is going upside down.

Jacob: The green car is upside down.

Professional: But look inside the box. It looks like it has a truck, not a car. Maybe a special kind of truck.

Mother: It looks like a four-wheel drive. That's a big pickup truck.

Jacob: Hey look at what on the wheel.

Mother: Oh, I don't know what's on the wheel.

Jacob: Here look at that. More on the wheel.

Professional: Mom, you can't see it from there.

Jacob: Look. Here that blue one (pointing to car in the box).

Professional: Jacob, those are hubcaps. There are hubcaps on the wheels.

Analysis of Session

In discussion of the therapy session, we can analyze which goals are being addressed during this interval of therapy. The goals are indicated by number and refer back to numbers indicated in Tables 9–3 to 9–6. This scenario helps to show the integration and overlap of multiple goals in the natural interactions, just like the cookie dough theory. The mother uses the simple activity of washing hands to work on listening in a natural setting while she stands behind Jacob and at times has the water running creating a poorer auditory signal or degraded signal (Goals 1, 6). She facilitates comprehension and expression within short phrases and sentences for a variety of morphemes, particularly plurals, contracted negatives, and present progressive verbs with the auxiliary verb (Goals 1, 2, 3, 4, 6, 9, 10, 11, 13, 14a and c). She is facilitating new vocabulary receptively and expressively as they wash, scrub, rub, and rinse. She acoustically highlights to take advantage of reinforcing the plurals in words that are naturally learned in plural form; e.g., *hands*, *bubbles* (Goals 1; 2; 3; 4; 6; 7; 8; 10; 14a, b, c, g; 15, a, b, c, g)

The transition from washing hands to going to play has a multielement instruction, including some familiar language and stereotypic phrases (Goals 3, 4). When they begin with the toys hidden in the bag, the mother and the professional support Theory of Mind by illustrating that they know something that he doesn't know and will give clues. In the interactions, they use thinking words and multiple elements in the clues to expand Jacob's auditory memory (Goals 3, 4). This activity allows for easy incorporation of a variety of morphemes and language structures as the adults use language forms to facilitate and correct the errors that Jacob makes. This is particularly noted for the receptive and expressive language and auditory feedback loop for plurals, the use of *is*, negatives, and question forms (Goals 2; 3; 4; 8; 9; 10; 11; 12; 13; 14a, c, g; 15a, c, g; 16; 18). At several points in the session, the professional models enhancing hearing. She does this particularly with regard to the plural form with /s/. This works on attending to and discriminating the phoneme /s/, attending to the word-final sounds, the auditory feedback loop, and the comprehension and expressive use of plurals (Goals 1c, d, e; 2; 7c, d, e; 8; 9; 10; 14c).

Summary

The professional considers the knowledge base, guides and coaches the parent, and teaches strategies to promote further development at this stage of grammatical errors in communication. This will help support the child to achieve all or most of the skills as outlined in Tables 9–1 and 9–2 and the targeted goals from this stage of language development from Tables 9–3 through 9–6. The achievement of these goals will provide a strong basis for the child with hearing loss to progress to the next level of listening and spoken language abilities. Behaviors that are indicative of the child emerging into the next stage of development are indicated in Table 9–13.

Table 9–13. By the End of the Communication With Childlike Errors Stage, the Child Should:

> Speak with complex, grammatically correct language.
>
> Use language consistently to converse and express themselves.
>
> Follow a conversation of an appropriate subject/language, maintain the topic, and use a discourse format to tell a story or explain something.
>
> Know a variety of words of multiple meanings (e.g., *too/to/two, trunk, hare/hair, fly* [noun and verb]).
>
> Use irregular plurals and past tenses.
>
> Understand passive-voice sentences, and subordinate and coordinate clauses.
>
> Use language with limited or no grammatical errors.

Discussion Questions

1. How do you determine if a child is at this stage?
2. How would you illustrate the chocolate chip cookie dough analogy to the parents of a child with hearing loss at this stage?
3. Select a goal from the one of the Tables 9–3 through 9–6. How would you explain to a caregiver to use a specific activity of daily living to target the goal? Consider and identify other goals that would be naturally included in that selected ADL.
4. What activities could you do with an older child to work on the goals at this level?
5. Consider a child with additional disabilities or needs and discuss an activity that you could work on to target a selected goal at this level.

References

American Speech-Language-Hearing Association (1997–2021). *Developmental norms for speech and language.* https://www.asha.org/public/speech/development/chart

Brown, V. L., Bzoch, D. R., & League, R. (2020). *Receptive-Expressive Emergent Language Test* (4th ed.). Western Psychological Services.

Carrow-Woolfolk, E. (1999). *Test for Auditory Comprehension of Language-3.* Western Psychological Services.

Cochlear Corporation. (2010). Integrated scales of development. In *Listen, learn, talk* (pp. 16–31). Cochlear Limited.

Dawson, J., Stout, C., & Eyer, J. (2005). SPELT-P 2, *Structured Photographic Expressive Language Test—Preschool.* Janell Publishing.

Go Fish [Card game]. (1984). U.S. Games Systems.

Klatte, M., Lachmann, T., & Meis, M. (2010). Effects of noise and reverberation on speech perception and listening comprehension of children and adults in a classroom-like setting. *Noise Health, 12*(49), 270–282.

Ling, D. (2003). The Ling Six-Sound Test. *The Listener*, 52–53.

Martin, N. A., & Brownell, R. (2005). *Test of Auditory Processing Skills* (3rd ed.). World Publishing. https://www.wpspublish.com/taps-3-test-of-auditory-processing-skills-third-edition

Robbins, M. (1971). *UNO* [Card game]. Mattel.

Rossetti, L. M. (1990). *Rossetti Infant-Toddler Language Scale*. LinguiSystems.

Storey, W. S. (1930). *Sorry* [Board game]. Hasbro.

Tsiakpini, L., Weichbold, V., Kuehn-Inacker, H., Coninx, F., D'Haese, P., & Almadin, S. (2004). *LittlEARS Auditory Questionnaire*. MED-EL.

Zimmerman, I. L., Steiner, V. G., & Pond, R. E. (2011). *Preschool Language Scales* (4th ed.). Pearson.

Chapter 10

Competent Communicator Stage

Sylvia Rotfleisch

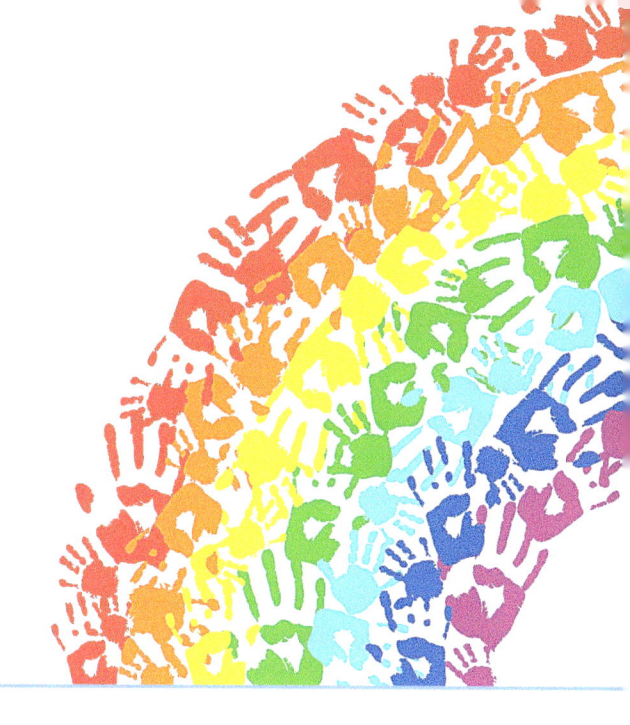

Key Points

- The child's listening and spoken language abilities are approaching levels of competence.
- At the competent communicator stage, the child will learn to listen in more challenging acoustic environments.
- The child's auditory feedback loop will develop and facilitate self-monitoring and self-correcting of appropriate phonemes.
- Flexibility related to language in both comprehension and expressive abilities will be addressed.
- Goals should be incorporated into a variety of natural experiences such as activities of daily living, conversations, playing with peers, and school activities.

Basic Characteristics of the Child Who Is a Competent Communicator

Listening

At this stage, the child with hearing loss is a competent listener, showing a variety of consistent auditory abilities that are integrated into listening and spoken language abilities. These abilities allow the child to be very functional in daily life in a variety of environments outside of the home. We see emerging abilities for the child to modulate voice intensity appropriately for a variety of environments with different acoustic situations and noise levels. Learning can be successful through listening, and there is evidence of new knowledge acquisition in both academic and other group situations. Social situations are more part of life experiences but are best with one-on-one interactions or small groups and quiet environments.

Self-advocacy is emerging as the child is learning to be responsible for communication breakdowns by using some initial and appropriate clarification and conversation repair strategies. Acoustically poor environments are still challenging for the child. In those situations, we expect the child to be the most successful when implementing a remote microphone for such environments. We see the child is able to follow complex instructions and is learning to listen in group situations (e.g., classroom, team sport sessions). These advanced auditory abilities typically evident and/or emerging in the competent communicator stage are indicated in Table 10–1. Skills listed are not sequential.

Language

At this stage of language development, the child with hearing loss will have language that closely approximates that of an adult who is a fluent native speaker. Limited errors are noted, though the child will continue to refine syntax and learn exceptions to most grammatical rules. More advanced language structures and uses are mastered, such as passive voice and figurative/nonliteral language. The child can easily communicate with children and adults. Vocabulary continues to develop both receptively and expressively. An ever-growing mastery of Tier 2 and Tier 3 vocabulary emerges related to specific academic domains. The child is learning to recount events, explain instructions and steps, easily converse on

Table 10–1. Auditory Abilities Evidenced by a Child Who Is a Competent Communicator

- Understands and carries out complex series of instructions with unrelated steps.
- Comprehends unstressed grammatical structures.
- Follows classroom directions like, "Put away your books, get out your pen, and draw circles around all the things you eat."
- Hears and understands most of what is heard at home and in school.
- May talk louder outside than inside.
- Talks in different ways, depending on the listener and place.
- May modify their language and use short sentences with younger children.
- Follows a topic and maintains a conversation.
- Can remember and retell a story or event to others telling what was first through to the end.
- Can identify initial sounds.
- Can understand and tell rhyming words.
- Can identify grammatical errors when listening to self or others.
- Listens in group situations.

Sources: Zimmerman et al. (2011); Carrow-Woolfolk (1999); https://www.home-speech-home.com/

a variety of topics, organize thoughts and present them in an appropriate sequence, include necessary detail, and use vocabulary specifically related to the topic (Peterson et al., 2012). Receptive and expressive language abilities evidenced or expected to emerge in this stage are included in Table 10–2. Skills listed are not sequential.

Speech

The child with hearing loss who has appropriate auditory access to the signal should show emerging mastery of phonemes in the expected sequence of development. The child's production will reflect their auditory access, perception, and hearing and listening experience. We expect speech productions to show emerging mastery at this stage, but we must keep in mind that, in typically developing children, mastery of speech sounds continues until 8 years of age and beyond (see Chapter 3, Table 3–11). It is not unusual for children to make mistakes with some of the later-mastered sounds, including phonemes such as /l/, /r/, /v/, /z/, /ʃ/, /θ/, /tʃ/, and /ð/ until the early teen years (Hustad et al., 2020).

Table 10–2. Language and Speech Skills Evidenced in the Competent Communicator Stage

Audition and Auditory Comprehension of Language	Expressive Language and Communication
• Comprehends smaller parts of speech. • Shows interest in "why." • Understands passive voice. • Expands vocabulary to include Tier 3—academic-related words. • Listens to short chapters when being read to and understands and recalls events and details. • Starts to understand some jokes and puns.	• Speaks in complete sentences of five words or more. • Refines syntax and emerging use of all grammatical structures. • Uses a variety of verb tenses. • Use of small parts of language—pronouns, articles, conjunctions, suffixes, prefixes. • Refines syntax and emerging use of all grammatical structures. • Uses a variety of verb tenses with auxiliary verbs. • Responds appropriately to different types of questions. • Responds to "What did you say?" • Uses sentences that have more than one action word, like *jump*, *play*, and *get*. • Masters most exceptions to grammatical rules. • Uses connected speech in an organized manner, appropriately sequenced and on topic. • Uses passive voice. • Begins to use figurative language.

Source: https://www.home-speech-home.com/

Goals for the Competent Communicator Stage

Developing an Appropriate Therapy Plan by Addressing Strengths and Areas of Need

The typical sequence of development will be followed to develop listening skills and appropriate speech and language abilities. All previous goals will be used as the basis for expanding to the next skills. Some goals from the communication with errors stage might not be mastered and might be carried over initially in this stage. Goals for the competent communicator stage focus on:

- facilitating listening in poor acoustic environments and for degraded auditory signals,
- reinforcing the auditory feedback loop for consistent use and self-monitoring of all appropriate phonemes,
- facilitating comprehension of flexibility of language, and
- facilitating competence in complex and flexible uses of language.

Select appropriate goals based on your assessment results that identify the child's strengths and needs (see Chapter 4). At this language level, standardized assessment tools are abundant.

Goals must be individualized within the stage to meet the child's needs. At this level, look for appropriate goals, for example, when determining goals related to advanced comprehension. One child might be able to understand jokes and puns based on multiple meanings of words but not understand jokes where idioms are incorporated or when words sound similar (e.g., for a humorous effect as in using *shellfish* for *selfish*, *berry* for *very*, "orange you glad" for "aren't you glad"). You might select goals for that child to address their literal way of approaching language and facilitate their comprehension of multiple meanings, idioms and figurative language (Goals 9, 10, 11, 14, 15). Another child with limited vocabulary might not understand the multiple meanings of words that make a joke humorous. You would select goals for expanding vocabulary by using words with multiple meanings or homophones (e.g., *too*, *to*, *two*) to help teach jokes and puns (Goals 7, 8, 10, 14).

Typical Goals for the Stage of Competent Communicator

Your selected goals continue to focus on expanding complex auditory skills through a degraded signal. Goals will support the mastery of communicative competence in comprehension and expressive abilities in complex and flexible uses of language. This mastery will be needed in addressing academic language and grade-level pragmatic uses of language (e.g., persuasive, biased, descriptive, procedural). The child will learn to apply those communicative competencies across all acoustic environments in their daily life. Auditory memory and the auditory feedback loop continue to support self-monitoring and self-correcting of both speech clarity and language structures. Understanding of the flexibility and nonliteral use of language will provide the foundational skills for the advanced communicator stage.

Typical, recommended goals for children with hearing loss at the competent communicator level are included in Tables 10–3 to 10–6. Goals are organized based upon defined skills related to the brain

Table 10–3. Auditory Goals for Understanding Sound as Meaningful in the Competent Communicator Stage

Auditory Attention, Detection, Discrimination, and Memory
1. Expand discrimination of open-set words and sentences at an age- and grade-appropriate language level.
2. Discriminate word-final consonants that differ by manner, place, and voicing.
3. Discriminate sentence material, including words and word endings, in good auditory situations and through a degraded signal (including background noise, phone, computer, and distance) when presented binaurally in a closed set of familiar language or lesser-known information with familiarization or preteaching of the topic with key words and then expanded to open set.
4. Attend, discriminate, and remember conversational turns when presented through a degraded signal.

Table 10–4. Auditory Feedback and Speech Production Goals in the Competent Communicator Stage

Auditory Goals for Development of the Speech Production System
5. Produce speech sounds correctly in single words and in conversational speech.
6. Facilitate and reinforce auditory feedback loop for self-monitoring and self-correcting of phonemes as identified as emerging, inconsistent, or with errors that are old habits.

Table 10–5. Auditory Goals for Language Comprehension in the Competent Communicator Stage

Auditory Recognition, Sequencing, and Comprehension
7. Expand auditory comprehension of new vocabulary at Tiers 2 and 3.
8. Demonstrate increasing comprehension for multiple meanings, including unknown and previously known vocabulary.
9. Comprehend and differentiate figurative language forms from literal uses of language.
10. Demonstrate comprehension of jokes by explaining them.
11. Demonstrate comprehension of idioms used at home and those from grade-level materials.
12. Comprehend an age-level/grade-level passage of multiple sentences when presented through audition only.
13. Comprehend sentence material and conversational partner's turn (including words and word endings) through a degraded signal (e.g., background noise, phone, computer, distance) in closed set and then expanded to open set.

Table 10–6. Auditory Goals for Developing Expressive Language in the Competent Communicator Stage

Auditory Retrieval and Expressive Communication
14. Can tell jokes and puns and explain why they are funny.
15. Use a variety of idioms appropriately in conversations and explain their meaning.
16. Use a variety of socially appropriate, advanced clarification strategies spontaneously for missed auditory information or to repair communication breakdown.
17. After listening to a grade-level passage, can correctly answer questions of reason (e.g., predictions, cause and effect, problem and solution, inferences).

functions necessary for learning to use audition for language development (see Chapter 3). The goals included in these tables should not be considered the definitive set of goals for all children at this stage. Neither should they be considered an exhaustive list of possible audition goals for the child with hearing loss at the competent communicator stage of language development. Goals must address the specific errors and needs determined during comprehensive assessment as well as from observation and informal diagnostic work.

How Do We Work on These Goals?

Professionals must have a knowledge base and multiple appropriate strategies (see Tables 10–7 and 10–8) applicable to the competent communicator stage to accomplish selected goals. The knowledge and strategies included in these tables are the basis for you to guide and coach the parent. The parent remains an important person to continue to support their child's listening and spoken language development. Knowledge areas and strategies applicable to the child at the competent communicator stage are identified in Tables 10–7 and 10–8.

Table 10–7. Knowledge Areas in the Competent Communicator Stage

- Hearing technologies being used
- Effective troubleshooting of technology
- Speech acoustics related to ongoing speech production
- Ling six sounds
- Sequence of development of speech phonemes
- Stages of development of complex receptive language
- Stages of development of complex expressive language
- Stages of literacy

At the competent communicator stage, you and the parent will talk to support conversational norms, have effective and natural conversations, facilitate advanced vocabulary development and multiple meanings, and expose the child to the flexibility of language using figurative and nonliteral language.

The parents will be learning and implementing strategies in therapy sessions. Support parents to use strategies (see Table 10–8) that will advance the child's language abilities. The parent who worked through the various stages of listening and spoken language is an effective language

Table 10–8. Optimal Strategies to Implement in the Competent Communicator Stage

- Chocolate chip cookie theory
- Activities of daily living
- Conversations
- Vocabulary enrichment
- Preteaching vocabulary for new experiences
- Modeling use of everyday idioms
- Modeling clarification strategies
- Teaching the unknown connected to the known
- Expanding world knowledge and the related language
- Elicit multiple events from stories and multistep instructions from personal experiences
- Elicit discourse and complex conversations
- Introducing jokes based on known words of multiple meanings, idioms, similar-sounding words
- Theory of Mind related to more advanced concepts, empathy, and conversational competence
- Conversations about social cues, underlying messages, and sarcasm

to master in this stage. All the strategies used when the child was mastering syntax are relevant as advanced language structures continue to evolve. Conversations should address Theory of Mind and its relationship to successful social interactions and fostering of friendships.

You will encourage parents to model the flexibility of language and explore social nuances of language. This is the perfect stage to play around with language, using expressions and jokes to show how language can be fun, funny and very punny!

Additional suggested activities for you to use and to guide and coach the parents are included in Table 10–9.

Targeting and Incorporating Goals

Auditory Attention, Detection, Memory, Discrimination, Auditory Recognition, Sequencing, and Comprehension
(Tables 10–3 and 10–5)

facilitator for their child and uses many different strategies consistently. Support and celebrate the success of the child and parent. You will introduce the parents to some new strategies and support the carryover into natural daily interactions. Help parents to understand knowledge related to the next skills in listening and spoken language for the competent communicator. The parent has become the professional!

Communication is easy to initiate and is successful at this stage. However, there are more complex conversations and communication strategies the child will need

Auditory Retrieval and Expressive Communication
(Tables 10–4 and 10–6)

Activities of Daily Living (ADL) and Life Skills

The child at this language stage learns to listen and follow more complex instructions as they are helping around the house with chores such as setting the table, washing dishes, and being independent with testing batteries and changing them for toys or their hearing technology.

Table 10–9. Guide and Coach Parents To:

Implement optimal strategies in the competent communicator stage (Table 10–8)

Listen! Talk, talk, talk!
- Speak in the language that is natural in the home.
- Tell and discuss stories from different perspectives.
- Continue to use precise vocabulary and don't accept *this*, *that*, *here*, and *there* as substitutes.
- Give their child clues and have them guess the mystery object.
- Discuss different solutions to a problem.
- Take turns making (or imagining) groups of items and have the other person figure out why they belong together.
- Make a family tree and talk about different relatives, their jobs, and where they live.
- Play word games such as I Spy or Twenty Questions (e.g., Describe something you see, like, "I spy something round on the wall that you use to tell the time." Let the child guess what it is. Have the child describe something. This helps the child listen and use words to describe an object).
- Use complex, multistep directions, like "Get your coat from the closet, put it on, and put my keys from the table in your pocket. Don't forget the grocery bags."
- Encourage the child to tell how to do something or get somewhere.
- Draw a picture that the child describes.
- Teach the power of storytelling and writing. Write down the child's story as they tell it.
- Discuss social cues and sarcasm.
- Use idioms and expressions to discuss literal and nonliteral use of language (e.g., "raining cats and dogs," "I have something up my sleeve," "you're pulling my leg").
- Keep teaching the child new words. Define words and help your child understand them. For example, say, "This vehicle is on the highway. It is a car. A bus is another kind of vehicle. So are a train and an airplane."
- Teach the child to ask what a word means when they don't know.
- Point out multiple meanings.
- Tell jokes and be punny and encourage their child to tell jokes.

Play, play, play!
- Play board games and card games. Teach the child to learn to follow rules, talk about the game, and teach somebody else to play the game.
- Use game language; e.g., *first, last, take a turn, win, tie, poor/good sport, die, dice, shuffle, deal, clockwise around the board*.

In real life
- Help their child master life skills (Table 10–10).
- Have the child help plan daily activities or special events (e.g., plan a meal and make a shopping list for the grocery store. Plan their birthday party. Ask their opinion, and have them make choices).
- Ask questions aligned with higher-order thinking skills: creating, analyzing, evaluating, and applying (see Table 3–13, Higher-Order Thinking Activities).

Table 10–9. *continued*

Read
- Continue to read to your child, even if they are able to read for themselves.
- Have the child read instructions (e.g., how to play a game, how to assemble something new, follow a recipe).
- Encourage child to read different materials at their age, grade, or cognitive level (e.g., magazines, newspapers, or news articles).

Theory of Mind
- Talk about what somebody else might think (e.g., What would your friend think if you didn't answer them because your hearing aid/cochlear implant wasn't working? What would your friend think if they were talking to you about a movie they saw but you started talking about what you have for lunch?)

Sources: https://www.asha.org/public/speech/development/01/; http://www.hanen.org/helpful-info/articles/tuning-in-to-others-how-young-children-develop.aspx; Hearing First Theory of Mind handout

So many useful life skills can be taught to even young children and should be seen not only as skills, but also as a jumping board for language that is easily used to incorporate the listening and spoken language areas being targeted (Table 10–10). Keep in mind that we are addressing language level, not age level. Select life skills as appropriate for the child with hearing loss depending on their actual age, and introduce them at previous language stages, at this stage, or the subsequent levels.

It is typical for a child to learn to tie their shoes as they are entering school, when they have the fine motor skills to do so and are at a good age to be able to introduce themselves. However, they are not able to do tasks that require reading and writing. Vocabulary is everywhere, as are more complex language structures and comprehension of issues as we transition to conversations about independence, household chores, and being a contributing member of the family unit and of society.

The parent can teach the child (even a young one) to set the table. Consider the child who is walking away to watch TV or have screen time. The parent calls out, "Over my dead body can you play a video game before the table is set and your homework is finished." The child might respond, "What did you say about playing my video game?" (Goal 16). The child and adult will continue and discuss setting the table, talking about what dishes and utensils are needed based on what the parent explains is on the dinner menu. The idiom "over my dead body" was used and should be clarified if necessary. For the child learning to discriminate place cues in phonemes, the parent might need to point out that the word is *ladle*, the utensil to serve soup, not *label* (Goals 1, 3, 4, 5, 6, 9, 11, 13). While setting the table, the parent could tell them not to use the "fork in the road," but the one in the dish drainer. They could joke that having strawberries for dessert is a "berry good idea" or ask, "What did one plate say to the other plate?" "Dinner's on me" (Goals 10, 11, 14, 15).

Natural Conversations

The child will be able to have more complex conversations at this level of

Table 10–10. Life Skills to Teach Children

Write a letter	Make a grocery list
Make a salad	Pick fruits and vegetables
Make a phone call	Test batteries
Number to call in case of an emergency	Change batteries in hearing technology, toy, or remote control
Complete a call in case of an emergency	
Plan a balanced meal	Care for a pet
Take a message	Make a plan to save and budget
Use a fire extinguisher	Do laundry
Play with a baby	Iron or steam clothes
Vacuum the stairs	Write a thank-you letter
Introduce himself/herself	Select a thoughtful gift
Wash a car	Make a smoothie
Hammer a nail	Peel potatoes
Clean the refrigerator	Put air in bicycle tires
Set the table	Wash dishes
Address and stamp an envelope	Sew on a button
Make scrambled eggs	Garden
Change ink cartridge in printer	Clean the bathroom
Clean a bedroom	Fix something
Write a check	Clean the kitchen
Change a lightbulb	Read and follow a recipe
Put staples in a stapler	Read a map
Jump rope	Give directions to a location
Call a store or restaurant	Make a bed
Follow instructions	Ride a bike
Explain instructions on how to do a task	Use a smartphone or computer

Source: https://growingchild.com/

language ability. Conversations begin to include discourse when the conversational partner has more to contribute. Or the conversation might be predominately discourse at times such as in academic settings. At this stage it is evident that goals from all areas (Tables 10–3, 10–4, 10–5, 10–6) are easy to incorporate in almost any appropriate activity or interaction. The chocolate chip cookie theory is at play as we naturally incorporate multiple goals while just talking to the child (e.g., Goals 3, 4, 7, 8, 9, 13, 14, 15, and 16).

This is a good time to begin working on conversational competence. Be certain to address how to follow the conversational partner's topic, change topics, repair communication breakdown, and use a variety of clarification strategies. You and the parent will introduce and facilitate these conversational skills and other ones appropriate to the child's identified needs. You should model strategies for clarification and conversation repair. For example, you can say, "I didn't hear what you said because it was noisy when the truck drove by." "What page in the book did you say I should look at?" "What do you mean when you say we need to be walking on eggshells?" "What does *controversy* mean?" "Ostensibly—you mean it's supposed to be?"

This is an appropriate time to have complex conversations related to Theory of Mind, as these topics naturally integrate executive function and Theory of Mind.

Raise issues related to Theory of Mind and their hearing loss. Raise questions to address and have the child think about how their friend will feel if they don't listen to what they say and always talk about what the child with hearing loss wants. What will the friend think if you misunderstand what they said because you didn't ask for clarification? Is it better to let somebody know that you didn't understand or risk a misunderstanding? What will someone think if you don't answer them? Is it better to let your conversational partner know that you can't hear well in certain situations or not?

Discussions about allowance and the conversations around money, the value of money, savings, charitable donations, and budgeting can start at this stage. Should all the children have to do chores? Does everyone in the family get the same amount of allowance? What will each family member have to do? What is fair for children of different ages? The child with hearing loss can discuss and negotiate their allowance or how they are able to earn money by doing different chores. The parent might discuss their family's perspective that chores are an expectation and not a way to earn money. These conversations touch on complex issues by addressing the family structure, rules, values, and mutual expectations. It can also demonstrate respect for others and differences in families' ways of dealing with a variety of aspects of family values and societal beliefs. This gives the adult and child the opportunity to begin to discuss why she doesn't get a new backpack or a very expensive electronic toy but her friend does. Keep in mind that the depth of these conversations is likely to be more a reflection of the child's age and cognitive level rather than the listening and language level.

Degraded signals are, more often than not, inevitable in most life and daily experiences. In these situations, the parent and child with hearing loss can work on troubleshooting to learn how to be more successful. Strategies will be taught and learned—these have been addressed in various parts of this book and include getting closer, establishing a closed set of language, familiarizing the child with some key vocabulary or elements of what will happen, and often using assistive technology.

It is advisable for the child to understand what will occur in a new situation that is possibly in an acoustically difficult environment. For example, explain the rules and key words before attending a baseball game in a noisy park or stadium or before going to a sister's dance recital in a school auditorium. They must know relevant vocabulary, learned in a good acoustic setting, to prevent potential errors in the perception and production of the words. If going to a baseball game, discuss the many related expressions such as *struck out, three strikes against you, ballpark, throw a curveball, touch base, on the ball,* and *hit a home run.* Talk about what the crowd might be yelling from the bleachers. Provide your child with the closed-set language to help them to understand the words in that acoustically difficult environment.

Activities allow the adults to focus on multiple goals when interacting with a child at this stage of listening and spoken language development. Activities discussed in Chapter 9 are appropriate at this stage, both as described and with more advanced variations.

Playful and Figurative Language

Look for opportunities to have fun with language and model this to the parent and child. Tell jokes every session and fit puns in everywhere you can. This allows for the flexibility of language to be a focus for the child with hearing loss. Use sarcasm, incorporate idioms, stumble on multiple meanings, tell jokes and puns, and explain the way we can play with language. Multiple meanings and idioms were introduced in natural situations when they came up in the previous stages, and now you should continue to model figurative uses of language. Opportunities for playing with words and language can be part of any conversation when you begin to think that way.

Joking and playful language might be difficult for some parents. You can provide support by giving the parents lists of multiple meanings such as the one in *The Reading Teacher's Book of Lists* by Kress and Fry (2015). Find resources for jokes, puns, idioms, and figurative language for the parents. Jokes are going to be different in different cultures. Discuss and explore the way this is conveyed in their home language.

You will need to introduce jokes, riddles, and puns to a child with hearing loss. This is difficult for some children with hearing loss, particularly for those who were older when they learned listening and spoken language. Find an easy joke to begin with based on language that the child can understand. An example of a first joke to introduce is, "What has wheels and flies?" If they are willing to guess, the child or parent will almost always say an airplane. They will often laugh or smile without really understanding what is funny when you deliver the punchline—a garbage truck. We discuss that *flies* could be a noun or a verb—typically they use that word both ways. You and the parent can discuss the element of humor and the unexpected or surprise meaning. You can go to other classic "fly" jokes where the customer says, "Waiter, there's a fly in my soup." Explore the many possible answers and why they are silly or funny. Explain why it is funny when the waiter responds by saying, "Shh! Everyone will want one." "That's because the chef used to be a tailor." "Don't worry, he can't drink very much of it." Or the slight variations: "Waiter, what's that fly doing in my soup?" "Looks like the backstroke" and, "What did the angry customer say to the clumsy waiter?" "Waiter, there's soup in my fly!"

Encourage the parent to find a joke when the child becomes aware of a multiple meaning. For example, when the child gets a new bicycle, there can be a conversation about the air in the tire. The pun that the bike can't stand up because it is too tired provides the perfect opportunity for explaining humor based on the multiple meanings. Discuss homographs, that the word tire can be a verb or noun (i.e., "you tire me out") and that a car has tires. Discuss the homophones *too* versus *two* versus *to*. Families can have a joke a day (or more) or put a joke in the child's lunch box. This also encourages conversation with peers at school, when the child has a joke to tell and/or learn with their peers. Be certain the child learns the vocabulary and expressions related to telling jokes such as the punchline, "I give up," and "Do you get it?"

Do Not Stop Reading!

Read books with more complex stories that will provide an opportunity to discuss the problem or conflict in the plot and opportunities to explore characters' feelings and reactions. Predictions and inferences are abundant in these books. Books with inferences built in are a wonderful opportunity for introducing more complex questions and predicting what might happen next.

And the Games Go On

Sports, physical activities, and games such as riding bikes, skateboards, or roller skates become additional situations to incorporate elements of listening and spoken language. When the child is learning these activities, use appropriate language to introduce, discuss, and learn the language related to the activity. Scavenger hunts are easily put together and the items can be collected or photographed. The items can be specific, themed, or based on an initial consonant, or clues can be given for the items. Children work independently or in teams with siblings or peers and can be provided with a variety of clues such as, find something: made of metal; spiky; smaller than a quarter; that smells good; borrowed; and that is your favorite color. Organized sports, whether individual or team sports, have the potential to facilitate a child's language in yet another domain. Parents and coaches are likely to be involved with the training in a sport, but the language can be examined and included in intervention in natural discussions with open-ended questions or conversation starters (e.g., "How was your weekend? Tell me about your soccer practice. There must be a lot of rules and new words while playing soccer; can we help you with them?).

Complex commercial board games are available that are geared at ages up to adulthood. The variety of board games is bound to allow the child to find games that are both challenging and of interest. There is no need to reinvent the wheel when there are many great games available. The adults only need to use their creativity to build in the listening and spoken language goals while keeping the child engaged.

A good basic plan is to take the time to learn the game. The written instructions are already structured in a very systematic way with appropriate sections. The child can either listen to or read the instructions to learn the game, and discuss the rules while those learning the game are asking questions to be certain all the rules are understood (Goals 3, 4, 7, 12, 13, 16, 17). Games can be introduced during intervention, continued at home, and then revisited in a subsequent session to use for other elements and goals. The child or parent could bring a game from home for the intervention session and give the opportunity to the child to teach the game and explain the rules to the professional.

The child can be guided with a series of questions to learn how to explain the rules of game through clear and appropriately sequenced set of instructions. When they teach the game, they learn to explain the object of the game, the procedure for each player's turn, and the scoring system if applicable. Different games deal with different language and concepts. Many games have inherent strategies, and Theory of Mind discussions regarding different players' strategies can be incorporated. Games listed here can be purchased in North America if desired, but any board or card game that is age appropriate can be used. The idea is to illustrate how games like these can be used for listening and speaking.

> Monopoly relates to real estate and uses concepts and vocabulary such as properties, utilities, rent, taxes, and mortgages (Maggie, 1904).
>
> Clue (Pratt, 1949) is a detective scenario involving solving a murder mystery by determining the location, weapon, and guilty person from the suspects through the process of elimination.
>
> Mousetrap (Glass, 1967) requires following specific steps for construction to "build a better mousetrap." What does that mean? And who moved the cheese?
>
> Chess is an advanced game to teach children, as they are cognitively ready, with different pieces, each specific move pattern, and an introduction to logic and strategies.
>
> Headbanz (Spin Master, 1991) uses picture cards that are held with a headband. The person is unable to see their picture and must ask questions of their opponents to determine the picture. This game provides an opportunity to teach logical thinking when asking questions.
>
> Sorry (Storey, 1929) is a game of revenge providing an opportunity to describe the numbers on the cards with clues of differing levels of complexity and vocabulary or math word problems. When the player picks up a card, before showing it to the opponents, they could provide a clue to the number using age- and grade-appropriate vocabulary (e.g., this number is the same as the number of people in your family. This number is less than 10, greater than 5, even, and divisible by 3). When you begin the game, put your head face down on the board, since there is a space for the cards that says "place face down." When playing Sorry, it is amazing how quickly one can go from being ahead to being stuck in start. This provides an excellent opportunity to be a good sport and learn that it isn't whether you win or lose, it's how you play the game.
>
> Scrabble (Butts, 1931) has set of specific rules and requires vocabulary, spelling, and strategy. When teaching this game, it is helpful to begin by playing collaboratively with everyone seeing each players' tile racks. That way, you can use listening and spoken language to explain and help each other and learn the rules while incorporating many goals targeted for the child at this stage. Start by using the tiles to demonstrate how to make words from letters even before placing them on the board. Provide detailed and specific instructions to the child, such as "Begin with the word *shelf*, remove the second letter

and put it at the end, then place the word *is* between the *f* and the *h*. What word did you make? *Selfish*. Play with the word. What letters can you add to name a kind of animal? *Shellfish*." Discuss connecting words vertically and horizontally, how to score double letter and double word points, what kinds of words are allowed, and how to challenge your opponent. Before placing down a new word, you could provide clues for the meaning of the word and have the child guess the word.

Card games can be fun and varied at this stage. Be certain the child has the basic understanding of how to play card games and the vocabulary that goes along with the deck of cards and initiating a game. If not, the specific relevant vocabulary will need to be addressed. There are many card games with a standard deck of 52 playing cards and many commercially available card games. Families might have their favorite games and relatives might be willing to teach more complex games. More complex games have more complex instructions to explain and understand. Games can involve tricks, trump cards, and bidding.

Scoring can be another aspect of the game. Learning how to score, listening to others reporting their scores, or having to report their scores to the person keeping track will target many of the goals for a child at this stage. Card games are explained in books, or instructions can be found online. Solitaire can also be taught using verbal or written instructions, which will also incorporate a variety of goals targeted at this level. Spades, Hearts, and Bridge are some very complex card games. They can promote social interactions and facilitate many aspects of listening and spoken language.

There are many word games, which do not typically need many materials. You can modify the game to be age and grade appropriate for the child. You should have a repertoire of word games that you can quickly incorporate into a session. They make for a great Plan B when needed.

Category games can be a continuation of games such as Going on Vacation and I Spy (see Chapter 9). Add components such as incorporating the alphabet or naming items by categories or attributes. Categories can introduce more complex vocabulary such as types of trees, string instruments, or currencies. A variety of commercial games, such as Outburst (1986), Outburst Jr. (1989), A to Z, A to Z Jr., and Scattergories (1998) use categories as a basic principle of the game. Players name items in some cases by letters of the alphabet. Rules can be modified to best meet goals or the child's reading level or understanding of initial consonants in the case of younger children. One can use the category cards in different ways for creating other word games. Another option would be to pick a category and have the player name items until they can't think of any more. Players could start with the alphabet written on a paper and keep track of which letters they used in naming items, and the first person to get all the letters wins. The game could be played in such a manner that opponents need to guess the category or define attributes when items that belong together are named. Another version of Going on Vacation could be that you need to name two items that meet the unknown criteria to be allowed on the airplane. Criteria for the items is decided by the "pilot" and are up to the imagination. They could be items that start with adjacent letters in the alphabet, or the person's initials, or have double letters in their spelling, or two items that start with the same letter.

Clever clues require thinking while listening to solve the mystery. In such games, one person thinks of a person, place, or thing and must provide multiple clues or information about the item. The opponents have to figure out what it is. The opponents must be able to hold these clues in their short-term memory and combine them to figure out the item. Provide challenging clues that use plays on words with multiple meanings. Twenty Questions for Kids by University Games is a board game that has great clues and uses language in flexible ways, such as "You can't hear my bark" or "I leave, but I don't go away" when the object is a tree. There are a variety of commercially available games that use this premise. Clues such as "I have no money, but I have bread" and "If you cut me, I won't bleed" are used for a sandwich. "I have lots of matches but I don't smoke," "My aces don't come in a deck," and "You don't need to make a racket to play me" are clues for the game of tennis.

Do You Potato Sack? is a verb variation of 20 questions. One player thinks of a verb that is designated as "potato sack" but does not tell anybody. The other players have to figure out what the verb is by asking questions that can be answered by yes or no. For example, "Do you potato sack in the house?" "Do you potato sack standing up?" "Do babies potato sack?" "Do you like to potato sack?" This promotes some logical thinking and requires organization of questions being asked.

In the word game What Belongs?, players must guess the category picked by the challenger. The challenger thinks of a category or attribute but doesn't say what it is. The challenger names an item from the category and the other players guess items and are told if it belongs or not. The game can be introduced with manipulatives to illustrate the principles. Begin with simple categories such as clothing, animals, foods, or household items. For example, the challenger decides to use "black and white animals" as the category and starts the game by saying *penguin*. Players take turns going in a circle. The first player guesses *flamingo*, maybe thinking "birds" is the category, but is told it does not belong. The next player, thinking "water animals," guesses *seal*. They are told it does not belong. Another player could guess *killer whale* and would be told it belongs. That player can guess another item to see if they are right. They guess *polar bear*, thinking it is an animal that lives in cold climates. But it does not belong. When play comes back to the challenger, another clue is provided (e.g., *zebra*). Play could stop when somebody figures out the category or could continue until every player solves the challenge. You can make the game more challenging by using complex defining categories such as things that start with the letter *B*, things that fit in a pocket, or crunchy food.

Anagrams can be played in many ways as a paper and pencil game or with any variations you create. Changing elements of this game allows you to incorporate many goals for this stage. Begin with a group of letters and try to make other words using only those letters. You can introduce the game with pieces of paper, tiles, or blocks that have letters, or write the letters at the top of a paper and work collaboratively to find words. Manipulate the situation to address goals targeted for the child. You can introduce new vocabulary words, give a definition to a word you have found, have the child listen to isolated words in an open set with a degraded signal, use words that have phonemes that are more challenging for the child to discriminate, or spell the word to be sure that child can discriminate the letters that are similar (e.g., *B, C, D, G, P, T, Z*). Playing this as a game allows for more repetitions of the activity for increasing practice in a way that is motivating (https://en.wikipedia.org/wiki/Anagrams_game).

Mastermind (1970) and Jotto (1955) are challenging codebreaker games using logic and the process of elimination. The nature of these games can provide wonderful opportunities for natural conversation and discourse. In Mastermind, the players try to solve for the color pattern of their opponent. Jotto is a word version of a codebreaker game. Each player secretly picks a five-letter word and has to figure out the other person's word. The game is played by taking turns guessing other five-letter words and being told how many letters in that word are in the opponent's secret word. Over several turns, one can determine the letters in the opponents' word. This requires some use of executive function, logic, and thought processes. When teaching and learning the game, each player can try to verbally explain what has been determined by the information they collect. This provides an opportunity to use complex and compound sentences to logically explain their reasoning process. The game can also be used to introduce new vocabulary, both in the discussion of how the game is proceeding and in an open set with the words presented to the child. Since the adult does not need to be competitive, words can be selected to practice phoneme discrimination with specific sounds that might be challenging for the child rather than to win the game.

Putting It All Together: Case History

Daniel is 4 years 4 months of age and was identified with a hearing loss at birth through the Newborn Hearing Screening. His current hearing age is 11 months due to the extended period of nonuse of hearing technology.

He received his hearing aids at 3 weeks of age and wore them consistently until 6 months of age. At 6 months, Daniel began pulling his hearing aids out. He fought to not wear them by pulling them out or screaming and crying when his parents attempted to insert them. This continued until Daniel was 1 year old. Daniel's hearing aids were reprogrammed, but he still refused to wear them. At this time, hearing aid use was discontinued per recommendation of the speech-language pathologist providing intervention. From 1 year to 3 years of age, Daniel did not utilize hearing aids.

At 3 years 1 month of age, Daniel was seen for a second opinion regarding his loss and hearing aids from an auditory-verbal therapist. At that time, his parents were concerned with his language abilities, his poor speech productions, and unintelligible speech. Consistent use of technology was a focus. With the assistance and insistence from the auditory-verbal professional, his parents, and his preschool classroom teacher, Daniel began to wear his hearing aids. He was wearing them all waking hours at the age of 3 years 2 months and he has been doing so since that time.

Daniel began weekly auditory-verbal therapy (AVT) sessions from the age of 3 years 1 month, when he began to wear hearing aids bilaterally.

He was assessed at the age of 3 years 3 months using informal observations, diagnostic therapy, and the Clinical Evaluation of Language Fundamentals—Preschool (CELF-P). Daniel's scores were mostly in the average range but his performance is indicative of gaps in his language development over time due to limited auditory access as he was not using hearing aids. Overall, his performance at that time indicated poor receptive and expressive abilities for the morphemes that are low-intensity grammatical markers. His areas of deficit reflected his lack of auditory access and were particularly apparent in /s/ morphemic functions and speech perception errors that interfered with development of present progressive verb tense, past tense -*ed* endings, irregular past tense, and pronouns.

Auditory Processes for Using Sound Meaningfully

Auditory Attention

Daniel demonstrates excellent attention to information presented through audition only. He attends to a variety of speech features including advanced skills such as the place cue information for a variety of manners of production. He is able to attend to and comprehend a variety of low-intensity grammatical morphemes including but not limited to: /s/ morphemic functions, negatives, verb tense markers, articles, conjunctions, and derivational suffixes.

Auditory Memory

Daniel is able to listen to several sentences or a short personal story and recall details to answer questions appropriately. He shows the ability to attend to five to six critical items and follow a series of complex requests. He will listen to a story from a book and recall multiple details, which he will include when retelling the story.

Auditory Discrimination and Identification

Daniel demonstrates consistent discrimination and identification of the suprasegmentals, vowels, diphthongs, and consonants by manner, place, and voicing. He demonstrates abilities to discriminate and identify the phonemes that he is inconsistently producing at this time (e.g., /w/ versus /l/, /s/ versus /ʃ/), which indicates he is making appropriate progress toward the development of these sounds. His production errors are in those discriminations that would be considered age appropriate.

The Compass Test was administered at this time. Daniel's total percentage of accuracy on the Compass Test was 96 percent. Discriminations that did not score at 100 percent were due to vocabulary knowledge. Daniel stated he didn't know the vocabulary word for two of the items in the test. His discrimination abilities per this assessment for speech features are:

Initial Consonants Different by Manner = 100% (8/8)

Final Consonants Different by Manner = 100% (8/8)

Final Consonants Different by Voicing = 100% (8/8)

Initial Consonants Different by Voicing = 88% (7/8)—did not know the vocabulary for one item

Initial Consonants Different by Place = 100% (8/8)

Final Consonants Different by Place = 88% (7/8)—did not know the vocabulary for one item

Auditory Integration

Daniel is able to follow an auditory-only conversation when engaged motorically or visually in a task.

Auditory Processes for Learning to Talk

Auditory Feedback

Overall, Daniel demonstrates excellent production of a variety of phonemes at a phonetic level with a few exceptions that are indicative of normal phonological development and a few that are indicative of emerging auditory attention and discrimination abilities. He demonstrates some inconsistencies in his productions, which are mostly place errors and are a more advanced auditory perception skill. At a phonologic level, his production of /s/ is often substituted with an /ʃ/. He is stimulable for the /s/ in isolation. He is inconsistent in the production in phonology. He typically uses /w/ for /l/ in words such as *lock*, *look*, and *lion*. He is able to produce a rapid string of the phoneme /l/ with some limited vowel variety. He will use /w/ and /r/ correctly and discriminates them. He has also been noted to make some limited errors with m/n, and p/t/k primarily in word-final position but also in word-initial position. Some of the word-initial errors (e.g., *meed* instead of *need*) are old habits. He is demonstrating emergence of several /s/ blends at a phonologic level spontaneously and, when he reduces the blend, he can easily correct it often without a model. He is not demonstrating consistent self-monitoring at this time.

Auditory Processes for Learning Language

Auditory Comprehension and Auditory Retrieval

Daniel is able to listen to a new story or book and demonstrate comprehension of the story and of new concepts presented (e.g., not telling the truth). He is able to re-tell a story, including details, from a book or a personal story with minimal prompts. Daniel is currently demonstrating comprehension and producing complex and compound sentences with syntax and uses a variety of age-appropriate morphemes. He consistently uses a variety of verb tenses including past tense *-ed* endings that are auditorily more difficult. He is developing some irregular past-tense forms as well. He uses and responds appropriately to a variety of question formats, including "why?" The following are typical examples of his spontaneous language recently gathered from AVT sessions and at home:

> We have two teachers so they take turns.
>
> I wonder how that light turns on.
>
> That means they are working so much.
>
> Daddy is supposed to take me.
>
> It's not ready.
>
> But I earned the field trip to the zoo to see the animals.
>
> We're talking about the hippopotamus.

I like the elephants too.

My super, duper favorite animal at the zoo was the rhino.

Mommy, why are you spelling *hippopotamus* and *elephants*?

I was making shapes in the glue and I accidentally got it on my elbow.

They had a baby and a mommy and daddy, and the mommy and baby went swimming, but not the daddy, he was eating grass.

Daniel's comprehension and expressive language skills were reassessed at 4 years 4 months using the CELF-P (Wiig et al., 2020). This assessment had been previously administered at 3 years 3 months. The scores for the subtests for both administrations are indicated in Tables 10–11 through 10–19.

Table 10–11. CELF-P Sentence Structure

Age at Administration	Scaled Score	Age Equivalent	Percentile	Growth in 13 Months
4 years 4 months	17	>7 y	99	>3 y 7 m
3 years 3 months	10	3 y 5 m	50	

Table 10–12. CELF-P Word Structure

Age at Administration	Scaled Score	Age Equivalent	Percentile	Growth in 13 Months
4 years 4 months	17	>7 y	99	>3 y 6 m
3 years 3 months	11	3 y 6 m	63	

Table 10–13. CELF-P Expressive Vocabulary

Age at Administration	Scaled Score	Age Equivalent	Percentile	Growth in 13 Months
4 years 4 months	11	4 y 8 m	63	>1 y 8 m
3 years 3 months	8	<3 y	25	

Table 10–14. CELF-P Concepts and Following Directions

Age at Administration	Scaled Score	Age Equivalent	Percentile	Growth in 13 Months
4 years 4 months	17	6 y 11 m	99	>3 y 11 m
3 years 3 months	9	<3 y	37	

Table 10–15. CELF-P Recalling Sentences

Age at Administration	Scaled Score	Age Equivalent	Percentile	Growth in 13 Months
4 years 4 months	12	5 y 5 m	75	>2 y 5 m
3 years 3 months	9	<3 y	37	

Table 10–16. CELF-P Word Classes—Receptive

Age at Administration	Scaled Score	Age Equivalent	Percentile	Growth in 13 Months
4 years 4 months	13	6 y 9 m	84	n/a

Table 10–17. CELF-P Word Classes—Expressive

Age at Administration	Scaled Score	Age Equivalent	Percentile	Growth in 13 Months
4 years 4 months	12	5 y 5 m	75	n/a

Table 10–18. CELF-P Word Classes—Total

Age at Administration	Scaled Score	Age Equivalent	Percentile	Growth in 13 Months
4 years 4 months	18	Not available	75	n/a

Table 10–19. CELF Preschool Scores

Subtest	Scaled Score	Age Equivalent	Percentile	Growth in 13 Months
Sentence Structure	17	>7 y	99	>3 y 7 m
Word Structure	17	>7 y	99	>3 y 6 m
Expressive Vocabulary	11	4 y 8 m	63	>1 y 8 m
Concepts and Following Directions	17	6 y 11 m	99	>3 y 11 m
Recalling Sentences	12	5 y 5 m	75	>2 y 5 m
Word Classes—Receptive	13	6 y 9 m	84	n/a
Word Classes—Expressive	12	5 y 5 m	75	n/a
Word Classes—Total	18	Not available	99.6	n/a

Auditory Memory, Auditory Comprehension

The Test of Auditory Processing Skills–3 (TAPS-3) was administered. This assessment is normed for ages 4 years through 18 years 11 months. This test was not previously administered. The subtests for auditory memory and auditory cohesion were administered to determine Daniel's auditory skills in these areas. Scaled scores between 8 and 12 are considered within the normal ranges. Table 10–20 indicates his scores, percentiles, and age equivalents for the subtests.

His scaled scores and percentile scores indicate that he is showing abilities in the average range and earlier for all of the auditory memory subtests. He shows a very high score for auditory comprehension. However, his abilities for auditory reasoning, which includes inferences and idioms, is in the low average range and clearly not similar to the levels for any of the other subtests.

The Children's Home Inventory for Listening Difficulties (CHILD) was administered with his mother as the respondent. This assessment has 15 prompts, each scored from 0 to 8 with words describing the different levels. The average of the scores for designated prompts within each category are included in Table 10–21. The different types of listening situations are listed in order from easiest to more difficult. They indicate that his auditory skills are developing in an appropriate way, from easier situations to more difficult environments and situations.

Descriptive explanations for the scores are as follows for those categories most applicable to Daniel. Items scored as the most difficult are indicated as follows:

2: tough going

3: sometimes gets it and sometimes doesn't

Table 10–21. CHILD Scores by Acoustic Environment

	Average
Quiet	5.75
Social Situations	4.4
Distance	3.3
Noise	3.2
Media/Degraded Signals	3
Average in all Environments	3.87

Table 10–20. Test of Auditory Processing Skills (TAPS) Scores

Subtest	Raw Score	Scaled Score	Age Equivalent	Percentile
Number Memory Forward	12	11	5 y 5 m	63
Number Memory Reversed	5	12	5 y 4 m	75
Word Memory	16	15	7 y 7 m	95
Sentence Memory	15	11	5 y 4 m	63
Auditory Comprehension	21	16	8 y 10 m	98
Auditory Reasoning	1	9	3 y 6 m	37

4: it takes work but usually gets done

5: OK but not easy

6: pretty good—hears almost all the words

Score of 2

Playing inside with a group of children

Score of 3

Understanding the dialogue from a TV show or video

Understanding in the presence of TV or noisy toy

Understanding speech in a noisy situation

Not speech reading

Calling from another room

Understanding phone conversations

Playing outside with other children

Summary

Daniel has shown excellent progress in development of his auditory and language skills. The CELF indicates significant gains in all areas as tested. The CHILD and the Test of Auditory Processing Skills (TAPs) indicate needs in the areas of auditory reasoning (inferences and idioms) and comprehension of degraded signals at lower levels. Daniel is an intelligent child who began to read at the age of 3 and is currently reading fluently.

The Intervention Session

Sessions with a child at this stage of language development can be very focused while remaining very conversational. In this session the professional introduces a joke based on multiple meanings and a conversation takes off from there. As you read through the session, note the child, professional, and mother are having a natural and easy conversation and that the goals are incorporated through the conversation and in the activity selected for the session.

Professional: I have a stuffed moose right here. Did I ever tell you his name?

Daniel: No, I don't think so. Or if you did, I forgot it.

Mother: No, if you told us, I would have remembered.

Professional: Want to guess?

Daniel: Muffin? Like from the book *If You Give a Moose a Muffin*.

Professional: Oh—good guess. I love that book. But not his name. Mom, any thoughts?

Mother: Bullwinkle, because we are both old enough to remember that TV show.

Professional: Another good guess, but not his name.

Daniel: OK, we give up.

Professional: Chocolate!

Mother (laughs and turns to her son): I love that. Do you get it?

Daniel: Yeah, he's brown like chocolate.

Professional: Yes—another good guess and that might be a logical answer. But it isn't funny. His name is like a joke. Mom asked if you get it. That is what we ask when we tell the punchline of a joke.

Mother: We don't do a lot of jokes.

Daniel: I don't know why jokes are funny. I laugh sometimes with my friends anyways so they don't know. It doesn't matter.

Professional: Well it does matter.

Daniel: I don't really understand them.

Professional: Well let's figure out this one and then talk about some more. Mom, do you want to explain it?

Mother: Sure! So, there are two kinds of moose. One is the animal, like the stuffed animal we are talking about. Do you know another one? You might, but I don't think you have ever had it.

Daniel: Had a moose?

Mother: The other mousse is a delicious dessert, like a pudding but usually lighter.

Professional: So why would it be funny that I call my moose Chocolate?

Daniel: Because he is brown like chocolate.

Professional: That is what you were saying before, but mom told you about the two different kinds of moose. What are the two kinds?

Daniel: An animal that lives in the wild.

Professional: Yes, with four legs and big antlers. And the other kind of mousse?

Daniel: Like a pudding treat.

Professional: So which kind of mousse would come in a chocolate flavor?

Daniel: The treat mousse.

Professional: Yes, but he's which kind of moose?

Daniel: He's a real moose, the animal.

Professional: Yes, but I'm calling him . . .

Daniel: Chocolate. . .

Professional: Because he is brown and because I'm making a . . .

Daniel: Joke. Oh! OK.

Professional: Yes, I'm making a joke (everyone chuckles).

Mother: Great figuring that out.

Mother: Do you know any jokes?

Daniel: Some dumb knock, knock ones—like interrupting cow.

Professional: Here's one. What has wheels and flies?

Daniel: An airplane?

Mother: Hmmmm, but that isn't really funny or a joke. I give up. That is what we say so the person tells us the punchline.

Daniel: Punchline? What is that?

Mother: I'm glad you ask when you don't know a word. The expression is *punchline*. It is the funny answer or last line in a joke.

Professional: So, the punchline is . . . a garbage truck.

Mother: Ha, cute.

Daniel: What?

Mother: Well, an airplane flies . . . but a garbage truck HAS flies.

Daniel: Oh, cuz of the garbage.

Professional: So, this joke was funny because we are using a word that could have more than one meaning. You might assume they mean one thing by the way the joke is worded but then the punchline uses the other meaning that was less likely to be assumed in the way the joke was told.

Daniel: Oh, OK.

Professional: So, let's think about it. Do you know words that have more than one meaning? How about two or three meanings?

Mother: She is joking around with you. Do you get it?

Daniel: Did you mean the word *too* or did you mean two meanings?

Mother: That is what she was kidding around about. You know the word *to* has . . . how many meanings.

Daniel: Oh yeah. My teacher taught us that. It has three meanings.

Mother: What are they? Can you define them?

Daniel: Well, there is the number two.

Professional: Great.

Daniel: When it is spelled with T-W-O the number...with two O's it kinda means *also*.

Mother: Ha, you played around with the word . . . *two* the number of O's for the word *too*.

Daniel: Hmmm—I did. Didn't realize.

Mother: Do you remember the third meaning?

Daniel: Yeah, but I don't know how to explain it.

Professional: If you can't define it, can you use it in a sentence? You just did.

Daniel: Sure. I don't know how to define the word.

Mother: Very clever! Or were you really telling us that you couldn't define it?

Daniel: No, I did that on purpose.

Mother: Nice!

Professional: Do you know other words that have more than one meaning?

Daniel: Probably, but I can't think of them right now.

Professional: You just used a word in that sentence that has more than one meaning.

Daniel: What?

Mother: Yes, you did. Say the sentence again. You said, you can't . . .

Daniel: Can't think of one now

Professional: You said you can't think of one.

Daniel: Oh, yeah, can't think of one right now. Right now, like at this time. But *right* not *left*.

Mother: What else?

Daniel: I don't know.

Mother: Think about it...but don't get stuck on the spelling. It is spelled differently.

Professional: Good clue, mom.

Daniel: Oh, *write*. Like I write with a pencil.

Professional: Yeah. You write with your right hand.

Daniel: Oooh! I get it!

Professional: I have a book with a bunch of these. Let me grab it. It is an easy book but it is kind of cute. Here (giving the book to the Daniel) (from Barretta, 2007).

Daniel: Dear deer . . .

Professional: Start here with the page with the moose. Since we were just talking about it.

Daniel: "The moose loves mousse. He ate eight bowls."

Mother: So, explain that. What are the different meanings?

Daniel: Well, the first moose is an animal that lives in the wild. And the second is a delicious treat.

Daniel: "Have you seen the eewee?"

Mother: That word is pronounced ewe.

Daniel: Oh. "Have you seen the ewe? He's been in a daze for days."

Mother: Ok. So, what are the two you's?

Daniel: The first ewe is like ummm, well like the only word I can think of is using the same word.

Mother: And if dad was here he wouldn't let you get away with that.

Professional: It is called a pronoun.

Daniel: Like you, I don't know.

Mother: A pronoun for another person.

Professional: But what is the second ewe?

Daniel: The ewe is a type of sheep.

Mother: What about *daze* and *days*.

Daniel: Isn't like a daze like a weird thing like you are mixed up?

Mother: Yes, and the other one?

Daniel: Like 24 hours? Seven of them in a week.

Professional: So, what day of the week is it?

Daniel: Wednesday.

Professional: OK, so you get this?

Daniel: Yeah, but didn't realize that was how jokes worked.

Professional: But now you do!

Daniel: I think so. It is really funny.

Mother: I'm going to get you that book!

Professional: Sure, you could get it probably at the library or online. But you can just find words with multiple meanings. Like when you defined mousse—you said it was a light pudding or lighter. Lots of meanings for *light*. You can talk about those on the way home or at dinner tonight.

Professional: Have you seen this book?

Mother: No, we haven't.

Daniel (reading): Why the banana split

Professional: What does that mean?

Mother: Make like a banana and split!

Professional: Anybody ever tell you that?

Daniel: Nope.

Professional: People sometime say, "I'm going to make like a banana and split." Going to leave. I'm getting out of here, leaving,

Mother: What's a banana split? You know that.

Daniel: A type of ice cream thing.

Professional: What's another expression or meaning of *split*?

Daniel: When you do the splits like in gymnastics.

Mother: Kind of, but cute expressions with two meanings. Like we were talking about with the words, but these are expressions.

Professional: So, this is a whole book of expressions that mean when somebody is leaving and are like jokes.

Mother: Fun! Let's read them. *Why the Banana Split* by Rick Walton (1999).

Daniel: "When the Rex came to town, everyone looked at his huge head high in the air and at his large sharp teeth. And they screamed. DINOSAUR! DINOSAUR! RUN AWAY! RUN AWAY! And they did. The jump ropes skipped town, and the astronauts took off. The bananas split, peeled out, slipped away."[4]

Mother: I love this book.

Daniel: "The frogs hopped train and that train made tracks. The basketball players went travelling." Oh . . . yeah like travel on the court. I know that from playing basketball. Or going away travelling somewhere like a vacation.

Professional: Do you get it?

Daniel: Yes! "While the baseball players struck out on their own . . . "

Professional: So, are they kind of funny?

Daniel: Yeah, kind of cute, and they have double meanings or multiple meaning words. "Good buy," said the shoppers.

Mother: So why is that funny

Daniel: Like they are leaving and saying goodbye.

Mother: But what is this buy?

Daniel: They are leaving...

Professional: No, different spelling. Right?

Mother: Look, B-U-Y. What kind of buy is that?

Daniel: Like buy this with some money?

Analysis of Session

In discussion of the therapy session, we can analyze which goals are being addressed in the described interval of therapy. The goals refer back to numbers indicated in Tables 10–3 to 10–6. This scenario helps to show the integration and overlap of multiple goals in the natural interactions. In this session, the conversation flows and is focused mostly on words with multiple meanings, jokes, and idioms. (Goals 7, 8, 9, 10, 14, 15). Throughout the session, the child is expected to be attending to the conversation and using his language skills and speech productions skills as best he can (Goals 1, 3, 5, 6). He is competent and there are no errors in his language or speech during this conversation. His mother explains expressions and words that he doesn't know and he asks for clarification (Goals 7, 16).

Summary

The professional considers the knowledge base, guides and coaches the parent, and teaches strategies to promote further development at this stage of communication. The use of natural conversations, interactions, and experiences will help the child to achieve all or most of the skills as outlined in Tables 10–1 and 10–2 and the outlined goals from this stage of language development in Tables 10–3 through 10–6. Development of the goals in daily life routines and interactions will ensure that the skills are used across all the child's environments and prevent isolated or splinter skills that need to be transitioned to natural experiences. The achievement of these goals will provide a strong basis for the child with hearing loss to progress to the next level of mastery of listening and spoken language abilities. Behaviors that are indicative of the child emerging into the next stage of development are indicated in Table 10–22.

Table 10–22. By the End of the Competent Communicator Stage, the Child Should:

> Have conversations using most conversational norms.
>
> Be a fully competent language communicator with an ever-growing vocabulary emerging in Tiers 2 and 3.
>
> Understand the use of words with multiple meanings in jokes.
>
> Understand some idioms and literal language versus figurative language.
>
> Consistently discriminate:
>   initial consonants differing by manner
>   final consonants differing by manner
>   initial consonants differing by voicing
>   final consonants differing by voicing
>   initial consonants differing by place
>   final consonants differing by place

Discussion Questions

1. How do you determine if a child is at this stage?
2. How would you illustrate the chocolate chip cookie dough analogy to the parents of a child with hearing loss at this stage?
3. Select a goal from one of the Tables 10–3 through 10–6. How would you explain to a parent how to use a specific activity of daily living to target the goal? Consider and identify other goals that would be naturally included in that selected ADL.
4. What activities could you do with an older child to work on the goals at this level?
5. Consider a child with additional disabilities or needs and discuss an activity that you could work on to target a selected goal at this level.

References

Barretta, G. (2007). *Dear deer*. Macmillan.

Butts, A. M. (1931). *Scrabble* [Board game]. Hasbro.

Carrow-Woolfolk, E. (1999). *Test for Auditory Comprehension of Language-3*. Western Psychological Services.

Glass, M. (1967). *Mousetrap* [Board game]. Hasbro.

Headbanz [Board game]. (1991). Spin Master Games.

Hersch and Company. (1986). *Outburst* [Board game]. Hasbro.

Hersch and Company. (1989). *Outburst Jr.* [Board game]. Hasbro.

Hustad, K. C., Mahr, C. M., Natzke, P. E. M., & Rathouz, R. J. (2020). Development of speech intelligibility between 30 and 47 months in typically developing children: A cross-sectional study of growth. *Journal* of *Speech, Language, and Hearing Research, 63*(6), 1675–1687.

Kress, J. E., & Fry, E. B. (2015). *The reading teacher's book of lists.* Jossey Bass.

Ling, D. (2003). The Ling Six-Sound Test. *The Listener,* 52–53.

Lowry, L. (2015). *"Tuning in" to others: How young children develop theory of mind. Hanen Early Language Program.* http://www.hanen.org/SiteAssets/Helpful-Info/Articles/tuning-into-others.aspx

Maggie, E. (1904). *Monopoly* [Board game]. Parker Brothers.

Martin, N. A., & Brownell, R. (2005). *Test of Auditory Processing Skills* (3rd ed.). World Publishing.

McWinney, B., & Snow, C. (1984). *The child language data exchange system.* Carnegie Mellon.

Meirowitz, M. (1970). *Mastermind* [Board game]. Hasbro.

Paffhouse, K. (2018). This handout provides tips for supporting a child's development of Theory of Mind. *Hearing First.* https://www.hearingfirst.org/m/resources/456

Peterson, C. C., Wellman, H. M., & Slaughter, V. (2012). The mind behind the message: Advancing theory-of-mind scales for typically developing children, and those with deafness, autism, or Asperger's syndrome. *Child Development, 83*(2), 469–485.

Pratt, A. E. (1949). *Clue* [Board game]. Parker Brothers.

Rosenfeld, M. M. (1955). *Jotto* [Board game]. Endless Games.

Scattergories [Board game]. (1998). Parker Brothers.

Sindrey, D. (2021). *Compass test of auditory discrimination.* Supporting Success for Children with Hearing Loss.

Storey, W. H. (1929) *Sorry* [Board game]. Parker Brothers.

Twenty questions for kids [Board game]. (2010). University Games.

Walton, R. (1999). *Why the banana split.* Gibbs Smith.

Wiig, E., Secord, W., & Semel, E. (2020). *Clinical Evaluation of Language Fundamentals—Preschool* (3rd ed.). NCS Pearson.

Zimmerman, I. L., Steiner, V. G., & Pond, R. E. (2011). *Preschool Language Scales* (4th ed.). Pearson.

Chapter 11

Advanced Communicator Stage

Sylvia Rotfleisch

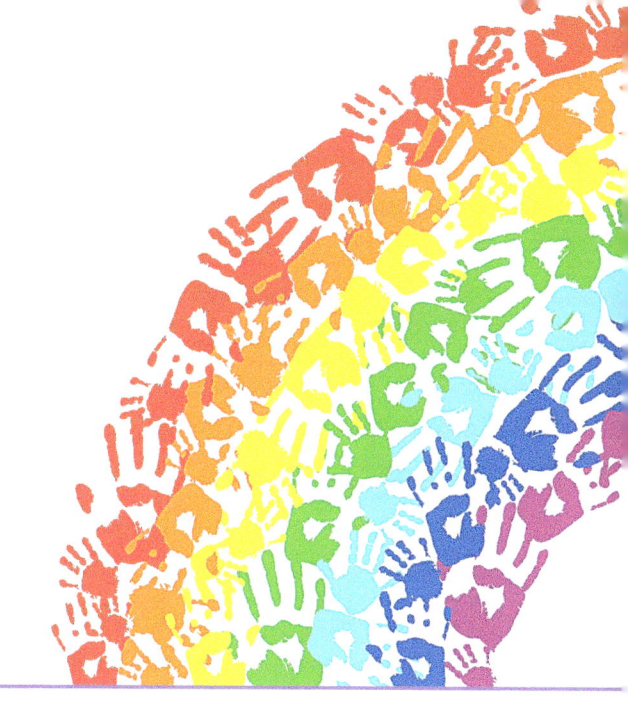

Key Points

- The child developing advanced language competence needs support to develop a variety of nuanced and important language skills.
- The child at this stage will help guide some of their goals and be a key decision maker in their sessions.
- Mastery of their auditory feedback loop across all acoustic environments will be addressed.
- The child at the advanced communicator stage will develop comprehension of nuisances of voice features that convey meaning.
- Nonliteral use of language is developed or expanded.
- Development of receptive and expressive conversational competence will be addressed in advanced areas such self-advocacy, clarification, jokes, and grade-level academics.

Basic Characteristics of the Child at the Advanced Communicator Stage

Listening

At this stage, the child with hearing loss is typically functioning independently without the support of their parents in social and academic situations. Interactions are successful through listening and natural communication strategies. Social situations are mostly successful. The child accepts their responsibility to successfully work and try to repair conversational breakdowns. A variety of appropriate advanced clarification strategies are being learned and used. The child will advocate with regards to the hearing loss in a variety of ways, including explaining the hearing loss, the use of technology and assistive hearing technology, preferential seating, and navigating the acoustic environment for success.

Improvement is noted in the ability to function auditorily in group situations (e.g., classroom, team sport sessions). There is improved ability to participate successfully in group conversations academically and socially but there continue to be challenging listening situations. Trying to guess or fill in the missing information based on language knowledge and communication competence can lead to misunderstanding nuances in a situation.

The child will understand that they will be most successful when implementing a remote microphone when the signal to noise ratio (SNR) is poor. Modulating voice intensity based on the acoustic environment is typically challenging. These advanced auditory abilities typically evident and/or emerging in the advanced communicator stage are indicated in Table 11–1. Skills listed are not sequential.

Language

The child with hearing loss at this stage is a competent spoken language communicator with a complete mastery of the semantics and syntax of language, which is used socially and in the school setting. They have a complementary repertoire of receptive and expressive vocabulary indicative of their level academically. Academic level will necessitate different language abilities such as oral presentations, cooperative group learning, debates, and participation in classroom discussions. This child is continuing to master advanced and nuanced language skills, which can include skills such as idioms, figurative language, jokes, puns, inferences, and sarcasm. Receptive and expressive language abilities evidenced or expected to emerge in this stage are included in Table 11–2. Skills listed are not sequential.

Speech

As previously addressed, the child with hearing loss with appropriate access to the auditory signal should be showing the correct sequence of development of speech sounds and typically should not have any articulation problems at this stage. However, the development of speech produc-

Table 11–1. Auditory Abilities Evidenced in the Advanced Communicator Stage

- Listens for specific purposes.
- Listens in group situations.
- Participates in classroom discussions in academic subject areas.
- Can listen and form an opinion or conclusion based on information provided auditorily.
- Effectively relies on the feedback loop for speech and language monitoring.

Sources: https://www.home-speech-home.com/; Carrow-Woolfolk (1999); McWinney and Snow (1984).

Table 11–2. Language and Speech Skills Evidenced in the Advanced Communicator Stage

Audition and Auditory Comprehension of Language	Expressive Language and Communication
• Understands multi-part complex instructions and explanations. • Understands words with multiple meanings. • Understands some jokes, puns, and riddles with word ambiguity. • Understands grade-level content material. • Understands inferences and common idioms. • Understands underlying social cues within language.	• Gives clear instructions and explanations. • Uses language effectively for a variety of functions. • Uses language to establish and maintain social situations. • Demonstrates full conversational competence, including but not limited to: initiates and closes conversations; maintains topic; takes turn appropriately; maintains eye contact; uses natural gestures; uses facial expressions as appropriate; expresses emotions through words and voice quality. • Tells a narrative with a theme, characters, plot, and emotion. • Uses figurative language/idioms in conversations. • Uses a variety of Tier 2 and 3 vocabulary in communications. • Uses advanced clarification strategies to be certain of comprehension and make self understood by others. • Uses a variety of conversational repair strategies. • Makes and plans an oral presentation. • Uses prefixes and suffixes consistently. • Participates in classroom/group discussions. • Tells jokes and uses puns.

Source: https://www.home-speech-home.com/

tion abilities for a child with hearing loss will reflect their auditory access and perception and hearing and listening experience. The phonemes expected to be mastered last are /θ/ and /ð/ (Templin, 1957) (see Chapter 3, Table 3–11). At this stage, the child with hearing loss has learned to rely on their auditory feedback loop and their speech perception and self-monitors and self-corrects their errors.

Goals for the Advanced Communicator

Developing an Appropriate Therapy Plan by Addressing Strengths and Areas of Need

The typical sequence of development will be followed to develop listening skills and appropriate speech and language abilities. All previous goals will be used as the basis for expanding to the next skills. Some goals from the competent communicator stage might not be mastered and might be carried over initially in this stage. Goals for the advanced communicator stage focus on:

- facilitating successful auditory functioning to successfully communicate across all acoustic environments with degraded auditory signals;
- reinforcing the auditory feedback loop for self-monitoring of speech production and monitoring volume across all acoustic environments;
- facilitating comprehension of nonliteral use of language and nuances of voice features that convey meaning; and
- facilitating advanced conversational competence with ability to address areas including self-advocacy, clarification, jokes, and grade-level academics.

Select appropriate goals based on your assessment results that identify the child's strengths and needs (see Chapter 4). At this language level, standardized assessment tools are abundant.

Goals must be individualized within the stage to meet the child's needs. At this level, you will look for appropriate goals, for example, when determining goals related to advanced comprehension. One child might understand jokes and nonliteral language but does not comprehend the combinations of language and social cues that signal language use such as sarcasm and exaggeration. You would select goals that expand nonliteral use of language and understanding of underlying messages (Goals 9, 10, 12, 16, 17). Another child might still be struggling with jokes and puns. You would select goals to address the inability to understand humor with further work with multiple meanings, idioms, and social nuances (Goals 9, 11, 18; see additional goals from Chapter 10).

Typical Goals for the Advanced Communicator Stage

Your selected goals continue to focus on expanding complex auditory skills through a degraded signal. Goals will support the mastery of advanced language abilities in social competencies of conversation, social language, nuances, and nonliteral and humorous uses of language. The mastery of these skills will be needed in addressing socially and grade-level appropriate pragmatic uses of language. The child will learn to apply those advance language competencies across all acoustic environments in their daily life. The advanced communicator stage allows for ongoing learning of language for social competence and advancing academics of education systems.

Typical, recommended goals for children with hearing loss at the advanced communicator stage are included in Tables 11–3 to 11–6. Goals are organized based upon defined skills related to the brain functions necessary for learning to use audition for language development

Table 11–3. Auditory Goals for Understanding Sound as Meaningful in the Advanced Communicator Stage

Auditory Attention, Detection, Discrimination, and Memory

1. Attend to appropriate language-level passages and discussions through audition only for comprehension tasks, including age- or grade-level academic vocabulary (see Goal 6).

2. Expand ability to attend, discriminate, and remember sentence material when presented through a degraded signal (e.g., background noise, phone, computer, distance) in closed set and then expanded to open set.

3. Facilitate expanded auditory memory skills for words and sentences including new age- or grade-level academic vocabulary.

Table 11–4. Auditory Feedback and Speech Production Goals in the Advanced Communicator Stage

Auditory Goals for Development of the Speech Production System

4. Reinforce and facilitate use of auditory feedback loop for self-monitoring and self-correcting productions of all phonemes.

5. Facilitate use of auditory feedback loop to monitor appropriate intensity of speech in variety of acoustic environments.

Table 11–5. Auditory Goals for Language Comprehension in the Advanced Communicator Stage

Auditory Recognition, Sequencing, and Comprehension

6. Demonstrate comprehension of a passage (see Goal 1) and related grade-level questions of reason (e.g., predictions, cause and effect, problem and solution, inferences).

7. Demonstrate comprehension of sentence material when presented through a degraded signal (Goal 2), beginning with closed set and expanded to open set.

8. Use advanced clarification strategies for communication breakdowns with peers and adults or when doesn't hear or comprehend verbal message.

9. Comprehend a variety of idioms (e.g., "You should keep an eye out for him").

10. Comprehend difference between literal and nonliteral language (e.g., idioms, simile, metaphor, hyperbole, sarcasm).

11. Understand puns and jokes, including those based on multiple meanings, idioms, and similar-sounding words (e.g., "How do you know when it's raining cats and dogs? You step into a poodle").

12. Understand sarcasm and underlying message beyond what is said through social cues, vocal tone, facial expressions, and gestures.

Table 11–6. Auditory Goals for Expressive Language in the Advanced Communicator Stage

Auditory Retrieval and Expressive Communication
13. After listening to a passage, discourse, or conversation (Goal 1), verbally respond to a variety of questions of reason (e.g., predictions, cause and effect, problem and solution, inferences).
14. Verbally explain sentence material when presented through a degraded signal (Goal 2), beginning with closed set and expanded to open set.
15. Expressively use a variety of advanced clarification strategies with adults and peers (e.g., "What does *primordial* mean?" "Excuse me, but I didn't hear what page is for social studies homework").
16. Spontaneously use a variety of idioms and can provide a verbal explanation (e.g., "You should keep an eye out for him").
17. Spontaneously use and can explain the difference between literal and nonliteral language (e.g., simile, metaphor, hyperbole, sarcasm) from grade-level materials.
18. Tell jokes and can explain why they are funny.
19. Demonstrate full conversational competence by appropriately: initiating and closing conversations; maintaining topic; turn taking; maintaining eye contact; using gestures and facial expressions.

(see Chapter 3). The goals included in these tables should not be considered the definitive set of goals for all children at this stage, neither should they be considered an exhaustive list of possible audition goals for the child with hearing loss at the advanced communicator stage of language development. Goals must address the specific errors and needs determined during comprehensive assessment as well as from observation and informal diagnostic work.

How Do We Work on These Goals?

Professionals must have a knowledge base and multiple appropriate strategies (see Tables 11–7 and 11–8) applicable to the child using advanced language. The knowledge and strategies included in these tables are the basis for you to guide and coach the parent. The parent remains an important person to continue to support their child's listening and spoken language development.

To promote the child's advanced language abilities, you and the parent will: talk to support conversational norms; support listening in difficult acoustic situations; facilitate advanced strategies for communication breakdowns; foster advanced, age- and/or grade-appropriate vocabulary development and multiple meanings; and foster the child's use of flexibility of language using figurative and nonliteral language.

As always, the professional is guiding and coaching the parent and the child is an active participant in the sessions. At this stage, it is likely that therapy will not be on a regular schedule such as weekly sessions, but on a schedule determined by the parent, child, and professional. Additionally, we find that other team members need to understand that advanced skills are important in the continued development of communication and that therapy does not stop at the level of competent communicator (Chapter 10).

The parents will be learning strategies and implementing them in therapy sessions. Support parents to use strategies (see Table 11–8) that will advance the child's language abilities. The parent who worked through the various stages of listening and spoken language is an effective language facilitator for their child and is using many different strategies consistently. Continue to support and celebrate the success of the child and parent. You will introduce the parents to some new strategies and support the carryover into natural daily interactions. You will help parents to understand knowledge related to the next skills in listening and spoken language for the advanced communicator. This parent has become the professional!

Knowledge areas and strategies applicable to the child at the advanced communicator stage are identified in Tables 11–7 and 11–8.

Table 11–7. Knowledge Areas in the Advanced Communicator Stage

- Hearing technologies being used
- Effective troubleshooting of technology
- Speech acoustics related to mastery of speech development
- Ling six sounds
- Sequence of development of speech phonemes
- Stages of development of complex receptive language
- Stages of development of complex expressive language
- Reading and fostering emerging foundations in literacy

Table 11–8. Optimal Strategies to Implement in the Advanced Communicator Stage

- Chocolate chip cookie theory
- Activities of daily living
- Conversations
- Vocabulary enrichment
- Pre-teaching vocabulary for new experiences and academic areas
- Teaching expanded understanding of jokes and puns
- Modeling use of everyday idioms
- Modeling and eliciting advanced clarification strategies
- Teaching the unknown connected to the known
- Expanding world knowledge and the related vocabulary from Tiers 2 and 3
- Eliciting multiple events from stories and multistep instructions from personal experiences
- Eliciting discourse and complex conversations
- Theory of Mind: more advanced concepts, empathy, and conversational competence
- Discussions about difficult listening situations
- Continuing discussions about social cues

Additional suggested activities for you to use and to guide and coach the parents are included in Table 11–9. Life skills (Chapter 10, Table 10–10) continue to provide opportunities to foster advanced listening and spoken language mastery.

Table 11–9. Guide and Coach Parents To:

Implement optimal strategies for advanced communication stage (Table 11–8)

Listen! Talk, talk, talk!
- Discuss current events.
- Help expand their child's interests: hobbies, crafts, sports.
- Use jokes and puns.
- Use idioms.
- Discuss social cues.
- Encourage their child to express opinions but understand other viewpoints.
- Use higher-level Bloom's taxonomy levels to encourage critical thinking.

Play, play, play!
- Play advanced games and discuss rules and strategies.

In real life
- Help their child master life skills (Table 10–10) at appropriate age and cognitive levels.
- Engage in activities requiring executive function.
- Involve the child in planning and organizing activities and events (e.g., Plan for their first sleepover away from home. Discuss and plan an outing or family vacation. Plan for a team get-together).
- Encourage the child to discuss options and make choices.
- Have the child express their opinions.

Read
- Continue to read aloud to the child to support more advanced language and higher-order thinking skills.

Theory of Mind
- Discuss good sportsmanship and being gracious whether they win or lose.
- Talk about what somebody else might think (e.g., consider what might be a good activity to plan with a friend; how to approach a friend who doesn't want to do the same activities as they do; ways to be kind or thoughtful to other people; how to write a thank-you note for a gift they don't like).

Sources: Compiled from ASHA https://www.asha.org/public/speech/development/01/; http://www.hanen.org/helpful-info/articles/tuning-in-to-others-how-young-children-develop.aspx; Hearing First Theory of Mind handout

Targeting and Incorporating Goals

Auditory Attention, Selection, Memory, Discrimination, Auditory Recognition, Sequencing, and Comprehension
(Tables 11–3 and 11–5)

Auditory Retrieval and Expressive Communication
(Tables 11–4 and 11–6)

At this stage, any activity will involve multiple aspects of listening and spoken language development, and goals can easily be incorporated into what happens in the child's life. The activities and areas to help target the selected goals are all examples of the cookie dough theory. Skills are integrated, not isolated.

Activities of Daily Living (ADL) and Life Skills

The child's age, interests, and grade level will guide the complexity of different experiences at home, which can become the focus of a therapy session. Planning and decision making involve executive function and will incorporate listening and spoken language skills. It can be a more routine type of experience such as grocery shopping or more unique such as planning a family outing or vacation.

Encourage the parent to use the experience of food shopping to expand listening and spoken language and target the child's selected goals. In the grocery store or an open-air market, the parent and child are learning to use strategies for an acoustically challenging environment where they are using daily life language. They will discuss where items are and what is on the list, and they will stumble upon new vocabulary and multiple meanings. Encourage the parent to find and use teaching and learning opportunities. As they select a spice, they can discuss that they will season their food when preparing the meal. However, we do not mean a season such as winter, spring, summer, or fall. Though it is hot in the summer, sometimes our food is hot. It might mean that it is seasoned and spicy, or hot as in temperature and we need the food to cool down before we eat it. This is an easy place to discuss that *hot* has multiple meanings and uses in expressions. It can mean spicy; a high temperature; the latest popular item; a very attractive person; when we are keen on an idea; or when we say that a person runs "hot and cold." Play with that language. Find a joke; for example, "Which is faster: hot or cold? Hot; you can catch cold."

Guide the parent to involve the child in planning a complex event, for example, when the family is planning a birthday party. Have the parent consider how the child can be involved in appropriate aspects of the planning and implementation of the celebration. They can begin with deciding when to schedule the party by consulting the calendar. Deciding on the location and the guest list could be a family conversation. All of these elements can involve discussions with many factors in the decision-making process. The child will listen and participate in these group conversations. Much of this vocabulary will be familiar, but there will be new vocabulary as well. The successful party needs a budget and maybe a theme, a menu, activities, and party favors. Invitations can be emailed or made or bought, stuffed and sealed in the envelope, and then stamped in the top right corner before being deposited in the mailbox or brought to the post office. Somebody will need to be responsible for keeping track of the RSVPs as the guests respond.

The new school year requires plans that involve the entire family. This is part of the annual cycle and could change the daily routines in the household. Executive functions are employed as discussions address shopping for school clothes or uniforms, supplies, transportation options to and from school, the schedule for morning routines, making a sack lunch, and the weekly schedule coordinated with other extracurricular activities. Do not forget times: homework time, mealtime, social time, screen time, and bedtime.

Allowance, budgets, chores, meal menus, play dates, behavioral consequences and punishments, getting a pet, and sleepovers are all areas of family life that will require conversations involving multiple complex factors and considerations. Each of these topics lends itself to extensive conversations and probably negotiations. Life skills (see Table 10–10) can be explored for those that are appropriate to the child. You can encourage parent to incorporate skills as targeted in the child's listening and spoken language goals or model some in therapy sessions.

Natural and Complex Conversations

Children are members of the household and should be functioning cooperatively within it. That in and of itself allows for listening and language use in conversations, discussions, lectures, disputes, negotiations, conflict resolution, and disappointments. Theory of Mind (Peterson et al., 2012) and executive functions are part of these complex conversations.

When the child with hearing loss is preparing for their first sleepover with a friend, the conversation can be brought up in therapy. The parent, child, and professional can explore the elements that needs to be discussed. The parent can explain and discuss the rules or rituals involved in such a rite of passage. Conversations will be extensive and will likely address topics such as what to pack to be away from home overnight, drop-off and pick-up times, telling the other parents about their hearing loss, food allergies, having phone numbers for emergency contact, and how to take care of their technology. Discuss with the child and parent when to take off their technology so they do not miss the conversations when the lights are out. The child could consider how to explain to their peers their ability to follow a conversation in the dark, with or without technology, and other scenarios. Intervention sessions should seem more like natural interactions that are part of daily life and one of many possible social situations.

Daily interactions will continue to be challenged by the environment and the situations that require listening in a degraded signal. The child with hearing loss at this stage of language abilities has an intrinsic understanding of sentence structure and of language overall and is better able to fill in the missing information. These daily situations allow for modeling and opportunities to ask for clarification using an expanding repertoire of advanced strategies. These opportunities allow the parent and child to further explore strategies to enhance the auditory signal, including placement to best access the signal being presented and to foster independence while implementing assistive devices.

Various interests and hobbies continue to emerge as the child gets older. An interest in crafts will require learning the instructions. The child might give or follow instructions for a variety of crafts and projects such as making paper airplanes, origami, needlecraft, drawing, painting, or calligraphy. Hobbies vary based on the child's age, interests, and exposure. Regardless whether interest lies in sports, learning magic tricks, gardening, photography, musical instruments, technology, or woodworking, listening and language are inherent in the activity.

Playful and Figurative Language

Jokes, tongue twisters, puns, rhyming words, and "sounds like" words continue to be very applicable at this point for continuing the development of listening and spoken language. Continue to work on jokes, idioms, and playing with words to expand the child's communicative competence and language flexibility.

Younger children might enjoy *Amelia Bedelia* books (Parish, 1963), which use words with multiple meanings that lead to amusing misunderstandings. You could approach idioms, jokes and puns by a topic (e.g., animals or food) for the week. Elephant jokes could be one way to start. Look for different types of jokes where the humor is based on the double meaning of a word (e.g., "How do you get down from an elephant? You don't; you get down from a duck"). Other jokes use an obvious but silly response. The response is not what is implied by the wording of the joke and makes it amusing (e.g., "What time is it when an elephant sits on your fence? Time for a new fence"). The more typical response to "What time is it?" would be the time of the day. Phrasing of a sentence to make the meaning ambiguous is another form of joke. Then there is Groucho Marx's famous line about the elephant: "One morning I shot an elephant in my pajamas. How he got in my pajamas I'll never know" (*Animal Crackers*, 1930). You can continue from the *elephant* or *down* theme and transition to idioms, such as the expression "feeling sad or down." A related joke: When your feather pillow splits, you would feel down for a while.

Puns can be punny and funny. Find puns and resources to share. You can make puns and teach the expression, no pun intended. Then consider the pun, "I put ten jokes in a contest to insure one would win. But no pun in ten did!" (Koster, 2012; Tearablepuns.org).

Explore expressions that are not literal. When talking with the child who has been learning baseball, you can discuss the different ways we can use many baseball-related expressions to mean something different. Consider expressions such as *struck out, three strikes against you, not even in the ballpark, out of left field, throw a curve ball, touch base, on the ball,* and *hit a home run*. But they should know that you will not find a meal at the home plate, or that umpires are fat because they always clean their plate. Some additional examples were provided in the previous section on ADL. Refer back to figurative and playful language section in Chapter 10.

Do Not Stop Reading!

Read books with more complex stories and different genres of books. Children at this stage may be reading independently or not depending on their age. Continue reading aloud. Trelease in *The Read-Aloud Handbook* (2019) tells us that it is not until the 8th grade when a child's reading level catches up to their listening level. The implication for children with hearing loss is significant. They are able to understand a more advanced text that has more advanced language, vocabulary, and figurative language including idioms, similes, and metaphors. For younger children, there are many beginner chapter books. For older children, consider some of the classics and popular novels for young adults. Reading aloud will help to build comprehension as they learn to listen to longer, more complex language and enriching, new vocabulary. Books are a wonderful way to begin discussions about difficult topics. Reading aloud will support the parent-child bond while fostering more advanced literacy, a love for learning, and world knowledge. Find books to spark and expand the child's interests. Explore different genres such as sci-fi, fantasy, the classics, mysteries, historical novels, thrillers, mythology, and so many more.

And the Games Go On

Children will continue with and learn new physical activities, team sports, individual sports, or just games they play when they are hanging out with their peers or learning in school. All of these require the constant integration of listening and receptive and expressive language.

Board games, card games, word games, and pencil-and-paper games abound and are constantly emerging. Keep looking for new games that meet the child's interest; these can be effective to meet specific auditory intervention goals. We encourage the professional to continue using the old, tried-and-true games, but be on the lookout for the new ones. No sooner will this book be published than a game will be considered vintage and new games will be the newest hot item that is flying off the shelves. Refer back to Chapter 10 for more examples of activities.

Words! Words! Words!

Children with hearing loss will typically depend on some pre- and post-teaching for vocabulary related to their school academics and Tier 3 words. We must help them to develop additional vocabulary related to specific activities, interests, current events, and world knowledge. Vocabulary related to the Olympics might emerge on a 4-year cycle but might continue to be used in daily conversations between the global sporting event. The child might be inspired and develop a new interest in events that they watched, such as horseback riding or gymnastics.

Language is growing and changing like a living organism, and children with hearing loss will need to learn more words constantly from a variety of sources. The child with hearing loss could pick up slang words and obscenities from peers and siblings but might need to have these words taught to them directly. They will need to keep up with the world and new, emerging words, particularly related to social media and technology, which are changing at a rapid rate, if not daily. This is yet another reminder that flexibility in language use is a skill to be developed and reinforced for children with hearing loss. Keep in mind and discuss that words that have changed meaning over time; e.g., *ghost*, from a supernatural phenomenon to the ending of a personal relationship. The word *binge* was used in the negative connotation for eating too much, but we now use it for bingeing shows or podcasts. *Tap* used to be a type of dancing, what you did with a cane, or movement with your fingers, but now it is how you pay with a credit card. During the coronavirus pandemic of 2020, some of the words Merriam-Webster (2020) added were: *self-isolate, contactless, physical distancing, work from home (WFH), iatrophobia,* and *intensivist.*

Putting It All Together: Case History

Isabel failed her newborn hearing screening and underwent multiple auditory brainstem response (ABR) and otacoustic emission (OAE) tests with varying results. One ABR indicated hearing loss and questionable auditory neuropathy. Additional sound booth testing indicated possible sensorineural hearing loss. She underwent an additional ABR at 12 months, which indicated a moderate hearing loss. At 14 months, she underwent bilateral tube placement but continued to have absent OAEs. She was identified with bilateral hearing loss at 14 months of age and aided binaurally at that time. Additional testing at 1 and a half years indicated bilateral moderate to severe hearing loss that appeared to be progressive. Genetic testing was suggested at that time to rule out syndromes. Testing indicated two known recessively inherited associated mutations in the Connexin 26 gene resulting in a nonsyndromic hearing loss. She showed little to no benefit from her hearing aids over the following months after being aided. School district provided services with the goal to promote the development of sign language, and Isabel attended a childcare program that supported signs.

Isabel was implanted in the right ear at 2 years 1 month and initially mapped at 2 years 2 months of age. After several months of cochlear implant (CI) use, the implant center suggested looking at therapy to help her use her CI and develop some listening skills. She had received speech therapy services from age 2 years 7 months to 3 years 11 months. Her mother reported her therapy focused exclusively on oral motor development and speech articulation, as the professional said her speech was unintelligible. Isabel made limited progress with her CI, per the implant center. Her mother changed service providers when Isabel was 3 years 11 months to be enrolled in auditory-verbal therapy (AVT). Isabel was implanted in the left ear and was initially stimulated at 5 years old.

Isabel is easily engaged and tries hard in sessions. She responds well to praise, modeling, and clear expectations. Mother continues to learn auditory-verbal (AV) strategies and implements them immediately. Progress has been noted consistently since she began AVT on a weekly basis. The mother reports good progress at home as well. This is supported by Isabel's testing completed at 5 years 4 months, which showed excellent progress in the development of language.

Auditory Processes for Using Sound Meaningfully

Auditory Discrimination and Identification

Isabel has been using her left CI only for activities in therapy and at home. Her discrimination abilities for words with her left CI only is below average as assessed using the Test of Auditory Processing Skills–3 (TAPS-3) (2005) (see Table 11–10). Error patterns noted were primarily for voicing, /r/, r-colored vowels, and word-final consonants.

She is demonstrating improved closed-set and bridge-set speech discrimination for familiar predictable language with her new CI. Isabel is developing some open-set discrimination skills with her left CI, but she still requires repetitions of language to understand all the key words and will miss the low-intensity grammatical markers.

Speech tracking was completed with a simple storybook, through audition alone with age-appropriate language, in quiet using a section of text of approximately 100 words. No repetitions were provided and words were scored as correct only if they were accurate. She scored 59% of words correct using her left CI only. She scored 97% correct in the binaural condition, which is an indication of her right CI abilities.

Auditory Memory and Comprehension

TAPS-3 (2005) is normed for ages 4 years through 18 years 11 months. The subtests for auditory memory and auditory cohesion were administered to determine her auditory skills in these areas. Testing was completed in the binaural condition, except for the word discrimination subtest, which was completed with her left CI only. Overall, her scaled scores and percentile scores indicate that she is showing abilities in the average range, with the exception of auditory reasoning and word discrimination, which are both below average. Both her mother and this professional felt that her performance on the word discrimination subtest was poorer than expected and that she was guessing or not attending at times. However, when completing an analysis of her errors, the results were indicative of specific error patterns, as mentioned earlier. It is possible that this score is slightly depressed. Table 11–10 indicates her scores for the subtests.

In therapy sessions, it has been noted that her auditory memory is currently affecting her ability to follow more complex instructions and to retain increasing

Table 11–10. Test of Auditory Processing Skills-3 (TAPS-3) Scores

Subtest	Raw Score	Scaled Score	Percentile	Age Equivalent
Word Discrimination LEFT CI only	19	5	5	<3 y 6 m
Auditory Memory				
Number Memory Forward	13	10	50	6 y
Number Memory Reversed	6	10	50	6 y
Word Memory	11	8	25	4 y 6 m
Sentence Memory	12	7	16	4 y 2 m
Auditory Cohesion				
Auditory Comprehension	20	13	84	8 y 4 m
Auditory Reasoning	1	6	9	3 y 6 m

amounts of information. In addition, it was noted that her lowest score was in the area of auditory reasoning. This subtest looks at inferences and idioms. Her raw score on this was 1, indicating difficulty with the easier items at the beginning of the subtest.

Auditory Processes for Learning Language

Auditory Comprehension and Auditory Retrieval

Isabel's comprehension and expressive language skills were assessed at the age of 5 years 4 months, using evaluations previously administered. At that time, she was demonstrating progress in comprehension and expressive abilities with progress of more than the time interval between evaluations. Growth of 1 year in the scores should be seen in an equivalent period of time as a measure of appropriate development. The Clinical Evaluation of Language Fundamentals—Preschool, Version 2 (CELF-P 2) (2020) and the Test for Auditory Comprehension of Language–3 (TACL-3) (2011) were administered at that time. These tests were previously administered and the scores over time are indicated in Tables 11–11 to 11–13.

At this administration, it was not possible to obtain a standardized score for the basic concepts subtest, as it is only scaled up to age 5 years. However, the subtest was administered as her score in the previous administration was low and the professional and mother determined that it was appropriate to check for growth over time. This subtest was not readministered at subsequent test intervals.

The TACL-3 (2011) was administered to look at the specific receptive skills that it assesses (i.e., vocabulary, grammatical morphemes, elaborated sentences). This is a test of comprehension of a variety of grammatical structures and morphemes that is normed on hearing children.

Analysis of the errors indicates excellent growth and development in all the areas assessed in the evaluation and at this time there are no indications of gaps in the sequence of development. Isabel's score in the area of elaborated sentences is the lowest score at this time but shows an improvement in the standard score from a 7 to a 9 and 1 year of growth in age equivalent score in a 7-month interval. Grammatical morphemes are an area where Isabel had very poor abilities historically and has continued to make improvements. At this time, Isabel has a score within normal limits and an increase in her standard score from 11 to 12, with a growth of 6 months in 7 months' time. Errors were noted with derivational suffixes and noun-verb agreement.

Isabel continues to show excellent improvement in her expressive use of grammatically complete sentences in spontaneous discourse. In the past few months, her language errors have improved and she is beginning to self-correct when she does make a mistake. Her errors are most typically noticed with word order in questions. The following are typical examples of her spontaneous language.

I want to do it.

Who is this for?

Try to run me over.

I watered the beans and they're growing.

Why can't I go to Sky High today?

Dad, why don't you have a shirt on?

Table 11–11. CELF Preschool 2 Scores by Subtest

CELF Preschool 2 Scores			
Chronological Age:	4 years 9 months	5 years 4 months	Change in 7-month interval
Sentence Structure			
Scaled Score	10	12	
Age Equivalent	4 y 8 m	5 y 9 m	+1 y 1 m
Word Structure			
Scaled Score	8	8	
Age Equivalent	3 y 11 m	4 y 5 m	+6 m
Expressive Vocabulary			
Scaled Score	8	8	
Age Equivalent	3 y 9 m	4 y 5 m	+8 m
Concepts and Following Directions			
Scaled Score	8	6	
Age Equivalent	3 y 11 m	3 y 11 m	No change
Recalling Sentences			
Scaled Score	5	8	
Age Equivalent	3 y 2 m	4 y 5 m	+1 y 3 m
Basic Concepts			
Scaled Score	6	n/a	
Age Equivalent	3 y 7 m	> 5 y	Over 1 y 5 m
Word Classes—Receptive			
Scaled Score	10	13	
Age Equivalent	4 y 8 m	6 y 9 m	+ 2 y 1 m
Word Classes—Expressive			
Scaled Score	13	12	
Age Equivalent	5 y 6 m	6 y 1 m	+ 7 m
Word Classes—Total			
Scaled Score	11	12	
Age Equivalent	4 y 4 m	> 7 y	Over 2 y 8 m

Table 11–12. CELF Preschool Scores

CELF Preschool Core Language Scores and Indexes				
Chronological Age:	4 years 9 months		5 years 4 months	
	Standard Score	Percentile	Standard Score	Percentile
Core Language	92	30	96	39
Receptive Language	88	21	102	55
Expressive Language	83	13	89	23
Language Content	85	16	91	27
Language Structure	86	16	96	39

Table 11–13. TACL-3 Scores

TACL-3 Age-Equivalent Test Scores: Subtests			
Chronological Age:	4 years 9 months	5 years 4 months	Change in 7-month interval
Vocabulary			
Standard Score	9	14	
Age Equivalent	4 y 3 m	6 y 6 m	+2 y 3 m
Grammatical Morphemes			
Standard Score	11	12	
Age Equivalent	5 y 3 m	5 y 9 m	+6 m
Elaborated Phrases and Sentences			
Standard Score	7	9	
Age Equivalent	4 y	5 y	+1 y
Total Language (Quotient)			
Standard Score	94	111	
Age Equivalent	4 y 6 m	5 y 11 m	+1 y 5 m

I didn't want to go to the pool today since it isn't sunny.

Dad, what are you doing today?

That's not fair because I really want to go to Sky High.

I'm not going to the beach today.

I want to go to my cousins' house after school.

I'm not going to Sylvia's house today.

I want a peanut butter sandwich.

Is Johnny having a chocolate and peanut butter sandwich?

She is able to use a variety of verb tenses, conjunctions, articles, pronouns, plurals, possessives, negatives, copula/auxiliary verbs, and question forms. She will use these structures with some errors and is typically able to correct them when requested. As she began to use question forms, more often she would ask, "Why I cannot go to the pool today?" or "Dad, why you don't have a shirt on?" At this time, she is able to consistently correct when prompted, without a model, but she does not yet self-correct and self-monitor more than about 60% of grammatical errors. These are more advanced stages of auditory skill development, which are being targeted currently in therapy sessions and at home.

Summary

Isabel has shown excellent progress over the past year in the development of her auditory abilities, which is reflected in improvement in the areas of speech and language skills as measured by informal and standardized assessments. Isabel has made good progress in the development of auditory skills with her left CI. At this time, it is not at the level of her right CI, nor at consistent speech perception levels or phonetic levels for a variety of speech features. Speech perception is about 60% for sentences.

It is recommended that she continue in auditory-verbal therapy to facilitate her auditory abilities in her left ear. AVT should also facilitate the development of the more difficult auditory skills with her right CI and binaurally, and language structures that have not yet developed consistently and more advanced language such as multiple meanings, inferences, and idioms. The goal is to facilitate and maintain age-appropriate auditory, speech, and language abilities.

Progress Over Time With Intervention

Intervention focused on the areas of need. Testing was done at appropriate intervals. The following tables show Isabel's continued growth in the areas targeted by this complete assessment. Testing results are indicated at 6 years 6 months (Tables 11–14 to 11–16), 7 years 9 months (Table 11–17), and 9 years 9 months.

Auditory Memory and Comprehension

The TAPS-3 (2005) is normed for ages 4 years through 18 years 11 months. The subtests for auditory memory and auditory cohesion were administered to determine Isabel's auditory skills in these areas. Testing was completed in the binaural condition for all subtests (Table 11–18).

The Test of Language Development—Primary (TOLD-P:3) (2008) is a test of expressive and receptive spoken language development and was administered at this time. This test is normed on hearing and typically developing children. The subtests are: Picture Vocabulary; Relational Vocabulary; Oral Vocabulary; Grammatical Understanding; Sentence Imitation; Grammatical Completion; Word Discrimination; Phonemic Analysis; and Word Articulation. Phonemic Analysis was not administered at this time. The administration of this test was completed over two sessions. This test was not previously administered. Isabel's scores are indicated in Table 11–19.

Table 11–14. CELF Preschool 2 Scores by Subtests at 6 Years 6 Months

Chronological Age: 6 years 6 months		Change in AE: 14 Months
Sentence Structure		
Scaled Score	12	
Age Equivalent	> 7 y	+ >1 y 3 m
Word Structure		
Scaled Score	11	
Age Equivalent	>7 y	+ >2 y 7 m
Expressive Vocabulary		
Scaled Score	8	
Age Equivalent	5 y 3 m	+10 m
Concepts and Following Directions		
Scaled Score	9	
Age Equivalent	6 y 3 m	+2 y 4 m
Recalling Sentences		
Scaled Score	8	
Age Equivalent	5 y 3 m	+10 m
Word Classes—Receptive		
Scaled Score	10	
Age Equivalent	6 y 9 m	approaching ceiling
Word Classes—Expressive		
Scaled Score	12	
Age Equivalent	6 y 11m	approaching ceiling
Word Classes—Total		
Scaled Score	11	
Age Equivalent	> 7 y	approaching ceiling

Table 11–15. TACL-3: Age-Equivalent Test Scores at 6 Years 6 Months

Chronological Age: 6 years 6 months		Change in AE: 14 months
Vocabulary		
Scaled Score	14	
Age Equivalent	8 y 6 m	+2 y
Grammatical Morphemes		
Scaled Score	11	
Age Equivalent	6 y 9 m	+1 yr
Elaborated Phrases and Sentences		
Scaled Score	9	
Age Equivalent	6 y 3 m	+1 yr 3 m

Table 11–16. Test of Auditory Processing Skills-3 (TAPS-3) Scores at 6 Years 6 Months

TAPS-3 Scores Subtest	Raw Score	Scaled Score	Percentile	Age Equivalent	Change in 1 Year
Word Discrimination—Both Cochlear Implants	30	10	50	7 y 6 m	+ > 4 yr
Auditory Memory					
Number Memory Forward	14	9	37	6 y 6 m	+6 m
Number Memory Reversed	9	11	63	8 y 2 m	+2 y 2 m
Word Memory	12	7	16	5 y	+6 m
Sentence Memory	13	6	9	4 y 6 m	+4 m
Auditory Cohesion					
Auditory Comprehension	21	12	75	8 y 10 m	+6 m
Auditory Reasoning	4	9	37	6 y	+2 y 6 m

Table 11–17. TACL-3: Age-Equivalent Test Scores at 7 Years 9 Months

Subtest	6 years 6 months Standard Score Age Equivalent (AE)	7 years 8 months Standard Score Age Equivalent (AE)	Change in AE Score Over 14-Month Interval
Vocabulary	14 8 y 6 m	9 7 y	–1 y 6 m
Grammatical Morphemes	11 6 y 9 m	11 8 y	+1 yr 3 m
Elaborated Phrases and Sentences	9 6 y 3 m	10 7 y	+9 m

Table 11–18. Test of Auditory Processing Skills-3 (TAPS-3) at 7 Years 9 Months

Subtest	Raw Score	Scaled Score (Previous Year)	Age Equivalent (Change Over 10 Months)	Percentile
Auditory Memory				
Number Memory Forward	18	11 (9)	10 y 3 m (+3 y 9 m)	63
Number Memory Reversed	11	12 (11)	10 y 1 m (+1 y 11 m)	75
Word Memory	16	10 (7)	7 y 7 m (+2 y 7 m)	50
Sentence Memory	19	9 (6)	7 y (+2 y 6 m)	37
Auditory Cohesion				
Auditory Comprehension	24	12 (12)	10 y 6 m (+1 y 8 m)	75
Auditory Reasoning	9	10 (10)	8 y 3 m (+2 y 3 m)	50

Table 11–19. Test of Language Development—Primary (TOLD-P:3) Scores at 7 Years 9 Months

Subtest	Raw Score	Standard Score	Percentile	Age Equivalent
Picture Vocabulary	15	8	25	6 y 6 m
Relational Vocabulary	15	9	37	7 y 6 m
Oral Vocabulary	17	11	63	8 y 6 m
Grammatical Understanding	23	12	75	8 y 9 m
Sentence Imitation	11	7	16	5 y 6 m
Grammatical Completion	19	13	84	9 y 3 m
Word Discrimination	25	10	50	7 y 6 m
Word Articulation	20	11	63	8 y 6 m

Chronological Age: 9 years 9 months. The TAPS-3 (2005) was readministered at this time to monitor her progress and growth over 1 year interval between test administrations. Her scores are indicated in Table 11–20.

The Test of Language Development—Intermediate (TOLD-I:4) (2019) is a test of expressive and receptive spoken language development and was administered at this time. This test is normed on hearing and typically developing children. The subtests are the following: Sentence Combining; Picture Vocabulary; Word Ordering; Relational Vocabulary; Morphological Comprehension; and Multiple Meanings. This test was not previously administered. Isabel's scores are indicated in Table 11–21.

The Intervention Session

Sessions at this stage of listening and language development are very conversational, with the child as a very active participant in their learning. The session begins with the parent raising issues regarding degraded signal and conversations about possible strategies. In sessions at this stage, it is not unusual to troubleshoot the more advanced goals and sometimes provide new strategies to try at home, as discussed regarding the volume of the TV. Notice the flow of the session moves to incorporate the goals addressing idioms and literal and figurative language

Mother: This school year, she is doing learning through the computer or tablet at school and at home. So how good an indicator are those online tests for checking her comprehension? So, for instance, she takes a test on a book she's read.

Isabel: Yeah, there are tests on books that I read. But I read it.

Mother: I am wondering if when she takes a test on a book she listened to and if she gets a 10 out of 10, does that mean she really got it all?

Table 11–20. Test of Auditory Processing Skills-3 (TAPS-3) Scores at 9 Years 9 Months

Subtest	Raw Score	Scaled Score (Previous Year)	Age Equivalent (Change Over 1 Year)	Percentile
Auditory Memory				
Number Memory Forward	20	11 (10)	13 y (+3 y 10 m)	63 (50)
Number Memory Reversed	13	12 (13)	13 y (no change)	75 (84)
Word Memory	21	8 (13)	15 y (no change)	25 (84)
Sentence Memory	18	6 (5)	6 y 6 m (+1 y 6 m)	9 (5)
Auditory Cohesion				
Auditory Comprehension	24	10 (10)	10 y 6 m (+ 1 y 4 m)	50 (50)
Auditory Reasoning	14	11 (11)	10 y 3 m (+ 9 m)	63 (63)

Table 11–21. Test of Language Development—Intermediate (TOLD-I:4) Scores at 9 Years 9 Months

Subtest	Raw Score	Age Equivalent	Percentile	Standard Score
Sentence Combining	6	<8 y	5	5
Picture Vocabulary	43	9 y 3 m	37	9
Word Ordering	15	9 y	37	9
Relational Vocabulary	14	9 y	37	9
Morphological Comprehension	15	8 y 3 m	25	8
Multiple Meanings	34	16 y 9 m	91	14

Isabel: Yeah, mom! That means "she got it all" (showing air quotes).

(Professional laughs)

Mother: I know that means you got the whole concept of the story. But is that a good indicator that she is hearing everything or do I need to go a little bit more in depth and into specifics of hearing?

Professional: When you are doing work on the computer, is it stuff you need to listen to and follow instructions or is it already there?

Isabel: Some of both.

Professional: And how much of that can you understand and hear? How much do think you are hearing?

Isabel: I can hear everything. I have some assignments that are just written but we have Zoom sessions where the teacher talks and the other kids are also talking. But they have to wait until it is their turn. The teacher makes sure we aren't talking at the same time or interrupting each other.

Mother: I'm not always sure, that's why I want to talk about this a bit for some ideas on how to figure that out.

Isabel: But I can hear it all.

Professional: Your mother isn't entirely sure of that. You know what we have told you about you don't know . . .

Isabel: Yeah, what I didn't hear—but I hear enough to understand what is going on and pass the tests. So, I must be hearing it all. Right?

Mother: We just want to be sure you are getting all of what you need to hear.

Professional: What if you don't always hear the *t* sound clearly or at the end of the word? You might misperceive the difference between *can* and *can't*. That is a very subtle difference in hearing but it completely changes the meaning of the sentence. Or if it's a new word and you aren't hearing one of the sounds correctly? Then you will think the word is different from what it actually is.

Isabel: So how do we know?

Mother: But what can we do? I know the audiologist does some testing like that.

Professional: Well, you could try doing some things to see how much she hears at different levels. (Turning to the Isabel) You OK with that? Like an experiment?

Isabel: So how do we prove that?

Professional: We can do it now but it is probably better for you to do it at home with your own tablet or TV or computer and whatever you use. You should be using some more advanced language level, open set language, and see how much you hear with the degraded signals and how much you are getting at different volumes. You could listen to part of the news or try to listen to a podcast on an unfamiliar topic. You're trying to figure out how much of the signal you are getting and if you are missing some through the TV, the computer, the phone—all these different ways that you are having to learn to listen and learn from your listening right now. Because there's a fine line sometimes between what seems like the right volume and what is the best functional volume for you to be listening at.

Mother: But she is convinced she hears it all but I want to be sure.

Professional: So, when you do that sort of listening, do you adjust the volume as you are listening by yourself?

Isabel: Yeah, my tablet is set at a volume that I can hear and I don't adjust it. The TV I change when I go to watch it if somebody else had been watching.

Professional: OK, so when you adjust the volume, do you need to raise it or lower it?

Mother: She is always making it louder.

Isabel: No, not really.

Mother: Actually, I think you always do with the TV unless the captions are on and then sometimes you don't bother. I think you play the TV pretty loudly.

Isabel: Not always.

Mother: Yes, sometimes I can hear it from upstairs!

Isabel: It's not that loud!

Mother: No, actually, it is and you need to acknowledge that. You need to be aware of those around you. And you don't always know if something is loud. You have a hearing loss, so things that sound loud to your sister or me don't necessarily sound loud to you.

Isabel: I know, but—

Professional: OK, she says she hears it from upstairs.

Isabel: But it isn't that loud.

Professional: OK, so we have a difference of opinion. So how do we figure that out to see how much you are getting different volumes? Sometimes in fact making it louder doesn't make it easier. The thought is that making it louder will help you hear it better but sometimes it doesn't and it actually makes it a bit distorted or less clear. We want to aim for clear and realize that isn't always louder. So how does it sound to you?

Isabel: Kind of medium. It's good. I can be listening OK and understanding.

Professional: OK, you've got it set at what seems like a good volume for you. Let's ask your mom what she thinks about the volume—if it seems loud or a reasonable volume?

Mother: I can understand it all and it seems clear, but I think it is a bit louder than I would have it set at.

Professional: OK—you feel it is a bit loud. But Isabel, you feel it is "kinda medium."

Isabel: Yeah, it's good.

Professional: So, we can do the experiment. First you will listen at the volume you think is good. Your mom will find something for you to listen to and then you repeat what you hear so we know how many of the words you are getting or what sounds you are missing. Then let's ask your mom to adjust the volume to a level that she thinks is comfortable and see how you do with that. Don't listen to the exact same sentences. So, you will listen at two levels and try to get a sense of if one is easier or not. You could also try at an even quieter volume to see how you do. Do you want to try it here or at home?

Mother: I think we could do that easily enough. What do you think?

Isabel: Yeah, OK.

Professional: I would suggest that you start by adjusting the volume to what you think is comfortable. Sounds like a plan!

Mother: So, when we started talking about listening at different volumes, I said, "There is a fine line sometimes between what the volume is that you think you should listen at and what you hear best at." What does that mean . . . there's a fine line?

Isabel: I don't know, I'm confused.

Professional: I think your mom had an idea to explain it to you.

Mother: So, let's use an analogy. You have been talking about analogies in literature at school. What if I draw a line between two items with a pencil or with a Sharpie—which one do you think would be easier to see, know is there . . . and kinda cross? If we were little people moving along here.

Isabel: The pencil line.

Mother: The pencil! So, the fine line is very fine, fragile, and delicate. It's really hard to tell which side is which because it isn't clear or easy to know. That is different from when people call something a hard line. It's like there. You know it is there. You know that clearly you can't go past that point.

Isabel: Umhum.

Professional: So that what she means by it's a fine line between what you think you can hear and what we know you can hear.

Isabel: I have a question.

Professional: OK . . .

Isabel: When I'm on YouTube and I can't always hear what they are saying, I put on the captions and I can follow it. So, I am understanding it.

Mother: Exactly my concern. But you don't have captions for the work from school. So, we need to prepare you for this. We will also reach out to the school to get your DM system.

Isabel: Sometimes it is too loud and I don't get it.

Mother: So that's what we are saying. We need to play around with this.

Professional: Play around? Play around. What? (Looking at Isabel) What does she mean?

Isabel: I don't know.

Mother: Practice, like fiddle around, get it right.

Isabel: Oooh.

Professional: You adjust it, you check it out. Doesn't mean you are playing like you are playing with a ball or a game. Right? And it doesn't mean that somebody is playing a fiddle.

Isabel: Mhmmm.

Professional: So, let me ask you a question. Do you prefer watching YouTube or TV with the captions or just listening and trying to understand? What's your preference?

Isabel: I have no clue what you just said. Can you repeat that?

Professional: Well, what did you understand about what I said, so that I don't have to repeat all of it?

Mother: What part did you get?

Isabel: I didn't understand any of it.

Mother: Well, did you catch any of the words?

Isabel: Something about watching TV.

Mother: Great, so you could say, "What were you saying about the TV?" Then we know you understood that part.

Professional: So, do you prefer to have the captions on when you watch TV?

Isabel: Somehow, I read the captions and listen and watch. I just watch it and I see the captions and I also see and read it and mostly I listen. But sometimes they make mistakes.

Mother: That is why we are asking the question. Do you prefer the captions being on or off?

Isabel: I prefer the captions being on.

Mother: OK, that is what we wanted to know.

Professional: OK. Good to know about the captions. Makes it easier and you know you're not missing anything. Do you notice sometimes you didn't catch something and then the caption helps?

Isabel: Of course, sometimes. But sometimes they make mistakes or misspell stuff.

Mother: I think that is what happens with captioning. Sometimes it's funny what the captions say when the captioners get it wrong. Sometimes we laugh when they get it wrong.

Professional: But you know what I think is fabulous? That you just said that sometimes you are reading it and notice the spelling mistakes.

Isabel: Yeah, I do! And sometimes they use the wrong word.

Professional: That is pretty impressive that you can tell when they made a spelling mistake.

Isabel: Sometimes the wrong word! And it is silly or doesn't make sense.

Mother: Or the thing that always cracks me up. Sometimes when I am watching a movie and there is music and they type, "dramatic music playing."

(Professional and Isabel both laugh)

Mother: Or they say, "heavy breathing."

Professional: Hold your horses. I don't see any cracks on your mom!

(Isabel chuckles)

Professional: Are you cracked? You just said it cracks you up? (Turning to Isabel) Is your mom full of cracks? She just said she cracks up. Is she broken? Does she need some glue?

Mother: I don't have any horses.

Professional: Hmmm. One expression at a time.

Isabel: Well, do you think I might have broken her back by stepping on those cracks in the sidewalks when I was a little kid?

Mother: No, I was fine!

(Everyone laughs a bit)

Professional: So, what does that mean when she said it cracks her up?

Isabel: She meant like it makes her laugh.

Professional: Yeah, that's the expression. It made her laugh, cracks her up. So, it's very interesting. We've talked about this lots of times before. That sometimes words mean more than one thing and sometimes expressions mean something different than the words seem to indicate. They aren't literal. Like "hold your horses." She doesn't have horses...just want her to slow down. Do you remember what we call those kinds of expressions?

(Isabel shrugs her shoulders)

Professional: Actually . . . I don't know if you can remember . . . if you never knew. Do you know what they are called?

Isabel: Is this for science stuff?

Mother: No, this is language. I don't know if you know this. Have you talked about expressions at school?

Isabel: You mean like figures of speech?

Professional: Yes, figures of speech or idioms.

Mother: I think maybe you know the word *idioms* from school.

Isabel: Yeah, I think so. Sounds familiar but I couldn't recall it.

Professional: So, I was thinking about a bunch of different idioms that have animals in them. Can we try a few? I think you might know some of them. I'm sure your mother uses some of them and they are easy.

Isabel: Sure.

Professional: So, if you can't sit still, what might someone say? Can you think of an expression with an animal?

Isabel: Hmmm. Can't think of one.

Professional: I'll give you a hint. Something in your pants . . .

Isabel: Oh, yeah, ants in your pants.

Professional: Can either of you think of one?

Isabel: I know one for when you eat too much. You pig out.

Mother: Yeah, good thinking. I think you know one, for when it is raining hard . . . with two animals.

Isabel: Raining cats and dogs!

Professional: Do you know how you know when it is raining cats and dogs?

Isabel: When it is raining really hard.

Professional: Right—that's what the expression means . . . but this is a joke. How do you know it's raining cats and dogs?

(Isabel shrugs)

Mother: I give up. (Turning to Isabel) Remember? That's what we say to somebody when we don't know the punchline. Then they can deliver it.

Professional: When you step in a poodle!

Mother: Ha! (Turning to Isabel) Do you get that?

Professional: Do you think that is funny?

Isabel: No, because there aren't really dogs.

Mother: Right. It is an expression, an idiom. There aren't literally cats and dogs falling from the sky. So, you don't get it?

Isabel: No. I don't.

Mother: What is funny about stepping in a poodle? Do you step in a poodle?

Isabel: No, you step in a puddle.

Professional: Yeah, but the punchline is "I step in a poodle."

Mother: Puddle. Poodle. Puddle. Get it?

Isabel: Ohh, oh oh!! Now I get it!

Mother: Great. So, why is that funny? So, explain it.

Isabel: Because you step in a puddle when it has been raining. It's a joke cuz poodle and puddle sort of sound the same.

Professional: Yeah, so what?

Isabel: And you say "raining cats and dogs" and poodle is a type of dog.

Professional: Yes!! Would it be funny if I said I stepped in a golden retriever? That's a dog.

Isabel: No, that is a real dog and not funny since it just doesn't make sense. It isn't really dogs falling from the sky. Just fooling around with how the words sound.

Analysis of Session

In discussion of the therapy session, we can analyze which goals are addressed in the described interval of therapy. The goals are indicated by number and refer back to goals indicated in Tables 11–3 to 11–6. Initial conversation in the session addresses issues of degraded signals and how to support the comprehension in such situations (Goals 2, 7, 13). In that conversation, an idiom is used and then the discussion moves to addressing idioms and literal and figurative language (Goals 9, 10, 15, 16). When the child misses an explanation, the professional and mother work to elicit and model more advanced clarification strategies (Goals 8, 14). Addressing new vocabulary or clarification of vocabulary by discussing the definition of *idiom* is incorporated into discussion of idioms, figurative language, and jokes (Goals 1, 3, 6, 9, 10, 11, 12, 15, 16, 17).

Summary

The professional considers the knowledge base, guides and coaches the parent, and teaches strategies to promote further development at this stage of communication. At this stage, the child should be involved and taking responsibility for their own learning and continued acquisition of advanced abilities in listening and spoken language. The use of natural conversations, interactions, and experiences will help the child to achieve all or most of the skills as outlined in Tables 11–1 and 11–2 and the outlined goals from this stage of language development in Tables 11–3 through 11–6. Development of the targeted skills in daily life routines and interactions will ensure that the skills are used across all the child's environments, including difficult listening situations. The incorporation of goals in a variety of settings prevents development of isolated or splinter skills resulting in generalization. The achievement of these goals will provide a strong basis for the child with hearing loss to become literate and to succeed in advanced academic situations. Behaviors that are indicative of the child achieving the advanced language skills are indicated in Table 11–22.

Table 11–22. By the End of the Advanced Communicator Stage, the Child Should:

> Use listening and spoken language comparable to that of an adult.
>
> Learn new vocabulary regularly and with ease from both Tier 2 and 3 in academic and daily life settings.
>
> Be a competent conversationalist and have emerging skills for public oral presentations.
>
> Understand social language and cues including jokes, puns, idioms, sarcasm, and inferences.

Discussion Questions

1. How do you determine if a child is at this stage?
2. How would you illustrate the chocolate chip cookie dough analogy to the parents of a child with hearing loss at this stage?
3. Select a goal from one of the Tables 11–3 through 11–6. How would you explain to a parent how to use a specific activity of daily living to target the goal? Consider and identify other goals that would be naturally included in that selected ADL.
4. What activities could you do with an older child to work on the goals at this level?
5. Consider a child with additional disabilities or needs and discuss an activity that you could work on to target a selected goal at this level.

References

American Speech and Hearing Association. (n.d.). *Developmental norms for speech and language.* https://www.asha.org/public/speech/development/chart/

Barber, L., & Barber, H. (2010). *Home speech home.* https://www.home-speech-home.com/

Carrow-Woolfolk, E. (1999). *Test of Auditory Comprehension of Language-3.* Western Psychological Services.

Hammill, D. D., & Newcomer, P. L. (2008). *Test of Language Development.* Penguin Random House.

Heerman, V., Director. (1930). *Animal Crackers.* Paramount Studios.

Koster, S. (2012). *Tearable puns.* https://tearablepuns.org/

Ling, D. (2003). The Ling Six-Sound Test. *The Listener,* 52–53.

Lowry, L. (2016). Hanen Centre. http://www.hanen.org/helpful-info/articles/tuning-in-to-others-how-young-children-develop.aspx

McWinney, B., & Snow, C. (1984). *The child language data exchange system.* Carnegie Mellon.

Martin, N. A., & Brownell, R. (2005). *Test of Auditory Processing Skills* (3rd ed.). World Publishing.

Merriam, C. (2020). *Merriam-Webster Dictionary.* Encyclopedia Britannica.

Parish, P. (1963). *Amelia Bedelia.* HarperCollins.

Peterson, C. C., Wellman, H. M., & Slaughter, V. (2012). The mind behind the message: Advancing theory-of-mind scales for typically developing children, and those with deafness, autism, or Asperger syndrome. *Child Development, 83*(2), 469–485.

Trelease, J. (2019). *Read aloud handbook* (8th ed.). Penguin.

Wiig, E., Secord, W., & Semel, E. (2020). *Clinical Evaluation of Language Fundamentals—Preschool* (3rd ed.). NCS Pearson.

Zimmerman, I. L., Steiner, V. G., & Pond, R. E. (2011). *Preschool Language Scales* (4th ed.). Pearson.

Index

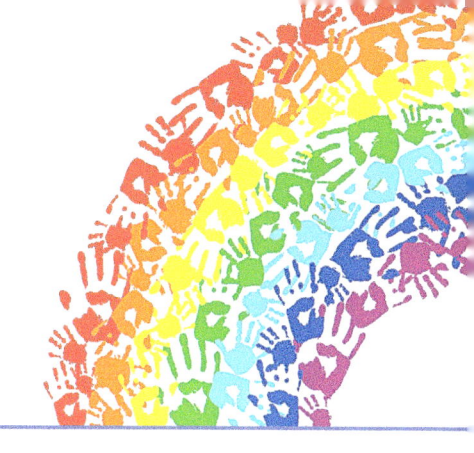

6-dB Rule, 7–8
6-dB Significance, 7

A

Acceptance of vocalizations, 135, 161
Acoustic correlates, 14, 16, 36–37, 42
  consonants, 17
  speech features, 32, 42
  vocalizations, 14
Acoustic cues for speech features, 20
Acoustic highlighting, 104, 120
  appropriate strategies , 50
Acoustic information
  high-frequency, 17
  invariant, 10
  low-intensity, 232
  variant, 13
Activities of Daily Living. *See* ADL
ADL (Activities of Daily Living), 60–63, 102, 113, 115–117, 134–137, 140–141, 161–162, 188–189, 217, 219, 232, 247, 277, 279, 281
  daily routines, 61, 122, 136, 141, 248
  formula, 62, 140, 142
Adult learning theory, 174
Advantages and disadvantages of language sampling, 108
Affricates, 15, 18, 20, 25, 31–32
  energy, 19
  manner, 11, 34, 159, 187
Amplification, 51
Articulation, 17, 42, 77, 83, 114
Articulation index, 53
ASHA-defined processes. *See* brain functions
Assessment of English language, 99–109
Assessments, 73, 76, 90, 92, 97–99, 101, 103–104, 107–109, 201, 227–229, 258, 260, 262
  complete, 226, 288
  formal, 71, 73, 101, 105, 226
  informal, 64, 71, 99, 105, 229
  ongoing, 97, 102
  phonologic, 90, 105
  standardized, 73, 168, 201, 288
  types, 99
Audiogram, 1–6, 10–11, 13–14, 17, 22, 24, 26–28, 30, 32–34, 38–39, 42, 49–51, 65, 76
  configurations, 39
  cookie bite, 39, 41
  corner, 39–40, 52
  downward sloped, 40
  functional audiogram, 30, 32–34, 38–39, 50
  reverse slope, 41
  sloping, 52
Auditory access, 4–6, 10–13, 16–17, 21–24, 26–27, 29, 32–39, 42, 45, 49–52, 59, 65, 70–73, 76, 130–132, 184–185, 231–232
  emerging perception, 59
  F_1, 16, 23, 29
  F_2, 29
  high frequency, 29, 104
  low and high frequencies, 39
  mid- and higher-frequencies, 38
  nasal murmur, 29
  new, 51, 72, 119, 130, 273
  optimal, 76
  sound and spoken language, 76
  vowels, 22, 29

Auditory feedback loop, 120, 147, 149, 159, 165, 202, 214, 216, 237, 244–245, 271–275
  child's, 184, 241
  self-monitoring of speech production, 274
  speech and language monitoring, 272
Auditory goals, 51, 132, 135, 139, 142, 178, 185, 207
Auditory information, high-frequency, 30, 42, 47
Auditory integration, 77, 100, 146, 149, 167, 169, 189, 259
Auditory processes, 76–78, 100, 114–115, 143–144, 166, 168, 198–199, 228–229, 258–259, 283, 285
Auditory rituals, 140, 158, 162
Auditory routines, 154
Auditory sandwich, 119, 188
Auditory sequencing, 77, 100, 199
Auditory signal
  degraded, 244, 274
  modifying, 4
Auditory skills, 21, 33, 45, 47, 64, 73, 89, 226–227, 229, 284, 288

B

Babbling, 42, 74, 79, 83–84, 90, 131–133, 139, 148, 150, 154, 156, 159–160, 165–167
  stages, 23, 39, 42, 82, 84, 132, 134, 156
Balance of low-frequency information, 35
Bilabial, 15, 17–18, 24, 36–37, 133, 156
Bilingual learners, 119
Bloom's Taxonomy Levels, 88
Brain functions, 76–78, 100, 133, 157, 185, 215, 274

C

CDS (child-directed speech), 21, 116, 135, 137, 141, 160–161
Checklists, informal, 73, 99
Child-directed speech. *See* CDS
Chocolate chip cookie theory, 113, 135, 139, 160–161, 165, 188–189, 217–218, 247, 250, 277, 279
  analogy, 113, 150

cookie dough analogy, 114, 135, 139, 142, 178, 208, 238, 268, 300
Clusters of energy in sounds. *See* formants
Coach parents, 50, 75, 137, 162, 190, 220, 248, 278
Coaching strategies, 66
Communication breakdowns, 57, 242, 275–276
Communicative intent, 72–74, 84, 117, 123, 131, 133–134, 139, 149–150, 163, 166, 193
Complex conversations, 247, 249, 251, 277, 280
Consonant features, 17, 26, 45, 136, 154, 182
Consonant manner, 14–15, 17, 20, 25–26, 35–37, 40–41, 45–46, 75, 120–121, 132–133, 154, 158–159, 181–182, 184–187, 215–216, 258, 268
  auditory cues, 24
  phonemes, 35–37
Consonant place, 11, 15, 17, 20, 24–25, 29–31, 33–34, 36–38, 41, 158–159, 182, 184–187, 215–216
  anatomical place, 15
  discrimination issues, 45
  information, 19, 25–26, 33, 38, 258
Consonant production, 35, 158–159, 186–187, 215–216
Consonant voicing, 11, 20, 37, 42, 133, 187
Consonants, 2, 10–11, 13–15, 17, 20, 22, 24–26, 32–35, 42, 44–45, 83–84, 90, 105, 120–121, 132–134, 144, 167–170, 176–178, 181–182, 186–187
  classification chart, 18, 35–37
  mastery consonants, 84
Continuants, 121
Conversational competence, 109, 247, 250, 273, 276–277
Conversational norms, 75, 104, 165, 246, 268, 276
Culture, 57–58, 60, 62–64, 104, 129–130, 153–154, 164, 181, 197, 220, 222
  adaptations, 67
  backgrounds, 63
  child's, 164
  cultural lens, 62
  diversity, 64, 142
  experiences, 62, 65

family, 57, 61, 211
family's language, 63
groups, 62, 65
heritage, 86, 100
interpreter, 63
norms, 62, 64
potential challenges, 63

D

Dangling carrot, 123, 161, 164
Detection, 3, 6, 17, 22–23, 27–28, 30, 38, 45–46, 49, 178, 186
Developmental milestones, 106, 130–131, 154–155, 182–183, 212–213
Difficult feelings, 56, 65
Diphthongs, 14–16, 19–20, 26, 31, 64, 105, 133, 136, 158–159, 186–187, 215–216
Discrimination, 6–7, 22–24, 38, 42, 45–46, 49–50, 89–90, 92, 119–120, 132–133, 177–178, 186–187, 193–194, 215, 258
Duration, intensity, pitch, (DIP) *See* Suprasegmentals

E

Ear shot/speech bubble, 5
Emergence, nasals manner, 42
ENUF, 56, 65
Environmental sounds, 76–77, 89, 130, 133, 158, 166–167
Error analysis, 24, 32, 35–36
Expectant pause, 117, 135, 139, 161
Expressive language, 72–73, 79–80, 101–102, 114–115, 160–161, 165, 168, 185, 188, 213–214, 228–229, 273, 276

F

Familiar sounds, 5, 53
Feelings, 56–58, 84–85, 99, 116, 162, 204, 253
Figurative language, 243–244, 252, 268, 272, 281–282, 292, 299
First words, 78–79, 81, 118, 129, 140, 154, 156
  common, 131
Formants, 9–10, 16–17, 20–23, 29, 38

Frequencies, 2–3, 5, 9–10, 12, 16–17, 22, 25, 28, 33–34, 38–39, 42, 46, 76
Fricative and affricate energy, 19
Fricative and affricate manners, 34
Fricative and affricate manners of production, 159, 187
Fricatives, 15, 17–18, 20, 24–25, 31–32, 34, 40–41, 44, 46, 49, 89, 92, 143, 202
  blowing, 92
  combination of stop plosives and fricatives, 15
  distortion, 44
  fricatives and affricates, 20, 25, 31–32
  higher-frequency, 38
  plosives and fricatives, 17
  turbulent noise, 20, 25
  unvoiced, 20, 29, 46

G

Garbage truck syndrome, 12, 23–24
Gestures, 79, 89, 98, 119, 131, 155, 161, 164, 166, 200, 275–276
Growth, 73, 76, 80, 87, 90, 94, 98, 199, 201, 260–261, 285, 288, 292

H

Hand cues, 119
Head shadow, 7
Hearing loss configurations, 34, 39, 52
Higher-order thinking, 86–87
  activities, 86, 88, 248
  skills, 248, 278
High-frequency language structures, 48
Home language, 59–60, 62, 64, 102, 130, 154–155, 252
Homographs, 124, 252
Homophones, 124, 244, 253
Humor, 85, 252, 274, 281

I

Identification, 7, 17, 23–24, 29, 32, 55–56, 58, 73, 76, 92, 258
Idioms, 244–247, 249, 252, 262–263, 267–268, 272, 274–276, 281–282, 285, 288, 298–300

Idioms *(continued)*
　addressing, 292, 299
　approach, 281
　common, 273
　comprehension, 245
　everyday, 247, 277
　multiple meanings, 252
IDS (infant-directed speech), 21, 23, 116, 122, 126, 135–137, 141, 151, 153, 157, 160–161
Imitations, 27, 105, 117, 123, 143, 158–159, 164–167, 174, 186, 195, 208
Infant-directed speech. *See* IDS
Inferences, 75, 214, 221, 246, 253, 262–263, 272, 275–276, 285, 288, 300
Instruments
　norm-referenced, 98
　standardized, 97, 99, 102
Intensities of sounds, 167
Intensity of speech
　acoustic environments, 275
　ambient noise conditions, 5
International Phonetic Alphabet. *See* IPA
Intervention, 55, 58–60, 63, 70, 72, 74, 83, 86, 103, 109, 253, 288
Intonation, 14, 21, 42
　patterns, 61, 92, 144, 147
　poor prosody, 29, 44
Invariant energy, 10, 25
　properties, 10
IPA (International Phonetic Alphabet), 17, 105

J

Jargon, 83, 131, 139, 156, 168, 171, 174, 200
Joint attention, 115–116, 118, 135, 146, 149, 161, 177, 207
Jokes and puns, 75, 80, 85, 243–249, 252–253, 263–268, 271–277, 279, 281, 298–300

L

Labiodental, 15, 18
Language, 59–66, 74–79, 94, 113–115, 117–120, 122–123, 141–142, 153–156, 159–164, 179, 181–185, 189–194, 196–197, 211–215, 222–223, 226–227, 241–249, 251–254, 271–274, 279–285

　delays, 63, 151, 179, 226
　error patterns, 34
　figurative/nonliteral, 242, 246, 274–276
　literal, 268
Language, parent input, 58, 60, 66
Language development, 45–46, 49–50, 65–66, 92–93, 107, 109, 185, 215, 217, 219, 229, 231, 246, 292–293, 299–300
Language samples, 64, 98–99, 102–103, 105, 108, 230
Language sampling, 97, 102–103, 106–109
Larynx, 14, 17
Laterals, 15, 18, 26, 31–34, 199
　discrimination, 41
Learning, 21, 52–53, 57–58, 60–61, 77–78, 93–94, 99–100, 115–116, 146–147, 149–151, 154–157, 164–165, 177, 192–194, 241–242, 246, 253, 281–282, 292
　strategies, 135, 157, 186, 218, 277
Levels of expectation for growth, 87
Ling, 1–3, 5, 7, 9–10, 12, 14–17, 23, 25–29, 33–35, 44–45, 47, 53, 105, 109, 135–136
Ling sentence, 49
Ling Six-Sound Test, 27–29, 53, 94, 106–107, 109, 143, 151, 179, 208, 239, 269
Linguaalveolar, 18
Linguadental, 15, 17–18
Linguapalatal, 18
Linguavelar, 18
Lips, 15, 17, 23
Liquids. *See* laterals
Listener, new, 21, 119, 129, 136
Listening, 1–2, 4–34, 49–50, 55–56, 58–62, 64–67, 69–73, 75–78, 97–110, 113–150, 153–154, 156–158, 163–166, 168–178, 181–182, 184–238, 241–242, 244–268, 271–272, 274–300
Literacy, 66, 73, 76, 135, 151, 161, 164, 188, 217, 246, 277
　advanced, 282
Localization, 158
Long-term acoustic speech spectrum, 3
Loudness, 2, 5, 9, 77
　perceived, 7
Low frequencies, 2, 11, 25, 29, 36, 39, 42, 135, 161
Low-frequency information, 11, 35–36

M

Manner and place, 17, 36
Manners and places of production, 198
Masking, 12, 24, 29, 50
Mastery of speech sounds, 213, 243
Mean Length of Utterance. *See* MLU
Mentor parents in material selection for activities, 61, 299
Metaphors, 275–276, 282
Microphone, remote, 242, 272
Mid frequencies, 22, 25, 29, 41, 45
Mid- to high-frequency information, 38
MLU (Mean Length of Utterance), 79–80, 98, 103, 109, 151, 183
    child's, 103, 185
    complex, 104
    language sampling, 106–107
    milestones, 79
Modalities, 28, 42, 50–51
    additional, 185
    primary, 42
Modeling clarification strategies, 247
Morphemes, 11, 24, 26, 81, 102–104, 182, 184–186, 188–189, 203–204, 212–216, 218, 227, 230, 232, 237
    advanced, 211
    analysis of morphemic functions, 46
    bound, 104
    Brown's morphemes, 91
    development, 78, 184, 187–188, 215–217
    functions, 46–47, 49, 71, 93, 230, 232, 258
    grammatical structures, 74, 184, 188, 208, 212–214, 218, 227, 230–231, 285, 287, 290
    initial, 46, 161, 181, 183–184, 188–189, 201, 204, 235
Multiple meanings, 124, 222, 238, 244–248, 252, 256, 263, 266–268, 273–276, 279, 281, 288, 292–293
Music, 7, 60, 79, 115, 130, 143, 167, 297

N

Narrating, 56, 117, 122, 140, 195
    incorporating, 163
Nasal, 12, 15, 18, 20, 26, 30–32, 40–41, 44–45, 121, 168, 185
    invariant acoustic information for nasal murmur, 10
    manner, 17, 33
    murmur, 10–11, 19–20, 25, 29, 31–33, 35–36
    murmur and voicing, 36
    nasal plosive discrimination, 41
    nasal sounds, 17, 32, 143
    resonance, 17, 35, 143, 158–159, 186
Nasal cavity, 15, 17
Nasalization, 44
Nasals and laterals discrimination, 41
Natural conversations, 59, 246, 249, 257, 268, 299
Natural interactions, 118–120, 135, 157, 165, 174, 189, 207, 218, 232, 237, 267
Negatives, 74, 93, 186, 208, 215–217, 237, 258, 288
Noise, 3, 5–6, 12, 50, 52, 66, 130, 133, 138, 174, 182
    ambient, 6
    background noise, 3, 5, 77, 102, 229, 245, 275
    common environmental noise levels, 52
    level, 3, 6, 241
    ratio, 3, 50, 65
    reducing, 59

O

Octave, 3
    band frequencies, 52
    bands, 3, 9, 25
Overhears, 164, 182

P

Pair, cognate, 17, 178
Palatal, 15
Palate, hard, 15
Paraphrase, 89
Parents
    guide, 59, 61, 75
    support, 157, 186, 218, 246, 277
Past-tense verbs, 24, 45
    endings, 231
    irregular, 46–47, 49, 81, 91, 93, 224, 231–232, 258–259

Past-tense verbs *(continued)*
  learning, 45
  regular, 46, 81, 91
Pitch, 2, 10, 14–15, 19, 21–22, 84, 115, 120–122, 131–133, 143–144, 147, 150, 156
  high, 21, 121
  higher, 10
  lower, 197
  natural, 14
  perceived, 14, 19
Plosives, 15, 17–18, 20, 24–25, 31–33, 35–38, 40–42, 44–46, 49, 89, 132
  confusion of nasals and plosives, 44
  F_2, 20
  final stop plosives, 26
  higher-frequency, 39
  nasals and plosives, 40–41, 45
  place cues, 46
  place cues unvoiced plosives, 33
  plosives and affricates, 20
  stop, 15, 17
  unvoiced, 20, 29, 31–34, 46
  word-final positions, 228
Plurals, 24, 46, 71–72, 91, 93, 183, 186–189, 200–202, 204, 207, 213, 216–217, 229–231, 234–235, 237
  irregular, 74, 80, 224, 238
  regular, 202
Poor intelligibility and error patterns, 19
Poor perception, 35
Pragmatics, 63, 104–105, 114–115, 149, 151, 155–157, 160, 166, 174, 200, 207
Praise for parents, 116
Preliminary words, 142, 165
Prepositions, 45, 47, 49, 74, 81, 161, 163, 182–184, 186–189, 195, 197, 208, 215–217, 230–231
Problem-solving skills, 60, 86
Production, self-correct, 216, 275
Prognostic indications, 39
  cookie bite audiogram configuration, 41
  corner audiogram configuration, 40
  downward sloping audiogram configuration, 40
  reverse slope audiogram configuration, 41
Pronouns, 45, 47, 74, 79–80, 91, 93, 182, 186, 200, 213, 215–217, 231–232, 266
Prosody. *See* intonation
Protoword, 71, 74, 150, 154
Puns, 243–244, 246, 252, 272–275, 277–278, 281, 300

Q

Questions, 21, 85, 87–89, 99–101, 104–105, 115, 151, 174, 182–183, 190, 195–196, 212–214, 220–221, 223–225, 229–231, 248, 253–254, 256, 296–297
  answer, 200, 230, 246, 258
  complex, 87, 253
  forms, 185, 216–217, 231, 237, 288
  intonation contour, 145, 148, 172
  open-ended, 59, 85, 165, 196, 253
  simple, 155, 187–188, 229
  yes/no, 183, 190, 195, 200, 224

R

Rainbow audiogram, 1–21, 24–25, 27–41, 45, 47, 49, 51, 53
  features, 32
  figure, 36–37
Receptive language, 61, 72, 79–80, 114–115, 132, 134–135, 139, 144, 161, 167–168, 188
Red flags, 1, 76, 87, 151, 179, 208, 227
  possible, 24, 50
Rephrasing, 57, 89
Resonance
  natural, 14, 19
  oral, 143
  pharyngeal, 21
  throat, 16
Rhymes, 79–80, 131, 154, 161, 164, 186, 191, 193, 196, 215, 222
  nursery, 21, 190
Rhythm, 14–15, 105, 130, 164, 190–191, 193
Routines, 6, 61, 130, 140, 162–163, 183, 191, 201, 220, 231
  basic, 201
  bedtime, 163
  daily, 62, 131, 140, 163–164, 169, 191, 280
  morning, 280
  natural, 55, 161
  teach classroom, 87

S

Sarcasm, 21, 23, 75, 247–248, 272, 274–276, 300
Second formants, 10, 16–17, 22, 25, 30, 32, 38, 49
  higher-frequency, 17, 22, 38
Segmentals, 14–15, 35, 105, 136–137, 140
Self-advocacy, 86, 93, 242, 271, 274
Self-determination, 86
Self-monitoring, 214, 241, 244–245, 274–275
Semantics, 77, 272
Semivowels, 15, 18, 20, 26, 92, 121, 154, 168, 199
Sensory modalities. *See* modalities
Signal in relation to ambient, 3
Signal to noise ratio. *See* SNR (Signal to noise ratio)
Signals, degraded, 182, 237, 244–245, 251, 257, 263, 274–276, 280, 292, 294, 299
Significant change in perception, 7
SNR (Signal to noise ratio), 3, 5–6, 50, 65, 272
Socialization, 65, 67, 85, 93
Songs, 115–116, 119, 136, 138, 140, 151, 154, 161–162, 164, 179, 182, 186, 222
  rhymes, 79, 161
  sing, 137, 162, 190, 220
  typical childhood, 140
Sound-object associations, 21, 135–136, 142–143, 149–150, 161, 165
Sounds
  high-frequency, 12–13, 21, 29–30, 39, 41
  high-pitch, 2, 84
  low-and mid-frequency, 38
  low-frequency, 12, 30, 143
  low-pitch, 84
  mid-range, 29
  unvoiced, 17, 24, 38
  voiced, 24
Speech, developing, 42
Speech acquisition, 105, 107
Speech bubble, child's. *See* ear ehot/speech bubble
Speech development, 50, 63, 65, 82, 113, 132, 156, 179, 217, 277
Speech features
  acoustics, 34, 46
  high-frequency, 11, 29, 44
  low-frequency, 33, 43
  mid-frequency, 43
  segmental, 84
  suprasegmental, 156
Speech intelligibility, 94, 149, 216, 268
  poor, 42
Speech perception, 12, 34, 42, 66, 73, 78, 178, 226, 238, 273, 288
Speech production system, 75, 108, 133, 139, 159, 164, 187, 193, 216, 245, 275
Speech sounds and features, 74
Spoken language growth, 60, 73
Stage
  babble, 82, 156
  vocalizations, 135, 139
Stages model, 69–70
Stages of children's vocalizations and sounds, 82
Stages of language acquisition, 1
Stereotypic phrases, 61–62, 80, 130, 134–135, 140–141, 154, 156–159, 161–165, 167, 189, 191–192
Strategies
  appropriate acoustic, 50
  auditory maximizing, 135, 161
  communication repair, 63
  conversation repair, 242
  conversational repair, 273
  highlighting, 50
  serve and return, 104, 139
    pausing, 165
Submarine analogy, 3–5, 7, 27, 53
Suprasegmentals, 11–12, 14–16, 19–23, 26, 30–32, 38–41, 45, 82–84, 120–121, 131–133, 142–146, 158–159, 167, 181–182, 186–187, 215–216
  DIP (duration, intensity, pitch), 11, 15, 19, 21, 23, 121–122, 132–136, 154, 156–159, 161, 184, 186–187, 215–216
  features, 16, 140, 154, 174, 207
  poor control, 41

T

Teach parents, 50, 122–123
Technology, 4–5, 28, 30, 33, 38–39, 50, 52–53, 59, 71, 76, 129–130, 135–136, 138, 158, 280–282

Theory of Mind (ToM), 84–85, 162, 191, 221, 223, 225–226, 247, 249, 251, 254, 269, 277–278, 280
  thinking words, 85, 188, 217, 232, 237
Three-act play, 122, 161, 163, 166, 188–191, 204, 217, 231–232, 234
ToM. *See* Theory of Mind
Tone of voice in words, 79
Transitions
  formant, 10, 19, 25
  phoneme perception, 165
  phoneme perception to production, 165
  vowel-to-consonant, 10
Turn taking and communication skills, 174
Two-word combinations, 200, 204

U

Utterances, 83, 98, 102–104, 123, 139, 182–183

V

Variable energy levels, 9
Variant energy, 10, 25, 50
  components, 10
  consonants, 25
Velar, 15, 24
Velopharyngeal port, 15
Verb tenses, 93, 103, 122, 161, 187, 212–213, 216, 223–224, 234, 243, 259
Vibrations, vocal cord, 19–20
Vocabulary, 79–80, 101, 123–125, 159–161, 191–193, 222, 225, 227, 229, 242–243, 248–249, 253–255, 258–259, 282, 290–291
  development, 81–82, 123
    advanced, 246
  efforts on Tier, 81
  grade-appropriate, 276
  milestones, 78
  preteaching, 217, 247
  tier, 75, 81–82, 124, 213, 242–243, 245, 268, 273, 277, 282, 300
Vocabulary stagnation
  avoiding, 232

  preventing, 123–124
Vocal cords, 15, 17, 22, 24
Vocal folds, 15, 26
Vocal rhythm, 77
Vocal system, 14–15
Vocal tones, 89, 132, 134, 154, 275
Vocal tract, 10, 83
Vocalizations, 14–15, 31–32, 79, 83–84, 129, 131–135, 139, 144–145, 149, 153, 156–157, 166, 169
Voiced, 15, 18, 20, 37
Voicing for consonant production, 215–216
Voicing Fricative, 46
Voicing of consonant production, 158–159, 186–187
Vowel and consonant, 25
Vowels, 9–17, 19–26, 29, 31–33, 38, 40–42, 44–46, 49, 82–84, 90, 121, 134–136, 142–144, 146–150, 154, 156, 158–159, 170–171, 174–177, 181–182
  acoustic energy for vowels, 23
  confusion, 22
  detection, 30, 32, 42, 49
  discrimination, 29–30, 32, 34
  F_1, 23
  F_2, 23, 31, 33, 38
  F_2 range, 23
  high-frequency, 41, 159, 187
  low-frequency, 21, 25, 133
  neutral mid-frequency, 84
  vowels and diphthongs, 15, 19, 31, 133, 158–159, 186–187, 215–216
  vowels and nasals, 185

W

Whispering, 13, 22–24, 120–121
Word approximations, 71, 74, 90, 92, 154–157, 159–160, 162, 165, 167–168, 172, 174, 178, 181–182, 184
  facilitating initial, 132
  first, 70, 131, 154, 164
Words, new, 118, 183, 190–194, 196, 199–200, 218, 220, 222, 248, 253, 255

[Created with TExtract/www.TExtract.com]